THE DIET DOCTOR'S WIFE'S COOKBOOK

with a few comments from her husband

Gabrielle Nagler, M.A.
and
Bill Nagler, M.D.

The Diet Doctor's Wife's Cookbook
with a few comments from her husband

For further information on mail order sales, wholesale or retail discounts, distribution, translations and foreign rights, please contact the publisher.

Note to the reader: Before following any of the diet or nutritional advice in this book, seek supervision and approval from your personal physician. The nutritional information contained herein is derived from material provided by the United States Department of Agriculture (USDA), the US Food and Drug Administration (FDA), and food suppliers and manufacturers.

Diet Results
16311 Middlebelt
Livonia MI 48154
U.S.A.

Telephone 734-422-8040
Toll Free 800-511-9769
Fax 734-422-8588
www.dietresults.com

First Edition February 2002
10 9 8 7 6 5 4 3 2 1

Acknowledgements

This cookbook came to fruition with the help of many people. In a way, I feel compelled to thank practically every single person I've ever eaten with. But given the limitation of time, space and memory, I will try to be a bit more practical.

Good food has always been an important part of my life and much of that has to do with my mother. She made most things from scratch, even my baby food. She grew her own herbs, strawberries, rhubarb and tomatoes, and was known for her adventurous culinary spirit. Childhood friends talk about how my mother introduced them to foods they had never previously heard of. Two of them had their very first artichoke at my mother's table.

I also have fond memories of helping my mother in the kitchen, especially preparing for parties and holiday dinners. She put me to work at a very young age and at times under strange conditions. One year, in the midst of an untimely blackout, we made over 75 cabbage rolls by candlelight.

My brothers, Aubrey and Michael, also helped me develop an appreciation for food and cooking. I used to love to watch Aubrey make whole wheat bread. He kneaded the dough with such speed and strength; it was like witnessing a great sporting event. As for Michael, there was no greater entertainment than watching him eat. It may sound strange, but when I was a little girl, Michael would wake me up soon after my parents had gone to sleep, and ask me to keep him company while he made himself a bedtime snack. His enthusiasm for food was something to behold. The quantity he could consume was legendary and his food combinations were amusingly creative.

Although my father doesn't cook, his influence has also been very strong. He helped me to become aware of the relationship between food and health, long before it was fashionable. He gave up red meat over 30 years ago. And soon after, he urged my mother to stop preparing fish caught from the polluted Great Lakes. Because of him, we only drank bottled water.

My Grandma Libby and Grandpa Harry offered something totally different. They contributed to my great love of farm-fresh fruits and vegetables. They used to take my brothers and me for Sunday drives to the farm stands in Leamington and Essex County to take advantage of the local harvest. They could both give you a dissertation on how to choose the best melon, ear of corn or tomato. My grandmother in particular would moan with pleasure as she sampled freshly plucked produce before making her well thought out selections. She was a careful, simple cook who knew the importance of using fresh, high quality ingredients.

I would also like to mention the friends and family members who hosted beautiful gatherings filled with warmth, hospitality and wonderful food. Each host had their signature dish that is indelibly marked in my memory: Grandma Sarah's potato muffins (bubalach), Aunt Susie's Hungarian cherry soup, Mrs. Kahane's pull-apart cake, Auntie Helen's challah, Judy Bernstein's wheat berry salad, Mrs. Putterman's cinnamon twists, Mrs. Rosenzweig's coleslaw, Simone Whiteman's couscous, Anita Moeller's white bean pasta, Bella Schaefer's manicotti, Debbie Stollman's pickled fish, Luanne Lemmer's ratatouille and Paula Weberman's flair for just about anything.

The list of the great cooks in my life goes on. Thank you to June Bearg, Ruth Berger, Dan Matthews, Arlene Steen, Laurie Rotman, Lesly Wade-Woolley, Ruthy Bodner, Peter Avery, Mary Ann Neary, Merla Wolk, Elsebeth Kolstrup, Gladys Bauer and Huldah (I don't know Huldah's last name; she took care of me when I was a child). The memories of your culinary creations still inspire me.

And then there is a small group of women who are not only great cooks, but also great cooking companions. Thank you Enid Markson, Carla LaBret, Rita Dates, Bozena Gidrol and Constance Singham for sharing your kitchens and epicurean talents with me.

Another group I would especially like to thank are the people who exposed me to some of the finest dining the world has to offer. Thank you Uncle Bob and Aunt Marilyn, Sue Hirsh, Diane and Earl Grant, Tullio and Rosemary Meconi, Joanne McKenzie, David Fingold, Paul and Malka Fingold, Connie Putterman, Arlene Rauwitscher, Julian Hurwitz, Eleanor Smith and Diane Lampe.

I would also like to thank those who introduced me to the multi-diverse splendor of Asian cooking: Claire Hong, Serene Tan, Nelly Kwa, Lily Low, Jean Kee, Mark Stevens, Eliyahu Solomon, Brian O'Neil, Robert Carnick, Bill Idsardi, Robert Bell, Ed Sitarski, Maggie Conn and Malcolm MacDonald. Other noteworthy eating companions are Aryeh and Yakov Stollman, Melvyn Dias, Sabrina and Margie Ullmann, Marion Kreitz and Margaret Hardwick. Thank you for sharing wonderful meals with me.

Thank you to Sandy Shatz for *The Moosewood Cookbook*, a birthday gift that helped launch me on a journey of vegetarian possibilities, and to Stewart Arneil who inspired me to stay on that journey. A very special thank you to my fairy godmother, Michele Flay, for suggesting that I try the macrobiotic plate at the Blind Faith restaurant in Evanston, Illinois in 1992. If not for that experience, this book would never have been realized.

Thank you to Sundardas Annamalay, Ai Mee Chua, Herman Aihara, Cornelia Aihara, Michio Kushi and Wendy Esko for sharing your knowledge of macrobiotics and showing me how to improve my health and sense of well-being.

Thank you to my neighbor Laura Roberts. I can hardly believe the great luck of living right next door to a macrobiotic, organic vegetable gardener whom I can relate to on so many levels. You are a great friend and a marvelous teacher.

Thank you to the cooking instructors at the Food Network, the Kushi Institute and the Vega Center for sharing your wisdom and technical skills.

For your endless inspiration, thank you to the countless writers and editors of the culinary magazines and cookbooks of the world. Thank you as well to the wonderful professional and home chefs who have delighted my palate throughout the various stages of my life.

I would also like to thank the people who helped me complete the actual production of this cookbook. Thank you Sue Vlangos for reviewing the manuscript throughout the course of its development. I don't know what I would have done without your tireless commitment and keen attention to detail. Thank you Billie Nagler for your insightful comments and help with the glossary and index. Thank you Shannon Bennett and Kelly Zombirt for your contribution to the enormous proofreading effort. Thank you Gordon Roberts, Tony and Gretchen Chaudhuri, and Todd and Peggy Nagler for your discriminating eyes and invaluable photography skills.

Thank you Sol Ta Triane for reminding me to be light and playful in every aspect of life (including the writing of this cookbook).

And last, but certainly not least, thank you Bill for your willingness to share this project with me. Your generosity is boundless.

Table of Contents

PART III

PART I

The Diet Doctor

Everybody always wants to know how much I weigh and what I eat, although they are usually too embarrassed to ask. But that's all right. It's only human nature. People just want to know if I practice what I preach.

So I'll confess. I'm fifty-one, five foot nine, and I weigh one hundred and fifty-five pounds. And the diet I live on is not the diet I use to help most of my patients lose weight. But it wasn't always that way.

The diet I use for weight loss is basically very low fat and high protein. When my patients follow my advice, and more often than not they do, they lose weight, and a lot of it. Most of my patients lose anywhere from five to ten pounds the first week on my program, and ten to twenty pounds every month. They eat fish until they grow fins, and salad until they sprout a bushy tail.

My diet is designed for exceptionally quick weight loss under my medical supervision. It is the fastest and best way I know to drop a whole bunch of weight in a hurry.

And after my patients reach their goal, I make a few changes in their diet to help them maintain their weight loss. Basically, I recommend following my low fat, high protein diet during the week, and splurging a bit on the weekend. This plan seems to work quite well if you stick to it. My guess is that most of my patients assume I maintain my weight by eating this way. The truth is, in some ways I do and in some ways I don't.

To start, I certainly don't eat much fat. As I tell all my patients when they start my program, fat is absorbed by your body six times faster than protein or carbohydrate. This means that every ounce of fat you eat is burned off before any of the fat on your body that you may want to get rid of.

In plain English, the more fat you eat, the slower you are going to lose weight, and even worse, the greater your risk for heart attack, stroke and cancer.

I feel better living on a low fat diet. I think most people do. Certainly there is evidence to suggest that cultures that follow low fat diets, such as the Japanese, have a higher average life expectancy than cultures that follow higher fat diets. The low fat diet of the Japanese may also contribute to their relatively low incidence of breast cancer, stroke and heart disease.

But, diet alone is not the answer to keeping weight off. Regular exercise is key. I sweat my brains out on my elliptical machine, forty-five minutes a day, five days a week. In every single weight loss study that I know of, exercise has proven to be the single most important factor in keeping weight off. The studies are conclusive. If you choose to lose weight without exercise, you have a 98% chance of putting every ounce you have lost back on, and maybe then some. If you choose to lose weight with exercise, and keep exercising, the numbers flip. You have a 98% chance of keeping off every ounce you have lost for good.

But following a low fat diet and exercising 5 days a week is not all I do. At least not anymore.

* * * * *

Seven years ago I made a major shift in my diet, a shift that dramatically improved the quality of my life. I feel better now, at fifty-one, than I have ever felt in my life. And I owe much of it to Herman Aihara.

Herman was as close to a guru for me as I ever thought possible. And believe me, I'm not the guru type. The whole idea turns me off. But that's another story.

For thirty odd years, Herman ran the Vega Center, a macrobiotic retreat in Oroville, California. He spread the gospel of brown rice, miso soup and seaweed. He never made much money, and plowed every last cent he made back into his center, getting people excited about macrobiotics. Folks would fly in from all over the world to spend anywhere from a few days to a few months to hang out with him. He'd talk about his theories of acidity and alkalinity, his thoughts on longevity and balance in life, and his love of salmon fishing and cheesecake.

In 1998, at age seventy-seven, Herman died of a heart attack. Until his dying day, he was the most vital, light-hearted man I ever knew.

*****

The macrobiotic people make a lot of dramatic claims. They talk about increased longevity, eliminating chronic illnesses like arthritis and diabetes, and even curing cancer. They share endless moving stories of their successes. But unfortunately, they don't have sound medical data to support their claims.

Sound medical data or not, I can say with a great deal of certainty, that when I followed Herman's diet, I felt much better. The only problem was that I couldn't stand the taste of the food.

On a macrobiotic diet, you live on brown rice, miso soup, beans, seaweed, pickles and vegetables. That's it. I'm not kidding. And when that is all you get to eat, you are going to suffer a lot. Believe me. I did.

Now, if you've been diagnosed with a serious illness, and you believe a diet of brown rice, miso soup, beans, seaweed, pickles and vegetables is going to save your life, that's one thing. But if you're just trying to get through the day and feel as good as you can, that's a whole other kettle of seaweed.

* * * * *

My introduction to macrobiotics was seven years ago, this Christmas. Gabrielle and I spent a week at the Kushi Center in Beckett, Massachusetts. It was quite an experience for us. We were the only two people in our class of fourteen, who hadn't been diagnosed with, or married to a person with cancer. Many of our classmates were terminal. Their doctors had little-to-nothing to offer. Most of the people we were with had come to the Kushi Center that week looking for a glimmer of hope. Macrobiotics was a last attempt to extend the quality and length of their lives, or the lives of their loved ones.

I don't know how many of our classmates found what they were looking for that week. I hope they all did. They were a terrific group of people. All I know is that after a week of living on macrobiotic food at the Kushi Center, I felt better than I had in a long, long time.

I always, always used to get colds. If you looked at me sideways when you had a cold, or worse, sneezed in my direction, I'd be sick the next day, and for weeks after. And when I wasn't sick, I had a chronic sore throat, stuffy nose, and sneezed constantly, usually feeling as if I were on the verge of getting a cold. And at least once every two months, I would be hit for a week or two with the genuine article.

But after four days of Kushi rice and seaweed, my chronic pre-viral symptoms disappeared. For the first time in years, I woke up in the morning feeling refreshed. I no longer had my usual morning experience of standing in the shower and moaning to myself that I don't feel well. I felt just fine. I could barely recognize myself.

* * * * *

From a medical perspective, the changes in the way I felt were particularly interesting. It certainly wasn't psychological, as I was extremely skeptical about the dramatic claims the macrobiotic people were making plus I found the food so intolerable that I was loathe to find any benefit. The Kushi Center was not a happy experience for me. It seemed that my general state of well-being had improved in spite of myself.

Digging into the medical literature, it became quite clear what was responsible for my newfound "wellness". It was as simple as A, B, C, or more precisely, as A, E, G and M. Immuno Globulins A, E, G and M are produced by the body in response to the presence of allergens.

There is a huge body of medical evidence suggesting that many of the foods present in the typical American diet cause allergic reactions. And dairy products may be the chief offenders. When a person allergic to dairy ingests milk, cheese, yogurt or ice cream, their body releases immuno globulins A, E, G and M. These immuno globulins attack the milk chemistry as if it were a dangerous foreign invader like a virus or bacterial infection. The dairy is not treated like a food or a nutrient, but more like an enemy that needs to be eliminated from the body.

Lactose or dairy allergies show up in a variety of symptoms. The most common are abdominal discomfort, severe gas, headaches, constipation and diarrhea. Dairy consumption has even been linked to the occurrence of certain chronic illnesses. Studies have shown that eliminating dairy products from the diet may reduce and in some cases completely alleviate symptoms of rheumatoid arthritis, psoriasis and chronic sinusitis.

From an evolutionary standpoint, our body's inability to handle dairy products makes perfect sense. We've been on the planet as Homo sapiens for nearly 600,000 years. But we've only been domesticating animals for about five thousand years. So our milk-drinking history (except for mother's milk) is relatively short. Five thousand out of six hundred thousand years is likely not a sufficiently long period of adjustment. One could argue that our bodies have not had enough time to adapt to drinking the milk of another species. It is no wonder that medical studies document allergic immune responses to drinking milk. Cow's milk is good for calves, not people.

Some cultures of the world have a particularly short milk drinking history. It wasn't until the 20th century that the Inuit began introducing dairy products into their diet. Until then, they lived almost exclusively on fish and blubber. Of all the ethnic groups on the planet, they have likely had the least amount of time to adapt to milk drinking.

Although the degree of lactose intolerance does vary among individuals, it is a fairly normal condition for most of the world's adults. According to the medical literature, only Caucasians of northern European origin retain the ability to digest lactose after childhood. I believe that it is safe to say that 80% of American adults have some degree of lactose intolerance.

Macrobiotics deals with this problem head on by eliminating all dairy products from the diet. As a matter of fact, most animal products are considered taboo except for an occasional 3-ounce portion of fish (which is only allowed if you are in optimal health), so beef, chicken, turkey, pork and eggs are out as well. Such dietary restrictions present a significant challenge as most Americans are serious meat eaters. Meals are centered on meat or poultry. As a result, fat consumption is generally high as is the incidence of fat-related illnesses such as cancer, stroke and heart disease. The longer living Japanese, on the other hand, consume only small quantities of meat and fish, which take a back seat to rice and vegetables.

The list of taboo foods on a macrobiotic diet continues. You also can't have sweets. That means no chocolate, no candy, no cakes, no cookies, no pie, no ice cream, nothing with sugar. Honey is out as well. Even fruit is questionable. So much so that the macrobiotic teachers love to quote an old Chinese proverb that basically reads "the family with the fig tree in their garden is doomed", meaning that if you eat too many sweets (figs), you will not lead a productive life.

From a medical point of view, limiting sugar consumption is well advised. Eating sweets pushes up your insulin level, which makes you crave and eat more sweets, which in turn pushes up your insulin level further, which not surprisingly makes you crave and eat even more sweets. So basically, if you really want to put on weight, the best thing to do is to eat sweets.

In addition to making the numbers on the scale go up, eating too many sweets can cause mood swings and energy fluctuations. By eliminating sweets from the diet, you may find that you become more even-tempered, less fatigued and possibly more productive (as the Chinese proverb predicts). You probably won't feel as hungry and you will likely have less tooth decay.

Another food group that the macrobiotic people have problems with, believe it or not, is a family of vegetables called the nightshades. This means no potatoes, tomatoes, eggplant, zucchini or peppers. According to macrobiotic theory, these vegetables are genetically engineered poisons, which exacerbate symptoms of arthritis and depression. The medical data do not support their claims, but I certainly can say from personal experience that after eating potatoes I feel sluggish and cranky. Gabrielle reacts similarly and also finds that her joints get stiff from food spiced with hot peppers.

And then there are a bunch of foods that you are only to have in moderation such as bread (even whole wheat), crackers and pasta. The medical literature is supportive in this case, since wheat gluten and yeast are common triggers of allergic reactions.

* * * * *

So there was some explanation for why I was feeling better at the Kushi Center. Eating macrobiotically for 5 days, I was no longer poisoning myself. I had eliminated dairy, meat, poultry, and sweets. And not one bagel passed my lips. I felt better because I was no longer eating food that caused my body to have an allergic reaction. So my chronic cold symptoms disappeared as well as my feelings of depression. It all made perfect sense. My body was purged of the usual toxins. My engine was clean. I was vital again.

But in spite of my newfound vitality, I still found it hard to get past the thought of enduring a daily diet of rice, vegetables and seaweed. It was a real struggle for me, but in the end, I came to realize that a macrobiotic diet was worth pursuing. I liked the idea that I was no longer eating food I was allergic to. I liked that I was feeling better than I had in years.

So I persevered. Over the next year, Gabrielle and I experimented with macrobiotics, and the same thing always happened. Every time we went macro for a few days, I felt better. Much better. But, unfortunately, the food wasn't getting any more appealing.

A year later, Gabrielle and I decided to give another macrobiotic center a try. We needed help. We wanted to see if there was any way we could hack the food. This time, we went west to hang out with Herman Aihara at the Vega Center.

Herman was a trip. He had breakfast with us every morning, and giggled through his bucktoothed smile while I suffered through mashed sweet potatoes on rice cakes. Herman was with us again at lunch, as I endured rice and seaweed soup. And occasionally he would join us for dinner, as I attempted to choke down brown rice, boiled chickpeas and kale. As the week went on, I kept feeling better and better. But I still was turned off by the food.

What was different this time though, was that I was quite charmed by Herman. He answered my incessant medical questions with patience and a sense of humor. The twinkle never left his eye. Macrobiotics to Herman was more a philosophy of life than a diet of rice and seaweed. There was nothing stern or judgmental about him.

Herman was not afraid to admit that he loved and ate food not on a strict macrobiotic diet. He rhapsodized about his love for cheesecake, and told us about how every Thanksgiving, he and his wife Cornelia would make a traditional turkey dinner with all the fixings for family and friends. He went into dreamy detail about the stuffing, cranberry sauce and pumpkin pie.

For the first time, I sensed that there might be some hope for me. I no longer felt that I was sentenced to a life of deprivation. I just had to figure out the right balance.

* * * * *

What was clear to me was that I really wanted to feel as good as I did on brown rice, miso soup and seaweed. So the macrobiotic diet was definitely in my future. What was also clear was that Gabrielle and I would have to come up with a way to make the diet palatable so we could still enjoy the pleasure of eating. We certainly had our work cut out for us.

Like I mentioned earlier, macrobiotics eliminates a lot from the diet. And given that Gabrielle and I are both serious food nuts, making the diet work was particularly challenging. You have to understand that we are obsessed with food. We love trying new restaurants, exploring specialty food shops and looking through cookbooks. Much of our daily chatter, both at work and at home, has something to do with eating.

Gabrielle and I debate the superiority of using fresh over dried pasta. We mark harvest dates for porcini mushrooms, truffles and Meyer lemons on our calendar. We spend a fortune on kitchen equipment. We don't even take our morning cup of coffee lightly. We spent weeks searching the internet before purchasing the consummate espresso machine. Finally we decided on an 8-cup Pavoni. No automatic coffee maker for us. After waiting a month for its arrival, it took us several additional weeks, and endless pounds of coffee, before extracting the perfect cup of espresso, rivaling the finest we have ever had, even in Europe.

The madness continues. When we go out of town, we spend hours at local markets, bakeries and gourmet shops. We love cookware, tableware, cooking classes and the Food Network. We obsessively comb the planet for the ideal version of this or that. I remember a two-year stint of searching for the ultimate brownie. We finally found the perfect rendition at the coffee shop at the Sir Frances Drake Hotel in San Francisco (it is seriously worth the trip), begged the baker for the recipe, and then made our own "necessary" adjustments. There are similar stories concerning the search for the ultimate recipes for chocolate chip cookies, lemon meringue pie, French macaroons, Szechwan hot-and-sour soup and Greek spinach pie.

So given our crazy obsession with food, we asked ourselves how we were ever going to manage living on a macrobiotic diet.

The answer was obvious. We had to find out how far we could stray from the macrobiotic diet and still feel well. We had to tinker with the program so that we could avoid the dreaded monastic, under seasoned, overly seaweedy taste of traditional macrobiotic cuisine.

Gabrielle got to work in the kitchen, and I got creative searching for quick and dirty solutions for instant gratification. My first project was to look for ways to make plain brown rice tolerable. Rao's Homemade™ bottled sauce was a terrific find. Rated as the number one pasta sauce by Consumer's Report, I thought I'd give it a try. The sauce is much better over pasta, but still gives brown rice a needed push. And even though tomatoes are not recommended on the macrobiotic diet, I don't see a problem with an occasional indulgence. I certainly don't feel any adverse effects. Gabrielle's killer Sesame Salt (see page 327) also satisfies my no-fuss requirements for adding a little welcomed flavor to plain brown rice, especially with a pinch of chopped scallion and ginger pickle (or any pickle for that matter).

With the rice situation under control, my next project was to experiment with animal protein. Avoiding beef for obvious health reasons, the choices were fish and poultry. Fish was not top of my list, so I gave chicken a go. But, as I suspected even before my introduction to macrobiotics, chicken made me feel cranky and anxious. I tried free-range chicken figuring it was a safer bet. Who needs the hormones and antibiotics. But unfortunately, the difference was not that significant. I still felt pretty low. Ditto for my reaction to turkey and eggs. Fish, on the other hand, didn't seem to bother me. As the macrobiotic people claim, it is the animal protein of choice. So I started to include more fish in my diet. I had it several times a week, far more often and in much larger quantity than recommended on the macrobiotic diet, and I felt just fine. I found that if I didn’t eat enough fish, I would feel a bit tired and sluggish. The recommended vegetable proteins (beans, tofu, tempeh and seitan) didn’t give me enough of an energy boost.

The next thing I investigated was my tolerance for baked goods. Not an easy task as I am a true lover of cookies, brownies and bagels. The macrobiotic people steer clear of all that stuff, the sweet baked goods in particular. Anything made with butter, eggs and sugar is off limits.

Truthfully, I didn't have high expectations on this front. As I mentioned earlier, it is no secret that refined sugar products trigger energy and mood fluctuations. And my reaction was totally predictable. Within minutes of eating a chocolate chip cookie or brownie, my energy would plummet and my mood would take a serious nose-dive. Given that I'm lactose intolerant, the butter would just make matters worse. And then of course, the egg content added fuel to the fire. So not so surprisingly, I have discovered that I don't do well with sweet baked goods. That doesn't mean that I never indulge. But when I do, I make sure that I have been good on my diet for a while. I find that when my body is garbage free, I am more resilient and can bounce back from a culinary indiscretion. My resilience is magnified if I follow my regular exercise program.

Unfortunately bagels and other yeasted products are not much better for me. My symptoms are sleepiness, lack of energy and a feeling of bleakness. If I eat too many bagels at a time, my mood gets so foul that my marriage is at risk. Gabrielle reacts differently, she gets short of breath and starts wheezing. In both cases, our symptoms last a day or two.

The hardest thing for me to have come to terms with is my reaction to dairy, especially ice cream. It usually takes no time at all for my sinuses to clog up, which brings on a full-blown headache. I get exhausted and lose clarity of thought. If I have a large quantity of ice cream or any other dairy product, I get uncontrollable diarrhea and severe gas. Plus, if I eat dairy for too many days in a row, I more likely than not develop pre-viral symptoms. And if I don't clean up my diet immediately, a cold will surely follow. Even so, I still love the stuff.

* * * * *

What I gradually have learned is that I can continue to feel well and still find things to eat that I enjoy. I stay away from bread, but can have pasta with tomato sauce in moderation. I now eat oatmeal and whole grains such as brown rice and barley. To satisfy my sweet cravings, I have fresh fruit but not too much (two pieces a day at most, or my chronic cold symptoms return), as well as root vegetables and tubers (carrots and sweet potatoes). I eat fish 3-4 times a week, otherwise it's beans, tofu or some other vegetable protein. Occasionally I grill a steak, just because I love it. And as long as I stay away from dairy products, poultry and eggs, I feel a heck of a lot better.

And eating this way has not made me gain any weight. I find that I can eat nice healthy portions and keep within my ideal weight range. I even use this diet to take weight off after trips or holidays. In fact, I eventually found a way to incorporate the principles of this way of eating to help my patients lose weight. You will hear more about this in the chapter on weight control.

* * * * *

As I was discovering what I could eat and not eat, Gabrielle was making great strides in the kitchen. She spent hours cooking, baking and experimenting, her nose always in a cookbook. She took cooking classes and watched the Food Network religiously. She grew our vegetables, dried our herbs and ground our spices. She took over a section of our basement for her pickling projects and filled our cupboards with every cooking implement imaginable. And finally after much trial and error, Gabrielle started coming up with some real winners. She was creating healthy, quasi-macrobiotic dishes in a true food lover's style. Her cooking was not only becoming palatable but downright awesome.

Gabrielle has found ways to make seaweed dishes I look forward to eating. Her miso soups have a serious gourmet quality, unlike any I've ever had. Her vegetable dishes could entice any meat-and-potatoes eater into considering new culinary possibilities. And believe it or not, Gabrielle has come up with macrobiotic desserts that taste like actual desserts, which is totally unheard of.

What I eat, more often than not, is in this cookbook. I eat more vegetables and grains than I ever have, as well as beans and vegetable proteins. I try to have a bowl of miso soup every day. And I feel terrific, most of the time. But that doesn't mean that once in a while I won't treat myself to some of my old favorites. Every time Gabrielle and I go to New York City, I stop in at Smith and Wollensky for a juicy steak, Dean and Deluca for Bouley breads, La Maison Du Chocolat for their chocolate sorbet, and Balthazar's bakery for their fruit foccacia. But like I said, most of the time, I eat Gabrielle's version of macrobiotics that you are now holding in your hands. I feel better than I've felt in years, thanks to Herman, and my wife.

Bill Nagler, M.D.
December 2002

The Diet Doctor's Wife

I met my husband in 1995 at his diet clinic. My mother had scheduled an appointment for a diet consultation. She had recently undergone surgery and was on a fairly high dose of cortisone, which had caused her to gain quite a bit of weight. Like many, I was suspicious of diet doctors so I asked my mother if I could tag along to check this guy out. I wanted to make sure that the highly recommended Dr. Nagler was not a quack. My mother's health was far from stable and I didn't want her to get into any more trouble.

When we met Dr. Nagler, I was relieved to discover that he too showed concern for my mother's medical condition. He took a thorough medical history, questioning her in detail about her symptoms and medications. He patiently answered all of our questions and helped to make us feel comfortable. He drew blood and took an EKG and blood pressure reading.

Dr. Nagler then proceeded to tell us about his high protein diet. He assured my mother that if she followed his program, she would lose weight, even on cortisone. My mother was thrilled. She desperately wanted to lose weight. She absolutely hated the way she looked.

The diet was pretty straightforward. Basically you could eat as much low fat protein as you wanted: lean beef, skinless chicken, fish and low fat cheese. Some vegetables were allowed but only in small quantities. High carbohydrate vegetables like carrots and potatoes were off limits, as well as bread, crackers and pasta. The diet seemed so easy to follow that I decided to try it myself. It was a way to support my mother and shed a few unwanted pounds at the same time.

To my surprise, the pounds just fell off. My mother was losing weight at a steady pace and so was I. We both felt great and were quite pleased with our progress.

In spite of the benefits of the weight loss, I was not at all happy with what I was eating. I admit that shifting to a high protein diet made me re-evaluate my eating habits. I was used to eating a lot of carbohydrates: pasta, bread, crackers, baked potatoes and fruit. My intake of protein was generally low, yet after being on Dr. Nagler's diet, I began to understand how carbohydrates can make you gain weight. But certainly, I could not be on a high protein diet forever. I craved vegetables and fruit, and most importantly, I needed more fiber since I was suffering from constipation. What I wanted was a healthy diet that would not cause me to gain my weight back.

I recalled my introduction to macrobiotics. It was 1992 at a vegetarian restaurant in Evanston, Illinois called The Blind Faith. I was with my cousin Michele who suggested that I order the macrobiotic plate. As she was always exposing me to interesting experiences, I thought why not give it a try.

When my meal came to the table, I was impressed by the ample portions and exciting variety. The macrobiotic plate included beans, brown rice, seaweed salad, pickled vegetables, pureed squash, steamed kale, as well as a bowl of piping hot miso soup. I ate every last morsel, delighted with the simplicity of the meal. And what amazed me was that in spite of the large quantity of food, I had a general feeling of lightness, as if I could sense the space between my cells. This was a completely new experience for me since historically I suffered from indigestion, especially after a large meal.

Later that year, I moved to Singapore on a 2-year teaching contract. During my stay, I had the opportunity to learn much more about macrobiotics. I studied under Sundardas Annamalay of the Youngson Institute of Natural Science.

Sundardas taught me about the health benefits of macrobiotics, and introduced me to a whole community of people who ate that way. I shared wonderful meals with these people as well as helped out in their kitchens. And lucky for me, Singapore hosted international conferences on macrobiotics, so I was able to attend lectures given by world famous macrobiotic teachers, including Michio Kushi.

I was intrigued and certainly had the experience that whenever I ate macrobiotically, I felt a lot better. I had more energy, better digestion and felt an unfamiliar sense of well-being. The only problem was that in Singapore I refused to step foot in my kitchen. The tropical climate was unbearable (I had no air-conditioning) and the thought of generating any more heat turned me off completely. I ate out 3 meals a day.

Even so, the virtues of macrobiotics were filed in the back of my mind. I promised myself that when I returned home, I would pursue the subject more thoroughly.

I told Dr. Nagler about my experience. He seemed quite interested and suggested that we go to the Kushi Center in Beckett, Massachusetts to enroll in one of their programs. By this time Dr. Nagler and I were dating. So from this point on, I will refer to him as Bill.

Bill and I enrolled in a five-day course at the Kushi Center, called The Way to Health. What we did not know was that this course was aimed at cancer patients. Most of our classmates were quite ill, some in the advanced stage of their cancer. The atmosphere was pretty grim. People were fighting for their lives and felt that macrobiotics was going to help in some way. The teachers were quite stern and strongly suggested that macrobiotics was our classmates' only chance of survival. Bill and I were taken aback. There was little to no scientific data to back their dramatic claims. Bill was particularly disturbed, given his professional background.

Even so, we decided to remain open and give this macrobiotic experience an honest try.

Throughout the five days, we ate a completely vegan vegetarian (no eggs or dairy products) and sugar-free diet. There were no restaurants or cafes around for miles, so cheating was nearly impossible. Although we did find a general store that sold very tempting junk food. The licorice whips and M&M's® looked almost too good to resist. Nevertheless, we controlled ourselves and bought nothing.

Each day at the Kushi Center, we were served an unusual variety of whole grains, vegetables and vegetable proteins. We were introduced to many new foods: burdock, tempeh, millet, various seaweeds and unusual condiments. In the daily cooking classes, we learned how to prepare miso soup, to use a pressure cooker to create rich tasting dishes without the use of much oil or fat, and to make desserts without eggs, butter or sugar. I found the meals nutritious, delicate and creatively executed. A new world was opening up to me.

Bill, on the other hand, was grumbling about the food. He absolutely hated everything that passed his lips. He found the taste of seaweed intolerable and complained that he was starving to death. The lack of protein was making him feel weak and sleepy.

Even so, as much as he hated to admit it, Bill could not help but notice some positive changes in the way he felt. His chronic sore throat seemed to disappear and his digestion had improved considerably. As for me, I found it easier to move my bowels and noticed that my eczema was starting to clear up. Best of all, for the first time in 33 years, I didn't feel sick after eating. That may sound overly dramatic, but it is true. For years, I had been plagued with indigestion. And 5 days at the Kushi Center made my lifelong problem disappear just like that. It seemed like magic.

Another surprising thing happened. Following the carbohydrate-rich macrobiotic diet, I was dropping weight without even trying. I sampled every dish. I had soup, grains, beans, vegetables, and dessert and still my clothes were getting roomier. There was something to this diet, data or not.

When we returned home, we tried to fit this new way of eating into our lives. I started cooking with ingredients that had never appeared in my kitchen before: brown rice, barley, millet, adzuki beans, tempeh, seitan, tofu, miso, collards, turnips, kale, burdock and seaweed. I repeated many of the recipes I learned at the Kushi Center. Bill hated everything I made. He would come home from the office and carry on about how much he loathed vegetarian food, and in particular, anything macrobiotic. Still he wanted to feel good and urged me to experiment and try to come up with something that didn't make him want to scream. It was hard going, especially since I didn't have a problem with my cooking. Of course, my preferences were mostly vegetarian to begin with.

As I started to get more comfortable with the macrobiotic diet, I began to spread my wings and get creative. I read every cookbook I could get my hands on: vegetarian, macrobiotic, French, Italian, Mexican, Middle Eastern, Southeast Asian, Chinese, Japanese, Fusion, you name it. I started adapting recipes, giving them a more vegan vegetarian esthetic, attempting to reduce the fat considerably. When a recipe that looked appetizing called for beef or chicken, I substituted a vegetable protein whenever appropriate. I looked for vegetarian dishes in non-vegetarian cookbooks to get ideas. I expanded my repertoire on fish (fish is allowed on a macrobiotic diet only if you are in good health). I was making stocks, confits and pickles, as well as canning our homegrown tomatoes. I combed through specialty food catalogues and surveyed gourmet shops for unusual oils, vinegars and other products. Anything to do with cooking or food became an obsession for me.

After a year or so, the fruits of my labor were finally realized. Bill and I were able to enjoy marvelous meals prepared in the comfort of our own home. We enjoyed dishes that rivaled some of our former favorites. We were able to eat well and stay trim without having to suffer through the regular feelings of deprivation and hunger associated with weight control. Plus the more we followed this dietary path, the better we felt. The increase in our fiber intake as well as the decrease in our consumption of animal protein and refined sugar helped us to overcome a lot of our chronic health issues. Bill was not as susceptible to flus and colds and was more even-tempered. My skin cleared up and my digestion was better than ever. And best of all, I no longer had a problem with constipation.

Convinced that we were onto something good, we dared to share our new cuisine with family and friends. We exposed our nearest and dearest to radical menu changes. The old standards of turkey and beef tenderloin went out the window. In their place were elaborate vegetarian soups and stews, and light fish dishes. We served desserts made without sugar, dairy or eggs. And we got rave reviews. No one left our table feeling protein or fat deprived and many were delighted by the different tastes and unusual preparations. We were encouraged to find out that our dinner guests could be satisfied with our extremely low fat, high fiber cuisine. Plus there were no complaints about having to endure fish or vegetable protein.

Although we were pleased with the food at home, Bill and I still enjoyed the idea of eating out and trying new things. "Visiting food," as Bill calls it, is one of our favorite forms of entertainment. We love exploring the breadth of culinary possibilities. But after shifting our diet, we found that eating out the way we used to left us feeling heavy and uncomfortable. Bill and I were discouraged. We still wanted to try exciting food preparations without feeling awful afterwards.

So we began to explore vegetarian restaurants. We tried dozens, locally and in our travels. But unfortunately, our search has, for the most part, been rather disappointing. Most dishes offered at vegetarian restaurants are heavy, uninteresting and not carefully prepared. We are also surprised at the high fat content.

As for non-vegetarian restaurants, many do offer vegetarian fare but the choice is often limited and not too exciting. And again, most cook with far too much cheese and fat. And very rarely are whole grains used.

We have found that our best bet is to eat in good fish restaurants where we can get grilled, broiled or poached fish. The thrill of fatty sauces no longer appeals to us, and we are getting wise to the unpleasant, heavy feeling that follows. Even so, we occasionally break out of our habitual pattern, and take a crack at a new restaurant or return to an old favorite just to get ideas for home creations.

Our disappointment and frustration with restaurant eating is a subject of constant discussion. We don't understand why it is so hard to find restaurants that serve tasty, creative and carefully prepared healthy food. We refuse to believe that our tastes are so strange that there is not a market for people like us. There are many vegetarian, vegan, macrobiotic and low fat food lovers out there. There must be. And there must be a restaurateur or two among them, interested in opening a restaurant that would cater to our culinary preferences. And if that aspiring restaurateur would be open to menu suggestions, all the better. Bill and I have a lot of ideas. As a matter of fact, a list of menu ideas for such a fantasy restaurant was basically how this book was conceived.

A few years ago, Bill and I were at one of our local restaurants. We were not particularly thrilled with the menu selection that evening. The fish of the day was baked in a cream sauce, there were no vegetarian soup choices, most of the vegetarian entrees were loaded with cheese and eggs, and to make matters worse, they were out of our favorite rice and bean dish. We tried to console ourselves by listing a bunch of things that we wished would appear on the menu, which Bill diligently crammed on both sides of a paper napkin. I took that napkin home and expanded on it and after many months of experimentation and research, came up with a few hundred recipes. And so, this cookbook was born.

Our original plan was to put together a healthy cookbook for food lovers. And of course, we secretly hoped that a great chef would be inspired by the recipes and open a restaurant with a menu to our liking, preferably in Ann Arbor and within 10-minute walking-distance of our house. But, we decided to do more than that. We thought we would share our story with you, and let you in on how this way of eating has changed our lives for the better. This diet has helped us to overcome most of our chronic health complaints plus it has given us a way to really enjoy food without gaining weight.

We hope you have fun with it. And if you want to open a restaurant, please let us know. We'll be there. In any case, bon appetit!

Gabrielle Nagler
December 2002

What We Eat

Bill and I are passionate about food. We spend hours at markets, gourmet shops, cafes, and bakeries. We are over-consumers of kitchen equipment and cookbooks. When dining out, we have been known to order much of the menu just to have a taste or an interesting experience. And throughout our explorations, there is continuous commentary. We love nothing more than to play games of discernment, critiquing cooking techniques and then proposing interesting revisions.

Despite our penchant for culinary exploration, our preferred esthetic is one of simplicity. We want to be "wowed" by what an herb does to a vegetable, or moved by the texture or consistency of a grain. We want fat and seasoning to be just the right amount to bring out flavor without taking over.

Much of our desire for simplicity is achieved by choosing quality ingredients, carefully combining those ingredients and selecting the correct low fat cooking technique. With these criteria in mind, we believe that food can delight the senses and nourish the body without creating extra padding. Plus, if you eat the way we suggest, and stick to it, you may experience a lot of positive health changes, such as:

Better digestion
Regularity
Better circulation
Easier menstrual cycle
Less joint pain
Less congestion
Softer skin
Clearer complexion
Better breath

Lower cholesterol
Better sleep
Better mood

The recipes in this cookbook reflect our passion for food and our strong desire for feeling well and looking good. The recipes include tasty and varied ingredients that are low in fat, high in fiber and rich in vitamins and minerals. What we are presenting is not a restrictive weight loss or health regime, but rather a new way of eating that celebrates the vibrant and irresistible flavors of fresh vegetables and whole grains.

The main food groups that are featured in this cookbook are:

Whole Grains
Fruits
Vegetables
Beans and Other Vegetable Proteins
Fish

As you already may have noticed, there are many food types that are missing from the above list, namely dairy, eggs, meat and poultry.

DAIRY

Although dairy is rich in calcium and high in protein, it is a food that many people are allergic to. Some of the allergic signs are indigestion, gas, sinus congestion, asthma, bad breath and drowsiness. And if you are allergic to dairy, there is reason to question whether your body can actually absorb the calcium from the dairy products you eat. Simply put, your body will likely consider dairy a foreign invader that needs to be eliminated. Your body won't expend the energy needed to assimilate the dairy for nutritional purposes. Instead, your body will make every effort to get rid of the infiltrator. That is why many people who suffer from dairy/lactose intolerance get diarrhea after eating ice cream or drinking a glass of milk. The calcium gets flushed down the toilet.

So if you cut out dairy products from your diet, where do you get the calcium you need to keep your bones and teeth healthy? Certainly you can take supplements if you want to, but there are also many non-dairy food sources of calcium to choose from. Many green vegetables such as broccoli, collards, kale and a variety of sea vegetables contain calcium. Calcium is also found in sesame seeds, sunflower seeds, almonds and tofu.

EGGS

Eggs are high in fat and for many, an allergenic food. In the United States, chickens are raised under such poor conditions that the quality of eggs is questionable. Chickens are injected with hormones and antibiotics to increase higher yields of egg production. Chicken coops are filthy and overcrowded. It is no wonder why salmonella contamination is such a problem.

If you must have eggs, we recommend free-range. Free-range eggs come from chickens raised without drugs and fed feed that contains no pesticides. Plus the chickens are not cooped up in such close quarters so they can enjoy more freedom of movement.

MEAT AND POULTRY

Meat and poultry are very high in protein and contain many essential vitamins and minerals. In spite of being so nutritious, meat and poultry are also high in fat and often full of hormones and antibiotics that you certainly don't want to ingest.

Although many people are trying to reduce their fat intake by cutting down on red meat, they still eat a lot of chicken and turkey. What we are recommending is eating less of the chicken and turkey as well. Better yet, cut out meat, chicken and turkey completely. But, if that's not realistic for you, we suggest that you try eating varieties raised without hormones and antibiotics. Free-range and Amish chickens are good choices. They are available in many grocery stores and upscale meat markets. Hormone-free meat is a little harder to find. Again, an upscale meat market is your best bet.

FISH

We recommend that you choose white, flaky fish such as flounder, halibut, cod, sole and red snapper for regular consumption. Higher fat fish such as tuna and rainbow trout should be eaten less frequently. Salmon, although relatively high in fat, is a wonderful fish due to its high omega-3 fatty acid content, which protects against heart disease. We prefer wild-caught ocean salmon over the farmed variety. The reason is that the farmed fishing industry uses chemicals and drugs that may be harmful to humans. The fear is that drug-resistant microbes may pass on to humans who eat infected farmed fish. Many believe that fish farming is also harmful to the environment since drug and chemical-laced waste is dumped into coastal coves and infected farmed fish are able to escape into the open waters, adversely effecting wild aquatic life.

Shellfish, although low in calories, should be eaten rarely. Shellfish is relatively high in cholesterol as well as a common allergenic food. Eating contaminated shellfish is a leading cause of food poisoning. In addition, much of the shrimp consumed in North America is farmed, creating the same potential health risk associated with farmed fish.

Great Lakes fish such as whitefish and walleye should be avoided altogether due to high levels of toxic chemicals and other pollutants.

FOODS TO EAT IN MODERATION

Flour products such as bread, crackers and pasta should be eaten in moderation. Although these foods are nutritious, they do not contain as much fiber as whole grains. And we all know that fiber is important to push wastes and toxins out of your system. A high fiber diet is also recommended by the American Cancer Association for the prevention of colon cancer.

Whole grain flour products are preferred over white flour products. First, white flour contains less fiber than whole grain flour. Second, the food value of white flour is relatively low. A great percentage of nutrients are lost in the refining process, which is the reason why white flour is often enriched with vitamins and minerals (only a small fraction of the nutrients lost are added back). Third, bleaches and chemicals are used in the refining process of most white flours. Lastly, many white flour products contain sugar, eggs, too much salt and chemical preservatives. If you are going to use white flour, make sure it is unbleached and not chemically processed.

So instead of having a daily serving of bread, adjust your thinking. Have a daily serving of a whole grain such as brown rice or barley instead. It's not that flour products should be cut out of your diet completely. Just don't make them your grain staple. Also, calorie for calorie, whole grains don't seem to make you put on weight the way bread and pasta do. The diet doctor will back me on this one.

Other foods to be wary of are sugar, alcohol and caffeine as they affect your moods and sleep patterns. Also, caffeine and alcohol consumption interfere with the absorption of many essential vitamins and minerals, particularly anti-oxidants which strengthen your immune system. Try herbal teas, grain coffees and non-alcoholic wines and beers for regular consumption. For sweet cravings, try a piece of fruit or one of the desserts in this cookbook. Artificial sweeteners should be avoided completely. Studies have linked their use with cancer, headaches and neurological disorders.

OUR DIET

Our daily diet consists of:

- Whole Grains
- Vegetables
- Vegetable Protein or Fish
- Miso Soup
- Pickles
- Fruit

Whole Grains

Whole grains such as brown rice, barley, corn, millet and wheat berries should be considered the staple of the diet. You should have at least one serving of whole grains at least once a day. Whole grains can be prepared in a variety of ways. They are wonderful served with vegetables, beans and fish.

Whole grain flour products such as whole wheat bread or rye crackers should be eaten less frequently. White rice should be eaten rarely. The reason is that much of the nutrition is lost in the refining process.

Vegetables

Have at least five servings of vegetables daily. To ensure the absorption of a variety of vitamins and minerals, eat from each of the five vegetables groups listed on the following page:

1) Green Leafy Vegetables: bok choy, chives, collards, dandelion greens, kale, leeks, lettuce, mustard greens, Napa cabbage, parsley, rapini, scallions, watercress

2) Round Vegetables: beets, broccoli, Brussels sprouts, cabbage, cauliflower, onions, radishes, rutabaga, turnips, winter squash

3) Root Vegetables and Tubers: burdock, carrots, celery root, daikon, Jerusalem artichokes, parsnips, sweet potatoes, taro

4) Sea Vegetables: agar agar, arame, hijiki, kombu, nori, wakame

5) Others: corn, cucumbers, green beans, green peas, mushrooms

Now, you don't have to follow this list to the letter. But do increase the amount of vegetables you eat in quantity and variety. Try sea vegetables. They are extremely rich in calcium and iron.

Most vegetables are fine for regular consumption. The only ones to eat in moderation are the nightshade vegetables: eggplant, zucchini, tomatoes, peppers and potatoes. Nightshade vegetables (and spinach) seem to aggravate symptoms of arthritis.

Bill and I eat eggplant, zucchini, tomatoes and peppers in the summer when they are in season, but not on a daily basis. We rarely eat potatoes; they cause the scale to go up almost immediately and make Bill really cranky.

Protein

In this style of cooking, the protein choices are mainly vegetarian. First on the list are beans. Any type of bean is fine. Soybean-derived tofu and tempeh are also very good sources of protein, as well as wheat-meat products like seitan. Last choice for protein is fish, which can be eaten 2-4 times a week. In any case, protein should not be considered the main feature of a meal. The focus is on grains, vegetables and miso soup. But not to worry, you won't leave the table hungry.

> Vegetable Proteins: beans (lentils, chickpeas, adzuki, navy, pinto, kidney), bean products (tofu, tempeh, miso), seitan
>
> Fish: halibut, haddock, sole, cod, red snapper, flounder, grouper, salmon, sea bass, striped bass (tuna on occasion and shellfish rarely)

Miso Soup

Miso is a fermented bean paste that is used in Japanese and macrobiotic cooking. There are many varieties. I tend to use the dark longer fermented miso in the winter, the red moderately fermented miso in the spring and fall, and the yellow young miso in the summer.

Miso is considered to have strong medicinal properties. In combination with brown rice, it promotes regulation of the bowels. Miso is also used to treat radiation sickness.

Miso soup is delicious and easy to make. It should be consumed at least once a day. Miso also adds flavor to stews, dips, gravies and sauces.

Pickles

A small serving of pickles aids in digestion. Pickles can be made from any of the recommended vegetables and should not be too spicy or salty. Overly salty pickles should be rinsed with water before eating.

Fruit

Too much fruit is like having too much sugar. In the long run, you will find that you will feel much better and be able to keep your weight down much more effectively, if you limit your fruit intake to only one or two servings daily. Less is best. Eat more vegetables instead.

Fruits should be in season and if possible, locally grown. Whole fruit is recommended over fruit juice since whole fruit has more fiber. Plus one serving of juice is usually extracted from several pieces of fruit. Fruit may be eaten raw, cooked or dried. Organic fruit is best. Dried fruit should be unsulphured.

Nuts and Seeds

Nuts and seeds may be consumed in small quantities, and infrequently. The best choices are walnuts, almonds, pumpkin seeds, sunflower seeds and sesame seeds. Super high-fat nuts such as Brazil or macadamia nuts should be avoided.

ORGANIC FOOD

Whenever possible we buy organic. We feel safer knowing that what we put in our mouths is not tainted with anti-fungal chemicals and pesticides. And in our own small way, we feel that the choice to eat organic contributes to the overall well-being of our planet, by keeping our waters a little cleaner, our animals a little safer, and our soil and vegetation a little healthier.

The Environmental Working Group lists certain conventionally farmed fruits and vegetables that have the most pesticide residues. They are strawberries, bell peppers (green and red), spinach, cherries, peaches, celery, apples, apricots, green beans and cucumbers. Avoid these if you can and buy organic instead. The conventionally farmed fruits and vegetables considered to have the least pesticide residues are avocados, onions, sweet potatoes, cauliflower, Brussels sprouts, grapes grown in the U.S., bananas, plums, green onions, watermelon and broccoli.

Another benefit of buying organic is that you are less likely to buy genetically engineered (GE) fruits and vegetables. The DNA in GE seeds is altered to resist certain diseases and pests. Some of the seeds are crossbred with other plant and non-plant species as well as chemicals and certain bacteria. The potential danger of this type of farming has lead to much debate around the world. Some studies have reported that GE bacteria can transfer potential cancer-causing agents. Certain GE vegetables are encoded with the DNA of Brazil nuts, theoretically creating a problem for people with nut allergies. There is growing public concern over the safety of GE corn, soy and canola. And GE farming may put the monarch butterfly at risk of extinction.

So our advice is to buy organic when you can. Organic fruits and vegetables as well as organic grains, flours, pasta, tamari, miso, oils and vinegars are available in many grocery stores, health food stores and specialty markets. For the home vegetable grower, there are many nurseries and seed companies that carry organic seeds.

WATER

Unfortunately our water supply is not as clean as it should be, especially around industrial areas. We recommend using water filters for home use and buying bottled water from natural springs when you go out.

Weight Control

Let me stick my nose in here and tell you how you can use the Diet Doctor's Wife's Cookbook to lose a little weight. As the title of this book suggests, I'm a diet doctor. I have been practicing weight loss medicine for over 20 years in the metropolitan Detroit area. My specialty is quick weight loss under medical supervision. I generally use medically safe crash diets to help my patients drop between five and ten pounds their first week, and at least five pounds every week after that.

But, I'm not talking about quick weight loss here. This section is aimed at those of you who are interested in losing weight slowly, one or two pounds a week, probably five to ten pounds every month. This section is for people who are not looking for a quick and dirty fix, but for a healthy lifestyle change. If you move in this direction, you will shed the pounds you want to lose and keep them off.

Before I get started, let me begin by saying that there is no secret to losing weight. There's no magic formula, miracle drug or special food. As your mother told you, in order to lose weight, you just have to eat less. It's as simple as that. You have to burn more calories than you consume.

Unfortunately, knowing what to do (that you should eat less) doesn't make you lose weight. And the reason is very simple. Eating less makes you hungry, which makes staying on a diet nearly impossible. Plus, when you are hungry, you generally crave sweets and starches. Eating sweets and starches raises insulin levels, which creates an increased cycle of hunger. The sad result is overeating and the pounds pile up.

In my clinical experience, the key to helping people lose weight is to deal with hunger and cravings, head-on. The following rules aim to keep those two demons at bay:

Diet Rule #1:
If you're not hungry, don't eat.

Believe it or not, one of the best ways to combat hunger is by not eating when you are not hungry. One of the worst things you can do, contrary to public perception, is to eat breakfast if you're not hungry. The reason is that as soon as you start to eat, your insulin level goes up which sets off the hunger cycle for the day. Breakfast does not start your metabolism or kick off fat burning. Your metabolism never stops. Eating just gives your body more calories and fat to burn.

Don't eat breakfast or anything at all if you're not hungry. The less you eat, the faster you will lose weight. You don't have to have three meals a day, nor do you have to eat every single thing recommended on your daily diet.

Diet Rule #2:
Drink at least 128 ounces of water a day.

The second most important thing you have to do to lose weight is to drink water, at least 128 ounces a day. Better yet, drink your weight in ounces of water. For example, if your current weight is 150 pounds, you should try to drink at least 150 ounces of water a day.

There are many reasons to increase your water intake. First, studies show that the average American is dehydrated. Second, about half the time you have the urge to eat, you are really more thirsty than hungry. Third, as fat is eliminated from the body through the urine and sweat, drinking water will help flush out fat without damaging your kidneys.

Last, drinking water makes you feel and look good. It does wonders for the complexion.

It's really quite remarkable, but most of my patients speed up their weight loss just by increasing their water intake to their weight in ounces. The sacrifice is just a few extra trips to the bathroom.

Diet Rule #3:
Exercise enough to break a sweat for 15-20 minutes per day.

Most Americans get no exercise, which is one of the reasons we are currently the fattest country on the face of the earth. (The other reason is that we eat too darn much.) If you take just 15 minutes a day and exercise hard enough to break a sweat, you'll probably drop about a pound a week. Exercise is an easy way to drop weight without altering your diet very much. And let's not forget the cardiovascular benefits. Plus, exercise increases endorphins, which are natural feel-good hormones that can also decrease feelings of hunger.

Note, that when I say exercise, I do not mean taking a brisk walk. I'm talking about fifteen minutes of serious sweat-inducing exertion.

Diet Rule #4:
Follow a special diet that works.

The truth is that just trying to eat less does not work well for most people. At least it does not work consistently enough over the long run for people to lose a significant amount of weight. My advice, based on over 20 years experience in the diet trenches, is that you follow a structured diet specially designed to decrease cravings and feelings of hunger. Doctor Nagler's 3-2-1 Program is just that kind of diet.

Doctor Nagler's 3-2-1 Program

If you are attracted to a diet rich in whole grains and vegetables, Doctor Nagler's 3-2-1 Program is for you. The nicest thing about this program is that most people find that they are not hungry. The reason is that the food choices are based on the macrobiotic system of balancing out cravings. The brown rice satisfies cravings for starches. The seaweed and greens radically diminish cravings for sweets. After a few days on this diet, carrots and squash will seem sweet enough. And you won't have to worry about constipation; the miso and brown rice combination is a magic bullet that will keep you regular.

Follow the simple diet below and you will lose weight. Remember, if you are not hungry, don't eat. If you are hungry, follow the instructions exactly.

Meal 1

1 cup brown rice
1 bowl miso soup
1-2 tablespoons non-sweet pickle

You must have all of these three foods for your first meal. Your brown rice can be eaten plain, or topped with a little soy sauce or sesame salt. Sesame salt (gomasio) can be prepared at home (see page 327 for the recipe) or bought in the macrobiotic section of a health food store. The miso soup can be prepared any of the ways indicated in this cookbook, but must contain seaweed (wakame, arame or kombu). Any pickle is okay, as long as it does not contain sugar.

The first time you get hungry each day, you must eat Meal 1 in its entirety. Don't skip any of the foods. The food combination is important. It is designed to limit your cravings.

Meal 2

cooked green vegetables
vegetable protein or fish

Only eat Meal 2 if you are hungry. You are allowed one serving (1-2 cups) of cooked green vegetables: cabbage, collards, kale, Swiss chard, mustard greens, bok choy or dandelion greens. Collards and kale are the best choices as they are rich in calcium. Your protein can be up to 8 ounces of beans, low fat tofu, tempeh, seitan or fish. Use any of the low fat preparations in this cookbook.

Meal 3

steamed vegetables

Only eat Meal 3 if you are hungry. Meal 3 consists of one serving (1-2 cups) of steamed vegetables: broccoli, carrots, cauliflower, turnips, parsnip or winter squash (refer to page 38 for a more comprehensive list). You may have any of the steamed vegetable preparations in this cookbook. Dipping sauce is allowed, preferably made without oil. Recipes for dipping sauces can be found in the Basics chapter.

Snack

cooked or stewed fruit

If you are still hungry after your 3 meals, you may have a single serving (1/2 cup) of cooked or stewed fruit, prepared without sugar or artificial sweetener. You can have a baked apple, apple sauce, fruit compote, stewed prunes, etc. A single serving only. No dried or fresh fruit. No pies, crumbles or cobblers.

If you are having a disastrous day, and are hungry and craving sweets, you may have another serving of steamed greens. If you have no energy, you may have another serving of protein.

Maintaining Your Weight Loss

If you follow the principles outlined in the What We Eat section (see pages 32-41), you basically are on an ideal maintenance diet. As a matter of fact, if you skip my 3-2-1 Program and just do maintenance, you will lose about a pound a month without even trying. Twelve pounds a year, doesn't sound like much until you put it in perspective. The average person who starts jogging 12 miles a week will also lose about 12 pounds a year. So in my opinion, the best way to lose a slow but healthy 25 pounds is to combine this way of eating with a cardiovascular exercise program.

But back to maintenance. If you want to keep your weight off for life, read the What We Eat section very carefully, and follow the guidelines below. The guidelines are simple, tried and true. You will not gain your weight back. Maintenance Rules 1-3 are the same as Diet Rules 1-3.

Maintenance Rule #1:
If you're not hungry, don't eat.
(see page 43)

Maintenance Rule #2:
Drink at least 128 ounces of water per day.
(see page 43)

Maintenance Rule #3:
Exercise enough to break a sweat for at least 15-20 minutes per day.
(see page 44)

Maintenance Rule #4:
Avoid fat.

Keep your fat intake low. Try to completely eliminate all butter and margarine from your diet. Vegetable oils should be used sparingly. Read over the low fat cooking techniques in the The Way to Cook section (see pages 62-65). Read labels carefully when you go out shopping to avoid unwanted fat.

Maintenance Rule #5:
Avoid sugar.

Avoid sugar and honey like the plague. Read labels carefully when you go out shopping to avoid unwanted sugar. Also don't eat more than one serving of fruit per day. Avoid artificial sweeteners as well. They may be low in calories but do stimulate your cravings for sweets throughout the day.

Maintenance Rule #6:
Avoid baked flour products.

It's almost impossible to keep your weight under control if you eat bread, crackers, pizza or pasta on a regular basis. And forget about cookies, cakes and pies. Baked flour raises your insulin level and makes you hungry, which leads to overeating.

Maintenance Rule #7:
Eat your greens.

Have at least one serving of cooked greens per day. Greens help to keep your cravings for sweets under control.

Nutritional Facts

We have indicated nutritional information for each of the recipes in this cookbook. In addition to including values for calories, fat, cholesterol, protein and sodium, we have added values for many essential vitamins and minerals. The reason is that we want to stress that the recipes in this cookbook are not only low in fat and calories but also loaded with nutrients. For example, many of the recipes have very high vitamin A levels. This is of particular importance, as medical studies have shown that the average American is vitamin A deficient, a condition that compromises immune response.

We have chosen to indicate weight rather than Percentage of Daily Value (%DV) for each nutrient, since percentage values are based on recommendations for "normal" healthy people with no illness, deficiencies, weaknesses, stress or toxic environmental exposure. Requirements vary from individual to individual because of genetic, lifestyle and other differences. For this reason, we also believe that the US Food and Drug Administration's Recommended Daily Intake values may be too low for some vitamins and minerals.

Recommended Daily Intake (RDI)

Potassium	3500mg
Calcium	1000mg
Iron	18mg
Zinc	15mg
Vitamin C	60mg
Vitamin A	5000 IU
Vitamin B6	2.0mg
Vitamin B12	6.0mcg
Thiamin B1	1.5mg
Riboflavin B2	1.7mg
Folacin	400mcg
Niacin	20mg

Fat

Americans are arguably the fattest people on the planet with a very high incidence of fat related illnesses such as heart disease, stroke, diabetes and cancer.

The average American diet is 35-40% fat. We are recommending radically cutting that level down to between 10 and 20 percent (25-45 grams of fat per day). The lower the better.

Cholesterol

Cholesterol is a waxy, fatty substance that can form deposits on the inside of artery walls. The deposits can cause narrowing or complete blockage of certain blood vessels, which can lead to heart disease.

Cholesterol is found in animal foods such as eggs, cheese milk, fish, poultry and meat. Cholesterol values vary among animal foods. For example, a single ounce of fatty red meat will have more cholesterol than a single ounce of whitefish. The US Food and Drug Administration (FDA) recommends that you have less than 300mg of cholesterol per day.

In addition to the dietary cholesterol found in animal foods, there is serum cholesterol, which circulates through the bloodstream. There are two types of serum cholesterol: HDL and LDL. HDL or "good" cholesterol helps the body to eliminate excess cholesterol, preventing its build up in the arteries. HDL levels should be high and can be elevated by exercise and weight loss. LDL or "bad" cholesterol is carried through the blood to the tissues and can potentially cause build up in the arteries. LDL levels should be low, and can be decreased by following a low fat, low cholesterol diet.

We recommend decreasing your intake of animal proteins. That includes baked goods made with butter and eggs. And when you do decide to eat an animal protein, make sure you choose lower fat versions like fish. We also suggest that you include more vegetable proteins in your diet such as beans, lentils, tofu, seitan and tempeh.

Saturated Fat

Saturated fats tend to raise LDL cholesterol in the blood. Saturated fats come from meat, poultry, milk products, butter and tropical oils. Saturated fats are also contained in many packaged foods. The FDA recommends that you consume no more than 20-25 grams of saturated fat per day. We recommend that you avoid saturated fats completely or at least try to keep them to a minimum.

Fiber

High fiber is recommended for decreasing the risk of colon cancer. The FDA recommends about 25-30 grams per day. We suggest that you increase those numbers, if you can.

Whole grains and vegetables are the best sources of high fiber. By whole grains, we do not mean whole wheat flour products such as whole wheat bread, crackers or pasta. We are referring to actual whole grains such as brown rice, barley, millet, and wheat berries.

Protein

You need protein in your diet to keep your muscles and organs healthy. Protein requirements vary according to sex and body weight. The FDA recommends that you consume between 50 and 65 grams of protein per day. We recommend that you choose vegetarian proteins (beans, seitan, tofu and tempeh) and fish.

Sodium

Many people have to watch their sodium or salt intake, particularly if they have high blood pressure. The FDA advises against consuming more than 2400mg of sodium per day. When reading the sodium values in this book, it is important to take into account the following:

1. The sodium content of salt is not indicated if a recipe instructs the cook to add salt according to taste. People's preferences vary enormously, so we have left the responsibility of salting up to the cook.

2. The salt content of cooked pasta, assumes that no salt has been added to the water. The reason is that it is hard to determine how much salt is absorbed by the pasta during the process of boiling. If you are on a low sodium diet, you may want to salt the water lightly or not at all.

3. Some recipes call for tamari or soy sauce, which are high in sodium. Low sodium varieties are available in most grocery stores.

Read nutritional information on all packaged foods. Sodium levels can be quite high. It is important to be realistic about serving size when you calculate sodium levels. You can eliminate some of the salt in bottled or canned goods by emptying contents into a colander, then rinsing with cold water and allowing the water to drain.

Vitamin B12

To prevent from becoming anemic, you have to include Vitamin B12 in your diet, or take B12 injections (oral B12 supplements are poorly absorbed). The food sources that we recommend for Vitamin B12 are fish and tempeh.

Yields

If a recipe yields a range of servings such as [serves 4-6], the nutritional information is calculated for the lowest number of servings. In other words, a salad serving 4-6 people will indicate nutritional information based on 4 servings. Likewise, a recipe that calls for 8-12 ounces of a given food item will have a nutritional count calculated for the lower value (8 ounces).

The Diet Doctor's Wife's Cookbook's Nutritional List

A nutritional analysis is included for each recipe in this cookbook, based on information from the US Department of Agriculture, the FDA, and food suppliers and manufacturers. Values are listed for the following categories:

Calories
Total Fat (g)
Saturated Fat (g)
Cholesterol (mg)
Sodium (mg)
Potassium (mg)
Total Carbohydrate (g)
Dietary Fiber (g)
Protein (g)
Calcium (mg)
Iron (mg)
Zinc (mg)
Vitamin C (mg)
Vitamin A (IU)
Vitamin B6 (mg)
Vitamin B12 (mcg)
Thiamin B1 (mg)
Riboflavin B2 (mg)
Folacin (mcg)
Niacin (mg)

Each recipe has a value for Calories, Total Fat, Saturated Fat, and Cholesterol, even if that value is zero. For all other categories, a value is only indicated if it is greater than zero or "trace."

The Way to Cook

COOKING EQUIPMENT

It is important to have good cooking equipment. The following is a list of what I consider essential for preparing the recipes in this cookbook:

Knives - A good set of knives is a must. At the very least, you should have a chef's knife, a paring knife, a cleaver for cutting large squashes, and a serrated knife. Ceramic knives are expensive but well worth it as they rarely need to be sharpened.

Knife Sharpener - Knives should remain sharp. An electric knife sharpener or a sharpening stone does the job.

2 Chopping Boards - I recommend using two chopping boards. One for vegetables and fruit, and another for fish.

Pots and Pans - Good quality, heavy, stainless steel or enamel pots will last a lifetime. You should have a small, medium and large pot, a pasta pot, a double boiler preferably with a steamer insert, a heavy stainless steel frying pan and a roasting pan.

Pressure Cooker - Pressure cookers are ideal for cooking grains, beans and soups. I would recommend a stainless steel, 6-quart pressure cooker to start with.

Heat Diffuser or Flame Deflector – A heat diffuser or flame deflector is very useful for cooking grains at a very low temperature.

Nonstick Frying Pan - Nonstick cookware is terrific for low fat cooking. Just remember not to use metal kitchen utensils as they can scratch nonstick surfaces.

Wok - Woks are wonderful for sautéing and steaming. The sloped sides create a broad surface area, which allows for more even cooking and less mess. I particularly like nonstick woks as they allow for lower fat preparations.

Bamboo Steamers – Bamboo steamers can be easily inserted in a wok. They come in various sizes.

Otoshibuta – This Japanese, wooden drop-lid is used in braising to ensure even cooking.

Colanders - Wire mesh colanders with handles are very convenient and come in various sizes. I would recommend a large, medium and small.

Wooden Spoons - Keep wooden spoons used for baking separate from ones used for cooking so that unwanted cooking odors are not transmitted to baked goods. Buy several spoons with long handles, making it less likely for you to burn yourself while stirring over a hot stove.

Tongs - Tongs with very long handles protect you from burning your arms and hands, particularly when turning hot roasting vegetables.

Wooden Skewers - Ideal for testing doneness.

Plastic Cooking Utensils (Spoon, Slotted Spoon, Spatula, etc.) – Essential for nonstick cookware.

Rubber Spatula – Use for scraping batter out of a bowl.

Whisks – Both metal and nonstick. I would also recommend getting a small whisk for preparing salad dressings.

Vegetable Brush - Great for cleaning carrots, turnips, squashes and other rough-skinned vegetables.

Vegetable Peeler – Necessary for removing skins from fruits and vegetables.

Zester – Used to remove lemon and orange zest.

Graters – Buy graters with large and small grates.

Ceramic Ginger Grater – A ceramic ginger grater with a surrounding moat to catch the ginger juice.

Salad Spinner – A fabulous gadget for drying lettuce leaves.

Kitchen Scale – I recommend a digital scale with both English and metric measurements.

Sieve – For sifting flour.

Rolling Pin – For rolling out dough and crushing nuts.

Measuring Cups – Get 2 sets, one for dry and one for liquid measurements.

Measuring Spoons – I recommend several sets.

Food Processor – It has endless uses. One of my favorite kitchen appliances.

Blender or Puree Wand – For purees. The wand can go directly in a pot, which makes pureeing super easy.

Electric Mixer (Hand or Standing) – A baker's must.

Baking Pans – 8" round, 8" square, loaf, 7" spring-form, muffin tins (regular and mini), jellyroll pans, baking sheets, 9" glass pie plate, 9" tart pan.

Parchment Paper - Important for low fat baking and roasting.

Suribachi and Surikogi (Mortar and Pestle) - A suribachi is a Japanese style mortar. The surikogi is a wooden pestle. The bowl interior of the suribachi is lined with unglazed narrow grooves, which make grinding quick and easy.

Electric Coffee Grinder - For grinding spices.

Food Mill – For making the smoothest tomato sauce.

Pickle Press - A convenient and efficient tool for making quick pickles.

Mandoline - Terrific for even and decorative slicing.

WASHING FOOD

Whether you buy organic or not, it is very important to wash vegetables, grains and beans thoroughly. It is also important to wash fish before cooking it.

Vegetables

Wash leafy greens under cold running water and then immerse them in a large bowl of cold water. Lift greens out of the water and place them in a colander to dry, or use a salad spinner.

Thick-skinned vegetables like carrots and turnips need to be scrubbed clean with a vegetable brush, while rinsing under cold running water. Unless they are young and tender, you should peel these types of vegetables before cooking, except if you are preparing a soup stock. Waxed vegetables like some squashes and cucumbers also need to be washed with a vegetable brush, and then the skin must be peeled and discarded.

Cauliflower and broccoli need to be immersed in salted or vinegared water (1 teaspoon salt or 1 tablespoon vinegar per quart of water) for about 10 minutes, to release worms and insects. Then the vegetables should be rinsed off thoroughly under cold running water. Depending on what is required in a given recipe, you may find it easier to cut the vegetables in smaller pieces before washing.

Cabbage may be cut in half or in quarters before running it under cold water. Separating the leaves is usually not necessary.

Mushrooms can be cleaned by rinsing under a light stream of cold water. For more fragile mushrooms (fresh shitakes), just wipe clean with a damp paper towel.

Most sea vegetables also need to be washed before cooking. Arame can be quickly rinsed under cold water. Hijiki needs to be washed more carefully as it can be gritty. You may want to pick through hijiki as well. Kombu just needs to be wiped with a damp rag or paper towel. Nori and agar agar require no washing at all.

To wash herbs, spray sprigs with water and allow to dry upright in a drinking glass.

Fruits should be washed whole under cold running water. To wash berries, first place them in a colander. Run cold water over them, making sure that the pressure is not too high so that the berries keep their shape. Line a baking sheet with paper towels. Set berries on the lined baking sheet, spaced 1-inch apart. Allow to dry.

Beans and Grains

Beans and whole grains (rice, barley and buckwheat groats) need to be sorted and washed before cooking. The best way to sort beans and grains is to spread them out in a jelly roll pan or a large roasting pan, so that each bean or grain is in view. Then you can easily pick out pebbles, twigs or clumps of dirt. After the beans and grains are sorted, place them in a large pot and cover with cold water. Swish the beans or grains around. The water will likely be cloudy. Drain. Repeat the washing procedure until the water runs clear. Drain.

Fish

Before you cook a whole fish, rinse it well under cold running water to get rid of dirt, traces of entrails and blood. After washing, thoroughly pat dry with a paper towel. Fillets need to be rinsed as well and then pat dry.

As salmonella may be passed on by handling raw fish, be sure to thoroughly clean your prep area and wash your hands well before handling other foods. If you have any open cuts, put on a Band-Aid or wear latex gloves.

Seeds

Sesame seeds need to be washed before cooking. After picking through for twigs and dirt particles, place the seeds in a pot and cover with cold water. Discard the seeds that float to the top and then drain. Cover with cold water again and drain. If the water is cloudy, repeat the washing procedure until the water runs clear. Allow the washed seeds to dry in a large, fine-meshed strainer.

KITCHEN BURNS

Lavender Oil

I burn myself a lot. I can't recall how many times I have touched a hot metal handle with my bare hands or bumped into a boiling pot. I have tried treating my burns by running the effected area under cold water and then using an ice pack, but have found that the pain lingers and blistering still develops. I have tried using aloe gel and Vitamin E oil to speed up healing and lessen the pain, but still find that I am dissatisfied with the results.

Thankfully, I have discovered a much more effective remedy, the essential oil of lavender. All I do is pour a few drops on the burn. The relief is instantaneous. If the pain comes back, I just add another few drops. And I don't blister.

The essential oil of lavender is available at most health food stores.

Long Handled Kitchen Utensils

To avoid burning myself, I like to use long handled kitchen utensils. Long handled wooden spoons are great for protecting yourself from rising steam, especially when stirring over a deep simmering pot. Long handled tongs are particularly good for turning roasting vegetables in a very hot oven.

Long Oven Mitts

I wear oven mitts that rise up to my elbows. That way if I reach into a hot oven and graze an oven grate with my forearm, I am less likely to burn myself.

LOW FAT COOKING

The style of cooking presented in this cookbook is extremely low in fat. You will notice that far less oil is called for than in comparable recipes. But don't worry. The reduction in fat does not compromise flavor.

Below are some of the low fat cooking techniques I use:

Boiling

Boiling is an ideal way to cook brown rice, basmati rice, Arborio rice, grains with a thin kernel wall (millet and buckwheat groats), and grains that are rolled or cut (rolled oats, barley flakes and polenta). Dense, long-cooking vegetables (beets, turnips and burdock) are usually boiled as well.

Don't discard the cooking water used for boiling vegetables. Add it to your soup stock instead. But before you do, remember to strain out any vegetable particles.

Steaming

Steaming is a very light, quick method of cooking, particularly in the warmer months. I recommend steaming vegetables separately to avoid unwanted mixing of flavors. If you are steaming a variety of vegetables, it is okay to use the same cooking water. Just steam the strongest tasting vegetables last. For example, carrots, cauliflower and broccoli should be steamed in the listed order.

Don't throw away the cooking water used for steaming. Add it to your soup stock instead. But before you do, remember to strain out any vegetable particles.

On the following page are 4 methods of steaming:

1) To use a collapsible stainless-steel steamer, add cold water to a pot to a level of 1-2 inches. Place steamer in the pot. Place vegetables in the steamer. Cover and bring to a boil. Steam until tender and a little firm. Cooking time depends on the type and size of the vegetable. Do not overcook.

2) Bamboo steamers are used in Asian cooking. They have a flat surface area, which makes them better suited for steaming larger foods like fish fillets.

   Bamboo steaming is safest if you place the steamer inside a wok. Pour cold water in the wok to a level of 1-2 inches. Place the bamboo steamer over the water. Place whatever needs to be steamed in the bamboo steamer and cover with the bamboo lid. Cover the wok as well and bring to a boil. Steam for the required cooking time. A bamboo steamer may also be safely placed inside a deep pot. Make sure that the sides of the pot are higher than the sides of the steamer. To begin steaming, pour cold water in the pot to a level of 1-2 inches. Place whatever needs to be steamed inside the bamboo steamer and cover with the bamboo lid. Fit the covered steamer inside the pot. Cover the pot as well. Bring to a boil. Steam for the required cooking time.

3) For double boilers with steamer inserts, fill the bottom pot with cold water to a level of 1-2 inches. Insert steamer. Place whatever needs to be steamed in the steamer and cover. Bring to a boil. Steam for required cooking time.

4) If you do not have a steamer, pour cold water in a pot to a level of 1-2 inches. Add vegetables, cover and bring to a boil. Steam for required cooking time. Do not discard cooking water. Add it to your stock instead.

Pressure Cooking

My introduction to pressure cooking was at the Kushi Institute in one of the Way To Health cooking classes. I had never seen a pressure cooker before, and had only heard horror stories about exploding tops and other complications. But after a few days of demonstrations in the Kushi kitchen, my fears were forgotten.

The pressure cookers today are very safe and easy to use, and are ideal for cooking grains, beans and soups. Pressure-cooking creates an intense, rich flavor without the use of added fat. And cooking time is often much faster than with other methods.

To use a pressure cooker, all you do is place ingredients in a cooker, no more than two-thirds full. Secure lid. Over medium heat, bring up to pressure (refer to your pressure cooker manual) and then lower heat. Cook for the required time. Wait until pressure releases before removing the lid.

Sautéing

In this cookbook, many recipes require sautéing with the use of very little fat. The challenge of low fat sautéing is to prevent food from drying out or sticking to the bottom of the pan. This can be accomplished easily by 1) using a brush to lightly coat the entire cooking surface with oil, 2) using nonstick cookware, 3) reducing the heat, and 4) adding small amounts of soup stock, water or cooking wine to your sautés after the initial browning. Using liquid seasonings like tamari or soy sauce instead of salt will also help.

Braising

Braising involves cooking with a small amount of liquid (water or broth) in a tightly covered pot. Before liquid is added, the vegetables are usually, but not always sautéed. The amount of fat used for sautéing in the braising recipes in this cookbook is minimal. Bitter leafy greens and dense vegetables, such as squash and turnips, taste lovely when braised.

SEASONING

You can use just about any natural seasoning with this style of cooking. Avoid bottled or prepared dressings with mystery chemicals or preservatives. Herbs, spices, mustards and vinegars are fine. However, seasoning should be light and gentle. Below are seasonings frequently used in this cookbook.

Sea salt - The sea salt referred to in this cookbook is the unrefined version, which is slightly grayish in color, not white like table salt. Table salt is refined sea salt that is iodized and doctored with anti-caking agents and crystal modifiers to make it more pourable. Unrefined sea salt, on the other hand, is obtained from the evaporation of ocean water, period. There are no additives. Unrefined sea salt is available in health food stores and gourmet shops.

Soy sauce (shoyu) is a fermented product made from wheat, soybeans, water and sea salt. Low sodium versions of soy sauce are available.

Tamari is a fermented product that is made from soybeans, water and sea salt. It is a wheat-free soy sauce. Low sodium versions of tamari are available.

Ginger juice - To make ginger juice, grate peeled fresh ginger root. Roll the pulp into a ball. Squeeze out the juice into a measuring spoon or directly into a pot or bowl. Small, easy-to-use ginger graters are available in specialty cookware shops as well as through macrobiotic mail order catalogues.

Brown rice vinegar - Brown rice vinegar is a fermented brown rice product.

Mirin - Mirin is a sweet cooking wine made from sweet rice.

Sake - Sake is a wine made from fermented brown or white rice.

COOKING OILS AND FATS

Oil is used in this cookbook, but in much smaller quantities than most recipes call for. If your pan gets too dry when you are sautéing, avoid the temptation to add more oil. Use water or broth instead. Lowering the cooking temperature also helps. Don't worry. The initial hit of oil will give you all the sautéed flavor you need.

The two oils I cook with most are grapeseed oil and extra virgin olive oil. Grapeseed oil is very light and does not impart a strong flavor. Extra virgin olive oil is wonderful for salad dressings and dishes for which an olive flavor adds just the right accent. I also use a modest amount of toasted sesame oil for flavoring Asian style dishes.

In baking, I use oil instead of butter or margarine. Flavorful nut oils such as walnut or almond work beautifully. Grapeseed oil is also a good choice (especially if you have nut allergies).

Although I have avoided the use of butter in this cookbook, in a few recipes, I use ghee. Ghee is clarified butter. As the milk solids are removed in the clarification process, ghee is easier on the digestion than regular butter. Ghee is a terrific choice when nothing but butter will do.

SWEETENERS

I rarely use refined *sugar and never use artificial sweeteners. The consumption of refined sugar leads to weight gain, moodiness and erratic energy fluctuations. Studies have linked the use of artificial sweeteners with cancer, headaches and neurological disorders.

When a sweetener is required in cooking or baking, I use fruit, fruit juice, brown rice syrup, barley malt, maple syrup or unsulphured molasses. Occasionally I use unrefined sugar as well as unrefined honey.

*Note: I use sugar syrup in the sorbet recipes. Natural sweeteners don't seem to work as well. Plus there is a small amount of confectioner's sugar in the Bisteeya recipe (page 222).

The Pantry

If you chose to cook the way I do, your pantry may start to look a bit different. Instead of loading up on canned goods, bottled sauces, boxed crackers, chips and prepackaged mixes, you will fill your cupboards with whole grains, beans and dried sea vegetables.

Your freezer will certainly not be as full, as you will no longer have a need for stocking up on meat, poultry, frozen vegetables and ice cream. Instead, you will be storing prepared vegetable proteins (tofu, tempeh and seitan) in your refrigerator. In addition, your refrigerator will likely contain a wider variety of fresh vegetables.

Below is a categorized list of the kinds of foods that you should have on hand:

DRY GOODS

1. Grains

Bill and I eat a lot of whole grains. Brown rice is our staple. We eat whole grain flour products (whole wheat bread, whole wheat crackers, etc.) on occasion. Whole grains and whole grain flour should be stored in airtight containers. If you have room, store flour in the refrigerator; it will stay fresh longer.

Rice - brown rice (short, medium and long grain), sweet brown rice, wild rice, brown rice crackers, brown rice flour

Barley – whole barley, barley flour

Buckwheat - buckwheat groats, buckwheat pasta, buckwheat flour, buckwheat flour products

Corn - popcorn kernels, cornmeal, corn flour, corn flour products

Millet - millet, millet flour

Oats - whole oats, steel-cut oats, rolled oats, oat flakes, oat flour

Rye - rye berries, rye flakes, rye flour, rye flour products

Whole Wheat - wheat berries, whole wheat pasta, whole wheat couscous, bulgur, fu, whole wheat flour, whole wheat flour products

2. Dried Beans

Beans are part of our regular diet. We recommend cooking with dried beans, which should be stored in airtight containers.

adzuki beans, black turtle beans, chickpeas, great northern beans, lentils, navy beans, pinto beans, red beans, split peas

3. Dried Fish

Bonito flakes are dried fish flakes used to make soup stock or condiments. They can be purchased at Japanese markets or in the macrobiotic section of many health food stores.

4. Dried Fruit

Dried fruit can be eaten as a snack or used to sweeten baked goods.

dried apricots, dried cherries, dried figs, prunes, raisins

5. Sea Vegetables

Sea vegetables are rich in vitamins and minerals. Arame, hijiki and wakame are particularly high in calcium. Sea vegetables usually come dried and may be purchased in Asian markets or in the macrobiotic section of most health food stores. Sea vegetables are also available through specialty food mail order catalogues.

agar agar, arame, hijiki, kombu, nori, wakame

6. Dried Vegetables

Dried shitake mushrooms add a rich meaty flavor to vegetarian cooking. They are found in Asian markets, gourmet shops and some grocery stores. They are also available through specialty food mail order catalogues.

CANNED GOODS

I usually have some canned goods on hand for times when I don't have the time to cook.

beans, dairy-free vegetarian soup, salmon, *tuna

*Note: Tuna is a relatively high fat fish and should be eaten in moderation.

PERISHABLE GOODS

1. Fruit

Fruit should be eaten in season, preferably locally grown. Below are the most highly recommended:

> apples, apricots, blueberries, grapes, lemons, melons, peaches, pears, plums, raspberries, strawberries, tangerines

2. Vegetables

This diet is rich in vegetables. Have a wide variety. Try something you've never tried before.

Beans - green/yellow beans, peas

Cabbage Family – broccoli, Brussels sprouts, cabbage, cauliflower

Greens - bok choy, celery, collards, dandelion greens, kale, lettuce, mustard greens, Swiss chard, turnip greens, watercress

Fresh Herbs - basil, chives, dill, oregano, parsley, rosemary, sage, thyme

Onion Family - garlic, scallions, leeks, red/white/yellow onions, shallots

Roots - burdock, carrots, celery root, daikon, parsnip, radishes, rutabaga, turnips

Squash - acorn, butternut, buttercup, cucumber, hokkaido, hubbard, kabocha, pumpkin

Tubers - Jerusalem artichokes, sweet potatoes

Others - corn, lotus root, mushrooms

3. Prepared Vegetable Proteins

We recommend that you include the following prepared vegetable proteins in your diet: seitan, tempeh and tofu. Seitan is a whole wheat protein, often referred to as wheat meat. Tempeh and tofu are made from soybeans. All three must be refrigerated. Seitan and tempeh can be purchased in health food markets. Tofu is more widely available.

seitan, tempeh, tofu

4. Fish

Fish may be eaten 2-4 times a week. The most highly recommended are:

cod, flounder, grouper, haddock, halibut, red snapper, salmon, sole, sea bass, striped bass

NUTS AND SEEDS

Nuts and seeds are used in both cooking and baking. Toasted sesame and sunflower seeds make nice condiments. Nuts may be eaten on their own as a snack, in moderation.

Nuts - almonds, chestnuts, hazelnuts, peanuts, pecans, pine nuts, walnuts

Seeds - pumpkin seeds, sesame seeds, sunflower seeds

PICKLES

A small serving of pickles is served with main meals. You can buy pickles in a health food store or make your own. A variety of pickle recipes are provided in this cookbook. Pickles can be prepared with a bit of sea salt, tamari or vinegar. They should contain very little spice and absolutely no sugar.

SEASONINGS

Many types of seasonings are used in this cookbook. In general, you will need to have the following on hand at all times:

> brown rice vinegar, fresh ginger root, miso, sea salt, soy sauce, tamari

I would also recommend that you store the following dried herbs and spices in your pantry:

> basil, bay leaves, caraway, cayenne pepper, cinnamon, cloves, coriander seeds, cumin, ginger, nutmeg, peppercorns (black and white), red pepper flakes, thyme, turmeric

COOKING OIL

The two oils I cook with most are grapeseed oil and extra virgin olive oil. Grapeseed oil is light and does not impart a strong flavor. Extra virgin olive oil has a slight fruity taste that is wonderful with French, Italian and Mediterranean style cooking. I also use a modest amount of toasted sesame oil to flavor Asian style dishes. In baking, I use nut oils (walnut or almond) and grapeseed oil. For nut allergies, you can substitute grapeseed oil or a light vegetable oil for nut oil.

PART II:

The Recipes

Salads

Jicama Salad

The Diet Doctor's Wife: Jicama is a low calorie vegetable that is filling, satisfying and slightly sweet.

1 jicama, peeled and cut in 1/4-inch thick strips
1/2 cup red onion, sliced in half-moons
juice of 1/2 lemon
2 tablespoons fresh cilantro, chopped
1/8 teaspoon sea salt
pinch of ground cayenne pepper

Combine ingredients.

[serves 4-6]

Nutrition Per Serving: Calories 74, Total Fat trace, Saturated Fat trace, Cholesterol 0mg, Sodium 68mg, Potassium 330mg, Protein 1g, Total Carbohydrate 18g, Dietary Fiber 9g, Calcium 37mg, Iron 1mg, Vitamin C 12mg, Vitamin A 223 IU, Vitamin B6 .1mg, Thiamin B1 .1mg, Riboflavin B2 .1mg, Folacin 6mcg

Carrot Salad

The Diet Doctor's Wife: This is a fresh, vibrant salad that is packed with Vitamin A. It is a wonderful accompaniment to almost any dish. I like to serve it with beet salad, lentils and mixed greens. Add some flat bread or crackers, and you have an easy healthy hors d'oeuvre, snack or light lunch.

1 pound carrots, grated or finely julienned
1 tablespoon fresh dill, chopped
1/8 teaspoon sea salt
1 tablespoon grapeseed oil

Combine ingredients.

[serves 6]

Nutrition Per Serving: Calories 50, Total Fat 2g, Saturated Fat trace, Cholesterol 0mg, Sodium 64mg, Potassium 235mg, Total Carbohydrate 7g, Dietary Fiber 2g, Protein 1g, Calcium 27mg, Iron 1mg, Vitamin C 7mg, Vitamin A 18973 IU, Vitamin B6 .1mg, Thiamin B1 .1mg, Folacin 9mcg, Niacin 1mg

Daikon and Carrot Salad

1 cup daikon, julienned
1 cup carrot, julienned
1/3 medium-size onion, thinly sliced in half-moons
1/8 teaspoon fresh green chili pepper, finely chopped
1 tablespoon freshly squeezed lemon juice
sea salt, to taste

Combine ingredients.

[serves 4]

Nutrition Per Serving: Calories 22, Total Fat trace, Saturated Fat trace, Cholesterol 0mg, Sodium 16mg, Potassium 168mg, Total Carbohydrate 5g, Dietary Fiber 1g, Protein 1g, Calcium 16mg, Vitamin C 10mg, Vitamin A 8581 IU, Vitamin B6 .1mg, Folacin 13mcg

Cucumber and Dill Salad

*3 pickling cucumbers or 1 Japanese cucumber, thinly sliced
1 tablespoon fresh dill, chopped
1/8 teaspoon sea salt
1 tablespoon white wine vinegar

Combine ingredients.

[serves 4]

Nutrition Per Serving: Calories 18, Total Fat trace, Saturated Fat trace, Cholesterol 0mg, Sodium 71mg, Potassium 200mg, Total Carbohydrate 4g, Dietary Fiber 1g, Protein 1g, Calcium 31mg, Iron 1mg, Vitamin C 7mg, Vitamin A 300 IU, Vitamin B6 .1mg, Folacin 15mcg

*Note: I have chosen unwaxed, thin-skinned cucumbers with small seeds for this dish. If using a regular cucumber, peel and seed before slicing.

Waldorf Salad

The Diet Doctor's Wife: Classic Waldorf Salad is made with a mayonnaise dressing. I use Sweet Sesame Vinaigrette instead, which is equally delicious and far more nutritious. And in my experience, much easier on the digestion.

3 tablespoons almonds, sliced or slivered
2 apples, cored and cut in chunks
2 stalks celery, chopped
1/3 cup raisins
3 tablespoons Sweet Sesame Vinaigrette (page 345)

Combine ingredients.

[serves 4]

Nutrition Per Serving: Calories 179, Total Fat 9g, Saturated Fat 1g, Cholesterol 0mg, Sodium 39mg, Potassium 301mg, Total Carbohydrate 24g, Dietary Fiber 3g, Protein 3g, Calcium 54mg, Iron 1mg, Vitamin C 6mg, Vitamin A 64 IU, Vitamin B6 .1 mg, Thiamin B1 .8mg, Riboflavin B2 .1mg, Folacin 14mcg

Grated Daikon Salad

The Diet Doctor's Wife: A tiny bit of this salad is very refreshing. Considered by the Japanese to be more of a condiment than a salad, grated daikon is traditionally served with fish as it is supposed to cleanse the body of lingering animal fat.

1 cup daikon, grated
1 teaspoon soy sauce
1 teaspoon freshly squeezed lemon juice
fresh chopped chives, for garnish

Place grated daikon in a colander and allow to drain for a few minutes.

Combine first three ingredients. Top with chopped chives to garnish.

[serves 4]

Nutrition Per Serving: Calories 6, Total Fat trace, Saturated Fat trace, Cholesterol 0mg, Sodium 49mg, Potassium 66mg, Total Carbohydrate 1g, Calcium 8mg, Vitamin C 7mg, Folacin 8mcg

Korean Chive Salad

The Diet Doctor's Wife: If you grow fresh chives in your garden, this recipe is an absolute must.

8 ounces fresh chives
1 1/2 tablespoons tamari or soy sauce
1 teaspoon garlic, crushed
1/2 teaspoon red pepper flakes
1/2 teaspoon Sesame Salt (page 327)
3/4 teaspoon maple syrup
3/4 teaspoon toasted sesame oil

Rinse and dry chives. Cut into 2-inch lengths.

In a mixing bowl, combine tamari, garlic, red pepper flakes, Sesame Salt, maple syrup and sesame oil until well incorporated. Add chives and mix gently.

[serves 6]

Nutrition Per Serving: Calories 23, Total Fat 1g, Saturated Fat trace, Cholesterol 0mg, Sodium 259mg, Potassium 126mg, Total Carbohydrate 3g, Dietary Fiber 1g, Protein 2g, Calcium 39mg, Iron 1mg, Vitamin C 22mg, Vitamin A 1654 IU, Folacin 41mcg

Citrus Salad

The Diet Doctor's Wife: The combination of fennel and orange makes me hum.

8 cups tender baby greens (bibb lettuce)
1 bulb fennel, thinly sliced
1/4 cup fennel fronds, finely chopped
4 mandarin oranges, peeled, seeded and membranes removed
16 green grapes, peeled, seeded and halved
1/2 cup Citrus Vinaigrette (page 345)

Evenly distribute vegetables and fruit among 8 plates. Drizzle with vinaigrette.

[serves 8]

Nutrition Per Serving: Calories 107, Total Fat 7g, Saturated Fat 1g, Cholesterol 0mg, Sodium 29mg, Potassium 321mg, Total Carbohydrate 12g, Dietary Fiber 2g, Protein 1g, Calcium 32mg, Vitamin C 33mg, Vitamin A 959 IU, Folacin 66mcg

Asian Salad

4 cups Napa cabbage leaves, shredded
1 cup carrots, grated or finely julienned
1 cup daikon, grated or finely julienned
2 ounces enoki mushrooms
1/4 cup Gingery Vinaigrette (page 343)
2 tablespoons fresh chives or scallions, finely chopped

Toss first 3 ingredients together, and evenly distribute among 6 plates. Divide mushrooms in six and place on top of vegetables. Add a drizzle of dressing and a sprinkle of herbs.

[serves 6]

Nutrition Per Serving: Calories 70, Total Fat 6g, Saturated Fat 1g, Cholesterol 0mg, Sodium 41mg, Potassium 250mg, Total Carbohydrate 5g, Dietary Fiber 2g, Protein 1g, Calcium 60mg, Iron 1mg, Vitamin C 28mg, Vitamin A 7164 IU, Vitamin B6 .1mg, Folacin 42mcg, Niacin 1mg

Field Greens

8 cups field greens
1/4 cup Balsamic Vinaigrette (page 340)
sea salt and freshly ground black pepper, to taste

Toss ingredients together and serve.

[serves 8]

Nutrition Per Serving: Calories 60, Total Fat 5g, Saturated Fat 1g, Cholesterol 0mg, Sodium 48mg, Potassium 201mg, Total Carbohydrate 3g, Dietary Fiber 2g, Protein 2g, Calcium 58mg, Iron 1mg, Vitamin C 39mg, Vitamin A 2968 IU, Vitamin B6 .1mg, Riboflavin B2 .1mg, Folacin 105mcg

Doc's Salad

The Diet Doctor's Wife: When I was growing up, my parents would take the family to The London Chop House in downtown Detroit to celebrate special occasions. What a treat it was to get all dressed up and feast on selections from the scrumptious menu. My favorite thing to order was the Doc Greene Salad, which I have recreated in the recipe below.

3 small heads bibb lettuce, washed and torn in bite-size pieces
1/2 cup hearts of palm, rinsed, drained and sliced
1/2 cup marinated artichokes, drained and halved
2 tomatoes, cut in wedges
1/2 avocado, peeled and cubed
1 pound cooked shrimp
1/4 cup Garlic and Chive Vinaigrette (page 342)

Combine the first 6 ingredients in a large bowl. Toss with the vinaigrette.

[serves 6]

Nutrition Per Serving: Calories 214, Total Fat 11g, Saturated Fat 1g, Cholesterol 115mg, Sodium 138mg, Potassium 951mg, Total Carbohydrate 13g, Dietary Fiber 3g, Protein 18g, Calcium 80mg, Iron 3mg, Zinc 2mg, Vitamin C 21mg, Vitamin A 1334 IU, Vitamin B6 .3mg, Vitamin B12 .8mcg, Thiamin B1 .1mg, Riboflavin B2 .1mg, Folacin 90mcg, Niacin 3mg

Middle Eastern Salad

The Diet Doctor's Wife: I look forward to making this salad in late summer when tomatoes, cucumbers and sweet peppers can be freshly plucked from our vegetable garden.

The Diet Doctor: Gabrielle and I try not to eat a lot of nightshade vegetables (tomatoes, peppers and eggplant). But, in late summer when they are locally in season, we simply can't resist. Since I've cut out these vegetables from my regular diet, I find that my arthritic symptoms have diminished considerably, as well as my moodiness. But an occasional indulgence doesn't seem to cause me any trouble.

*1 cup cucumber, seeded and cubed
1 cup tomato, seeded and chopped
1 cup sweet yellow pepper, seeded and chopped
3 tablespoons shallots, chopped
2 pinches My Zatar (page 335)
2 tablespoons Lemon Vinaigrette (page 341)

Put vegetables in a bowl and mix together.

In a separate bowl, combine zatar and vinaigrette, and whisk together. Add vinaigrette to the vegetables and toss together until all vegetables are coated with the dressing.

[serves 4]

Nutrition Per Serving: Calories 74, Total Fat 5g, Saturated Fat 1g, Cholesterol 0mg, Sodium 23mg, Potassium 246mg, Total Carbohydrate 6g, Dietary Fiber 1g, Protein 1g, Calcium 14mg, Iron 1mg, Vitamin C 80mg, Vitamin A 1380 IU, Vitamin B6 .1mg, Folacin 22mcg, Niacin 1mg

*Note: I prefer to use organic, unwaxed, thin-skinned cucumbers with small seeds for this recipe. If they are not available, I use regular cucumbers and remove the skin as well as the seeds.

Michele's Salad

The Diet Doctor's Wife: My cousin Michele serves this simple salad every time I come to visit. The avocado is what makes it special for me. Given a bad rap for its high fat content, the avocado is also very high in essential nutrients. So, I consider it a sensible treat if eaten in moderation.

The Diet Doctor: If you want to decrease the fat content, use less avocado or leave it out completely.

8 cups field greens
2 tomatoes, cut in eighths
1 small avocado, peeled, halved and sliced in 1/4-inch sections
3 tablespoons red onion, finely chopped
1/4 cup fresh dill, chopped
1/4 cup Basic Vinaigrette (page 342)
sea salt and freshly ground black pepper, to taste

Toss ingredients with the vinaigrette. Season to taste.

[serves 8]

Nutrition Per Serving: Calories 68, Total Fat 4g, Saturated Fat 1g, Cholesterol 0mg, Sodium 22mg, Potassium 449mg, Total Carbohydrate 7g, Dietary Fiber 3g, Protein 2g, Calcium 77mg, Iron 2mg, Vitamin C 48mg, Vitamin A 3359 IU, Vitamin B6 .2mg, Thiamin B1 .1mg, Riboflavin B2 .1mg, Folacin 126mcg, Niacin 1mg

Summer Harvest Salad

The Diet Doctor's Wife: This salad is not only delicious but also packed with essential vitamins and minerals.

1 cup raw beet, peeled and finely julienned
1 cup carrot, finely julienned
1/2 cup radishes, finely julienned
1 cup tomato, peeled, seeded and chopped
1 cup cucumber, peeled, seeded and finely julienned
8 cups lettuce, chopped
1 red bell pepper, cut in thin strips
6 tablespoons Sweet Sesame Vinaigrette (page 345)

Combine vegetables and toss with the dressing.

[serves 10]

Nutrition Per Serving: Calories 78, Total Fat 4g, Saturated Fat 1g, Cholesterol 0mg, Sodium 45mg, Potassium 335mg, Total Carbohydrate 8g, Dietary Fiber 3g, Protein 2g, Calcium 70mg, Iron 2mg, Vitamin C 49mg, Vitamin A 6000 IU, Vitamin B6 .1mg, Thiamin B1 .7mg, Riboflavin B2 .1mg, Folacin 110mcg, Niacin 1mg

Salad Nicoise

The Diet Doctor's Wife: I love Salad Nicoise. It is a light, nutritious meal that is very easy to prepare. I could eat it every day. I'm not kidding.

3 cups bibb lettuce, torn
4 small new potatoes, boiled until tender and halved
1 cup green beans, trimmed and steamed
1-2 tomatoes, cut in eighths or 8-12 cherry tomatoes
8 black olives
12 ounces canned tuna or cooked salmon
2 tablespoons shallots, chopped
3 tablespoons Basic Vinaigrette (page 342)

Divide first 7 ingredients among 4 plates. Drizzle with vinaigrette.

[serves 4]

Nutrition Per Serving: Calories 297, Total Fat 9g, Saturated Fat 1g, Cholesterol 26mg, Sodium 391mg, Potassium 1113mg, Total Carbohydrate 28g, Fiber 4g, Protein 26g, Calcium 52mg, Iron 3mg, Zinc 1mg, Vitamin C 38mg, Vitamin A 1183 IU, Vitamin B6 .7mg, Vitamin B12 2.5mg, Thiamin B1 .2mg, Riboflavin B2 .2mg, Folacin 66mcg, Niacin 14mg

Vegetarian Salad Nicoise

The Diet Doctor: This salad is a tasty and zero-cholesterol alternative to the classic Salad Nicoise.

3 cups bibb lettuce, torn
4 small new potatoes, boiled until tender and halved
1 cup green beans, trimmed and steamed
1-2 tomatoes, cut in eighths or 8-12 cherry tomatoes
8 black olives
8 ounces cooked chickpeas, white beans or lentils, plain or marinated
2 tablespoons shallots
3 tablespoons Basic Vinaigrette (page 342)

Arrange first 7 ingredients among 4 serving plates. Drizzle with the vinaigrette.

[serves 4]

Nutrition Per Serving: Calories 291, Total Fat 10g, Saturated Fat 1g, Cholesterol 0mg, Sodium 108mg, Potassium 1077mg, Carbohydrate 43g, Dietary Fiber 6g, Protein 9g, Calcium 71mg, Iron 3mg, Zinc 2mg, Vitamin C 39mg, Vitamin A 1451 IU, Vitamin B6 .5mg, Thiamin B1 .2mg, Riboflavin B2 .1mg, Folacin 160 mcg, Niacin 3mg

Gado Gado

The Diet Doctor's Wife: Gado Gado is a steamed vegetable and tofu salad, served with a spicy peanut dressing. It is a nutritious and perfectly light meal on a hot sticky summer night. I used to order it regularly when I was living in Singapore.

Peanut Sauce

2 shallots, chopped
2 medium cloves garlic, chopped
1 small red hot chili pepper, chopped
2 quarter-size slices of fresh ginger root
1 stalk lemongrass, tender section only, coarsely chopped
2 teaspoons grapeseed oil
1 tablespoon Thai fish sauce or soy sauce
1/4 cup unsalted and unsweetened peanut butter
2 teaspoons maple syrup
1 cup reduced fat coconut milk
juice of 1/2 lime or 1 teaspoon tamarind paste
sea salt and freshly ground white pepper, to taste
pinch of ground cayenne pepper (optional)

Place shallots, garlic, chili, ginger and lemongrass in a mortar. Pound to a coarse paste with a pestle. In a saucepan, heat oil over medium heat and cook paste for 2-3 minutes. Add remaining ingredients and whisk together until blended. Season to taste and cook for 1 minute. Remove from the heat. Remove lemongrass pieces.

Salad

10 ounces tofu, cut in 1-inch cubes and steamed or lightly sautéed
2 cups green beans, trimmed and steamed
2 cups cabbage, shredded and steamed
2 cups carrots, cut in 1/4-inch diagonal slices and steamed
2 cups potato, cut in 1-inch cubes and steamed
1 cup cucumber, sliced in 1/4-inch rounds

Arrange salad ingredients on a platter. Drizzle dressing on top or serve dressing in individual dipping bowls on the side.

[serves 8]

Nutrition Per Serving: Calories 147, Total Fat 7g, Saturated Fat 1g, Cholesterol trace, Sodium 20mg, Potassium 523mg, Total Carbohydrate 19g, Dietary Fiber 4g, Protein 5g, Calcium 42mg, Iron 1mg, Zinc 1mg, Vitamin C 24mg, Vitamin A 9171 IU, Vitamin B6 .2mg, Thiamin B1 .1mg, Riboflavin B2 .1mg, Folacin 38mcg, Niacin 2mg

French Dejeuner Salad

The Diet Doctor's Wife: When I was living in Montreal, I would often have lunch at a charming cafeteria called Quatre Saisons on Crescent St. Although most of the menu was appealing, I always ordered the same thing, the Dejeuner Salad. For me, the combination of poached leeks, salmon and avocado is a near perfect marriage of flavors.

The Diet Doctor: This is a nice filling salad that gives you a general nutritional boost. If you want to reduce fat, omit the avocado.

4 leeks, washed thoroughly and trimmed to the pale green just above the whites
2 small heads bibb lettuce, leaves separated
1 Belgium endive, leaves separated
1 pound poached salmon, cut in 4 pieces
1-2 tomatoes, sliced
1/4 avocado, peeled and thinly sliced
*1 cup cucumber, sliced
1/4 cup Dijon Vinaigrette (page 340)
fresh chopped parsley or dill, for garnish

Bring a pot of salted water to a boil. Tie leeks together with string and drop them into the pot. Simmer for 7-9 minutes until leeks are just tender. Drain and set aside.

Arrange lettuce and endive leaves on 4 plates. Top with salmon, tomatoes, avocado, leeks and cucumber slices. Drizzle vinaigrette over each salad. Sprinkle with chopped parsley or dill.

[serves 4]

Nutrition Per Serving: Calories 309, Total Fat 16g, Saturated Fat 2g, Cholesterol 44mg, Sodium 158mg, Potassium 1258mg, Total Carbohydrate 22g, Dietary Fiber 7g, Protein 22g, Calcium 168mg, Iron 4mg, Zinc 2mg, Vitamin C 37mg, Vitamin A 4055 IU, Vitamin B6 .5mg, Vitamin B12 2.5mcg, Thiamin B1 .4mg, Riboflavin B2 .3mg, Folacin 323mcg, Niacin 6mg

*Note: I prefer to use organic, unwaxed, thin-skinned cucumbers with small seeds for this recipe. If they are not available, I use regular cucumbers and remove the skin and seeds before slicing.

Cooked Salad

The Diet Doctor's Wife: In the winter, I hardly ever eat raw vegetables or cold salads. Instead, I toss cooked vegetables with a vinaigrette.

2 medium carrots
2 medium turnips or 1 small cauliflower
2 cups green beans, trimmed
1 tablespoon shallots, minced
1/4 cup Dijon Vinaigrette (page 340) or Basic Vinaigrette (page 342)
sea salt and freshly ground pepper, to taste

Cut carrots in 1/4-inch diagonal slices and then half lengthwise. Cut turnips in half and then in 1/4-inch slices. If using cauliflower, cut in small florets.

Steam vegetables separately, until tender. Alternatively, bring salted water to a boil. Add carrots and cook until tender. Remove with a slotted spoon and set aside. Add turnips to the boiling water, cook until tender, remove with a slotted spoon and set aside. Finally add green beans to the boiling water. Cook 2-3 minutes. Remove with a slotted spoon and set aside. Add cooking water to your soup stock if you'd like.

Place vegetables in a serving bowl. Sprinkle with chopped shallots. Add dressing. Mix gently and season to taste.

[serves 6]

Nutrition Per Serving: Calories 95, Total Fat 7g, Saturated Fat 1g, Cholesterol 0mg, Sodium 49mg, Potassium 241mg, Total Carbohydrate 8g, Dietary Fiber 3g, Protein 1g, Calcium 34mg, Iron 1mg, Vitamin C 17mg, Vitamin A 7204 IU, Vitamin B6 .1mg, Thiamin B1 .1mg, Riboflavin B2 .1mg, Folacin 23mcg, Niacin 1mg

Beet Salad

The Diet Doctor's Wife: Many cooks don't like to bother with beets because of the long cooking time. With a pressure cooker, there's no fear of that. In 8-10 minutes, beets are cooked to perfection.

1 1/2 pounds medium beets, trimmed
1 clove garlic, peeled and minced
1/2 teaspoon Dijon mustard
2 teaspoons red wine vinegar
2 tablespoons extra virgin olive oil
sea salt and freshly ground black pepper, to taste
1 tablespoon mixed fresh herbs (parsley, tarragon, chives), finely chopped

Wash beets and place in a pressure cooker. Add water to the level of 2 inches. Bring up to pressure over medium heat. Reduce heat to low and cook for 8-10 minutes depending on the size of the beets. Allow pressure to come down naturally. Remove beets and peel off skin. Cut beets into 1/2-inch cubes.

To prepare vinaigrette, whisk together garlic, mustard and vinegar. Whisk in the olive oil. Add salt and pepper. Taste for seasoning, adjusting if necessary. Pour vinaigrette over beets. Toss to coat. Add herbs and toss again.

[serves 4]

Nutrition Per Serving: Calories 111, Total Fat 7g, Saturated Fat 1g, Cholesterol 0mg, Sodium 97mg, Potassium 382mg, Total Carbohydrate 11g, Dietary Fiber 3g, Protein 2g, Calcium 22mg, Iron 1mg, Vitamin C 7mg, Vitamin A 92 IU, Vitamin B6 .1mg, Folacin 126mcg

Mom's Potato Salad

The Diet Doctor's Wife: I love my mom's potato salad. She uses a Dijon vinaigrette instead of mayonnaise and adds a hit of capers and garden fresh herbs.

The Diet Doctor: We've kept the servings small here. The reason is that too much potato can make you sleepy as well as aggravate feelings of depression.

1 pound new potatoes, boiled with skin, sliced 1/4-inch thick
1/4 cup shallots, chopped
1 tablespoon capers, rinsed, drained and chopped
2 tablespoons fresh parsley, finely chopped
2 tablespoon fresh basil, finely chopped
1/4 cup Dijon Vinaigrette (page 340)

Combine ingredients.

[serves 4]

Nutrition Per Serving: Calories 174, Total Fat 5g, Saturated Fat 1g, Cholesterol 0mg, Sodium 198mg, Potassium 414mg, Total Carbohydrate 24g, Dietary Fiber 11g, Protein 10g, Calcium 38mg, Iron 3mg, Zinc 1mg, Vitamin C 10mg, Vitamin A 4398 IU, Vitamin B6 .2mg, Thiamin B1 .2mg, Riboflavin B2 .1mg, Folacin 151mcg, Niacin 1mg

Mom's Garden Potato Salad

The Diet Doctor's Wife: Ever since I can remember, my mom has grown culinary herbs in her garden. She delights in the vital aromas and flavors. Her all time favorite is the nasturtium with its delicate peppery notes and charming beauty. She swoons (to use her words) over the perky lily-pad-shaped leaves and colorful edible flowers. As soon as nasturtiums break the soil, my mom looks for ways to incorporate them in her cooking. This potato salad is a perfect and delightfully delicious example.

The Diet Doctor: Keep your portions small. Potatoes make insulin levels skyrocket, which can lead to overeating and moodiness.

1 pound new potatoes, boiled with the skin, sliced thick
1/4 cup nasturtium leaves, chopped
2 tablespoons fresh parsley, finely chopped
2 tablespoons fresh chives, finely chopped
2 tablespoons Dijon Vinaigrette (page 340)
nasturtium flowers, for garnish

Combine first 5 ingredients. Garnish with nasturtium flowers, if desired.

[serves 4]

Nutrition Per Serving: Calories 137, Total Fat 5g, Saturated Fat 1g, Cholesterol 0mg, Sodium 32mg, Potassium 649mg, Total Carbohydrate 21g, Dietary Fiber 2g, Protein 2g, Calcium 14mg, Iron 1mg, Vitamin C 27mg, Vitamin A 621 IU, Vitamin B6 .3mg, Thiamin B1 .1mg, Folacin 21mcg, Niacin 2mg

Soups

Basic Vegetable Stock

The Diet Doctor's Wife: I always have this stock on hand. It is a great base for miso soup, as well as an essential ingredient for impromptu risottos and stews. Basic Vegetable Stock is perfect for adding low fat richness to a stir-fry. And with a pressure cooker, it can be made in no time.

6 kale leaves
2 leeks, white and pale green parts only, sliced in thin rounds
2 onions, cut in chunks
6 cloves garlic
2 carrots, cut in chunks
2 stalks celery, sliced
1 turnip, cut in chunks
1 cup winter squash, cut in chunks and skin removed
bouquet garni (2 bay leaves, 3 sprigs parsley, 1 sprig thyme)
*4-inch piece kombu (optional)
8-10 cups water

Put all ingredients in a pressure cooker. Bring up to pressure over high heat. Reduce heat to moderately low and cook for 10 minutes. Allow to cool and strain.

If you don't want to use a pressure cooker, you can bring the ingredients to a boil, then lower heat to simmer, uncovered, for 1/2 hour. Allow to cool and strain.

Store in an airtight container in the refrigerator for up to 5 days, or freeze.

[serves 8]

Nutrition Per Serving: Calories 20, Total Fat 0g, Saturated Fat 0g, Cholesterol 0mg, Sodium 25mg

*Note 1: If using kombu, don't discard after cooking. Kombu can be re-used to make relishes and other condiments that are wonderful with rice. Kombu can also be re-used to make Japanese Stock (page 95).

Note 2: You can also add to the stock by using the cooking water from boiling or steaming vegetables. Just remember to strain out the vegetable particles first.

Chinese Stock

The Diet Doctor's Wife: As much as I love the taste of Chinese food, I don't react to it well. It makes me feel so sleepy, probably due to the MSG, and the chicken and pork based broth used to flavor almost every dish. So if I want to enjoy Chinese food, I am forced to prepare it myself. And when I do, I always use this completely vegetarian broth.

2 scallions
1 carrot, sliced
2 stalks celery, sliced
1 cup cabbage, sliced
1 stalk lemongrass, lower 4 inches, coarsely chopped
2 thin slices fresh ginger root
1 clove garlic

Place ingredients in a soup pot with 9 cups of cold water. Bring to a boil. Reduce heat and simmer for 30 minutes, or pressure cook for 10 minutes. Strain, and store in the refrigerator for up to 5 days.

[serves 6-8]

Nutrition Per Serving: Calories 10, Total Fat 0g, Saturated Fat 0g, Cholesterol 0mg

Japanese Stock (Dashi)

The Diet Doctor: This is an exceedingly simple soup stock. Even I can make it.

*4-inch piece kombu
*5 dried shitake mushrooms
5 cups water

Wipe kombu with a damp cloth. Place all ingredients in a soup pot. Bring to a boil. Remove from heat and let steep for 1/2 hour. Strain and refrigerate for up to 5 days.

[serves 6]

Nutrition Per Serving: Calories 10, Total Fat trace, Saturated Fat trace, Cholesterol 0mg, Sodium 10mg, Potassium 48mg, Total Carbohydrate 2g, Dietary Fiber trace, Calcium 7mg, Vitamin A 2 IU, Folacin 8mcg

*Note: Do not discard the kombu or the mushrooms. They can be re-used to make soup stocks, stir-fries and pickles.

Bonito Dashi

The Diet Doctor: I love the miso soup you get in Japanese restaurants. But after indulging in a bowl, I can't wake up the next morning. I think it's the mystery chemicals in the bottled dashi base. Gabrielle's miso soup is just as tasty and doesn't make me feel so sleepy. Her secret is homemade Bonito Dashi.

4 cups water
2, 4-inch pieces kombu
1/4 ounce bonito flakes

Wipe kombu with a damp cloth. In a soup pot, bring water and kombu to a boil over medium heat. Just before the water reaches a boil, remove kombu. Save kombu to make condiments or to use in other stocks.

Add the bonito fish flakes to the stock and return to a boil. Immediately remove from the heat and skim off any foam. Let the mixture stand for 2 minutes.

Strain stock. Discard bonito fish flakes or use to make a second Bonito Dashi.

Refrigerate stock for up to 3 days or freeze for up to 3 months.

[serves 4]

Nutrition Per Serving: Calories 6, Total Fat trace, Saturated Fat trace, Cholesterol 3mg, Sodium 15mg, Potassium 2mg, Protein 1g, Calcium 9mg, Vitamin A 3 IU, Folacin 5mcg

Bean and Barley Soup

1 cup white beans, washed and soaked 8 hours
1 cup barley, washed and soaked 4-8 hours
1 stalk celery, diced
1 large carrot, diced
1 cup onion, chopped
1 bay leaf
1/2 teaspoon celery seed
1/2 teaspoon dried dill weed
4 cups water
sea salt, to taste

Drain beans and barley, and place them in a pressure cooker. Add celery, carrot, onion and herbs. Cover with water.

Secure lid and bring up to pressure over medium heat. Reduce heat to medium low and cook for 45 minutes. Remove from heat and allow pressure to come down naturally. Remove bay leaf. Season to taste.

[serves 8]

Nutrition Per Serving: Calories 178, Total Fat 1g, Saturated Fat trace, Cholesterol 0mg, Sodium 136mg, Potassium 636mg, Total Carbohydrate 35g, Dietary Fiber 8g, Protein 9g, Calcium 83mg, Iron 4mg, Zinc 2mg, Vitamin C 3mg, Vitamin A 2548 IU, Vitamin B6 .2mg, Thiamin B .3mg, Riboflavin B2 .1mg, Folacin 109 mcg, Niacin 1mg

Middle Eastern Lentil Soup

The Diet Doctor's Wife: This is a very nutritious soup that is so simple to make.

2 teaspoons extra virgin olive oil
1 medium onion, chopped
1 stalk celery with leaves, chopped
1 medium carrot, peeled and chopped

2 cups lentils, sorted and washed
8 cups Basic Vegetable Stock (page 94) or water
1/2 teaspoon sea salt
freshly ground black pepper, to taste
juice of 1 lemon
1 teaspoon ground cumin

Heat oil in a soup pot. Add onion, celery and carrot, and sauté for 5 minutes, until vegetables soften. Add lentils and stock. Bring to a boil, then reduce heat and simmer gently until lentils are soft, about 30-45 minutes.

Season soup with salt, pepper, lemon juice and cumin. Simmer a few minutes longer. Use a potato masher to break up the lentils or puree in a blender until smooth. Taste for seasoning.

[serves 8]

Nutrition Per Serving: Calories 187, Total Fat 2g, Saturated Fat trace, Cholesterol 0mg, Sodium 134mg, Potassium 511mg, Total Carbohydrate 30g, Dietary Fiber 15g, Protein 14g, Calcium 34mg, Iron 5mg, Zinc 2mg, Vitamin C 8mg, Vitamin A 2561 IU, Vitamin B6 .3mg, Thiamin B1 .2mg, Riboflavin B2 .1mg, Folacin 214 mcg, Niacin 1mg

White Bean Soup

The Diet Doctor's Wife: Bill does not believe that this is a vegetarian soup. He swears that he can taste a ham hock. But, he is mistaken. There is not a stitch of animal protein in this recipe. The secret is the chipotle pepper, which imparts a smoky, meaty flavor.

1 1/2 cups dried navy or great northern beans
1/2 head garlic, unpeeled
1 handful sage leaves
2 teaspoons extra virgin olive oil
3 red onions, peeled and chopped
1 bunch celery (including leaves), chopped
4 cloves garlic, peeled and chopped

1 dried chipotle pepper, crumbled
3 sprigs fresh rosemary, leaves chopped
2 tablespoons tomato puree, or 2 tomatoes, peeled, seeded and chopped
sea salt and freshly ground black pepper, to taste

Soak dried beans overnight or use the quick soak method. Drain beans well, place in a pressure cooker and cover with fresh cold water. Add garlic head and sage. Bring beans up to pressure over medium heat, then reduce to low, and cook for 40 minutes.

While the beans are cooking, heat oil in a large heavy saucepan and sauté the onions and celery over medium heat. When the onions are soft and translucent, add the garlic, chipotle and rosemary. Continue to sauté for 1-2 minutes. Stir in the tomato puree, and continue to cook for approximately 15 minutes.

Add beans and some of the bean cooking liquid to the onion and celery mixture. Stir to combine. Add more bean cooking liquid if the soup seems too thick. Season to taste.

[serves 10]

Nutrition Per Serving: Calories 136, Total Fat 1g, Saturated Fat trace, Cholesterol 0mg, Sodium 210mg, Potassium 468mg, Carbohydrate 24g, Dietary Fiber 9g, Protein 8g, Calcium 65mg, Iron 2mg, Zinc 1mg, Vitamin C 6mg, Vitamin A 67 IU, Vitamin B6 .2mg, Thiamin B1 .2mg, Riboflavin B2 .1mg, Folacin 127mcg, Niacin 1mg

Yellow Split Pea Soup

The Diet Doctor's Wife: While I was studying at McGill in Montreal, Canada, I would spend Saturday afternoons with family friends, Simone and Gabriel Whiteman. Simone, who is an outstanding Moroccan cook, would often prepare the tastiest split pea soup. This recipe is my vegetarian version.

1/2 pound yellow split peas, soaked 6-8 hours
1 stalk celery, chopped
4 cups water or Basic Vegetable Stock (page 94)
1/2 teaspoon cumin
1 tablespoon freshly squeezed lemon juice
1/2 teaspoon sea salt
freshly ground black pepper, to taste
fresh chopped parsley and coriander, for garnish

Place split peas, celery and water in a pressure cooker. Secure lid and allow to come to pressure over high heat. Reduce temperature to moderate heat and cook for 45 minutes. Remove from heat and allow pressure to release naturally. Remove lid. Add cumin, lemon juice, salt and pepper. Simmer a few more minutes. Puree the soup. Check for seasoning. Ladle into serving bowls. Garnish with herbs.

[serves 6]

Nutrition Per Serving: Calories 132, Total Fat trace, Saturated Fat trace, Cholesterol 0mg, Sodium 174mg, Potassium 404mg, Total Carbohydrate 23g, Dietary Fiber 10g, Protein 9g, Calcium 30mg, Iron 2mg, Zinc 1mg, Vitamin C 4mg, Vitamin A 133 IU, Vitamin B6 .1mg, Thiamin B1 .3mg, Riboflavin B2 .1mg, Folacin 108mcg, Niacin 1mg

Simple Vegetable Soup

The Diet Doctor's Wife: Bill calls this salad soup. It is particularly good at the end of June when Swiss chard, radishes and dill can be harvested from our vegetable garden.

2 teaspoons grapeseed oil
2 Swiss chard leaves with stems, coarsely chopped
2 carrots, peeled and coarsely chopped
5 red radishes with leaves, coarsely chopped
1/2 head cauliflower, cut in small florets
5 scallions, chopped
2-3 cups Basic Vegetable Stock (page 94)
1/4 cup mixed fresh herbs (parsley, dill, chives), minced
1/2 teaspoon sea salt

Heat oil in a soup pot over medium heat. Add chard, carrots, radishes, cauliflower and scallions. Cover and cook 2-3 minutes. Reduce heat to low and cook 4 more minutes. Uncover and add stock, herbs and salt. Bring to a boil and reduce heat to simmer for 15 minutes. Puree. Check for seasoning.

[serves 4]

Nutrition Per Serving: Calories 61, Total Fat 2g, Saturated Fat trace, Cholesterol 0mg, Sodium 312mg, Potassium 363mg, Total Carbohydrate 9g, Dietary Fiber 2g, Protein 1g, Calcium 43mg, Iron 1mg, Vitamin C 24mg, Vitamin A 11,112 IU, Vitamin B6 .1mg, Riboflavin B2 .1mg, Folacin 32mcg, Niacin 1mg

Creamy Onion Soup

The Diet Doctor's Wife: This is a much lighter version of the classic French onion and potato soup. The secret is that there is no potato. Cauliflower, turnip and carrot are used instead.

The Diet Doctor: The first time I had this soup I kept wondering what Gabrielle did to make it taste so rich. I even opened the refrigerator to look for a carton of cream. I didn't find one.

6 leeks
10 cups Basic Vegetable Stock (page 94), water or combination
2 medium onions
2 teaspoons extra virgin olive oil
6 shallots, peeled and halved lengthwise
10 cloves garlic, peeled and halved lengthwise
bouquet garni (6 sprigs parsley, 3 sprigs tarragon, 12 chives and 3 bay leaves, tied together with string)
1 medium cauliflower, cut in small florets
1 medium turnip, cubed
1 medium carrot, cubed
sea salt and freshly ground black pepper, to taste
fresh minced herbs (parsley, tarragon, chives), for garnish

Trim leeks separating the dark green portion from the white and pale green portion.

In a large stockpot, place the dark green portion of the leeks and the stock. Bring to a boil. Reduce heat to medium low, cover and simmer for 15 minutes. Strain broth and set aside.

Chop white and pale green portion of leeks. Peel onions and slice in thin half-moons.

In a large stockpot, heat oil and add chopped leeks, onions, shallots, garlic, bouquet garni and a pinch of sea salt. Cook on medium low, covered, until vegetables soften, about 10 minutes.

Pour broth over the onion mixture. Add cauliflower, turnip and carrot. Cover and bring to a boil over medium heat. Lower heat to medium low and simmer for 1 hour. Remove and discard bouquet garni. Puree the soup. Season to taste. Ladle into serving bowls and garnish with fresh herbs.

[serves 8]

Nutrition Per Serving: Calories 109, Total Fat 2g, Saturated Fat trace, Cholesterol 0mg, Sodium 78mg, Potassium 617mg, Total Carbohydrate 21g, Dietary Fiber 4g, Protein 4g, Calcium 151mg, Iron 5mg, Zinc 1mg, Vitamin C 85mg, Vitamin A 6148 IU, Vitamin B6 .3mg, Thiamin B1 .1mg, Riboflavin B2 .1mg, Folacin 139mcg, Niacin 1mg

French Onion Soup

The Diet Doctor's Wife: This is a rich satisfying soup that even the pickiest non-vegetarians will enjoy. The trick is the miso.

The Diet Doctor: I swear that Gabrielle puts beef in this soup, but she insists that she doesn't. I'll just have to take her word for it.

Soup

4 cups Basic Vegetable Stock (page 94)
1 tablespoon extra virgin olive oil
2 large onions, sliced in half-moons
4 cloves garlic, minced
1/4 cup brandy
1 bay leaf
2 sprigs fresh thyme
1-2 tablespoons red miso
1-2 tablespoons low sodium soy sauce
1 teaspoon Dijon mustard
5 slices toasted crusty bread or fu

Heat stock. In a separate soup pot, heat oil over moderate heat. Add onions and garlic until onions caramelize (about 30 minutes). Add brandy and simmer until alcohol cooks away. Add stock, bay leaf and thyme, and simmer for 30 minutes. Remove 1/4 cup of cooking liquid and whisk together with miso until fully incorporated. Add soy sauce and mustard to the miso mixture. Add miso mixture to the soup pot. Stir to combine. Check for seasoning.

Place one piece of toasted bread in each of the 5 serving bowls. (If using fu instead of bread, soak fu in a separate bowl according to the directions on the package. Squeeze out excess water and add fu to the soup pot. Simmer for 10-15 minutes. Just before serving, place one piece of fu in each of the 5 serving bowls.)

Tofu Cheese Sauce

3 ounces Tofu Cheese (page 210)
splash of freshly squeezed lemon juice
1/2 teaspoon Dijon mustard
1/2 teaspoon garlic, minced

Scrape miso off Tofu Cheese and set miso aside for another use. Combine Tofu Cheese with lemon juice, mustard and garlic. Puree.

To serve, ladle soup over the toasted bread or fu in each of the serving bowls. Top with a dollop of Tofu Cheese Sauce.

[serves 5]

Nutrition Per Serving: Calories 185, Total Fat 5g, Saturated Fat 1g, Cholesterol 0mg, *Sodium 523mg, Potassium 149mg, Total Carbohydrate 24g, Dietary Fiber 2g, Protein 5g, Calcium 57mg, Iron 2mg, Zinc 1mg, Vitamin C 4mg, Vitamin A 36 IU, Vitamin B6 .1mg, Thiamin B1 .2mg, Riboflavin B2 .1mg, Folacin 22mcg, Niacin 1mg

*Note: The sodium content of this dish is on the high side. Make sure to watch sodium intake for the rest of the day, and drink a lot of water. If you want to lower the sodium count in this recipe, omit the bread and Tofu Cheese Sauce.

Fresh Pea Soup with Tarragon

The Diet Doctor's Wife: When fresh peas are in season, this soup is an absolute must. Your family and friends will be wowed by the exquisite shade of green and magical combination of flavors. The natural sweetness of the peas highlighted by the delicate perfume of tarragon is truly beyond compare.

2 teaspoons grapeseed oil
1 onion, coarsely chopped
2 cloves garlic, minced
4 cups Basic Vegetable Stock (page 94)
*4 ounces Jerusalem artichoke, taro or yucca, peeled and chopped
1 1/2 pounds fresh or frozen sweet peas, shelled
1/8 teaspoon ground cayenne pepper
2 tablespoons fresh tarragon, chopped
sea salt, to taste

Heat oil in a saucepan. Sauté onion and garlic, and cook over gentle heat for 10 minutes. Add stock and Jerusalem artichoke. Bring to a boil and reduce heat. Simmer 15 minutes. Add remaining ingredients and simmer 10 more minutes. Puree. Taste for seasoning.

[serves 8]

Nutrition Per Serving: Calories 107, Total Fat 2g, Saturated Fat trace, Cholesterol 0mg, Sodium 18mg, Potassium 297mg, Total Carbohydrate 19g, Dietary Fiber 5g, Protein 5g, Calcium 29mg, Iron 2mg, Zinc 1mg, Vitamin C 36mg, Vitamin A 564 IU, Vitamin B6 .2mg, Thiamin B1 .3mg, Riboflavin B2 .1mg, Folacin 60mcg, Niacin 2mg

*Note: This soup is traditionally made with potato. I use Jerusalem artichoke or taro root instead, although the sweet, aromatic starchiness of yucca is my favorite. The only problem is that yucca is not readily available.

Cabbage Soup

The Diet Doctor's Wife: This recipe is based on my mother's sweet and sour cabbage soup. My version is vegetarian and just as yummy. I can eat a whole potful in just one sitting. Thankfully, it's not at all fattening.

The Diet Doctor: This soup is great for dieting. It's low in fat and calories, high in fiber, and has a mild diuretic effect. You can enjoy it in large quantities, guilt-free.

2 teaspoons grapeseed oil
2 cups onion, chopped
2 cloves garlic, minced
1 cup carrot, diced
1 cup celery, diced
bouquet garni (1 bay leaf, 6 sprigs parsley and 6 chives, tied together with string)
1 teaspoon ground caraway or 1 tablespoon caraway seeds
1 bay leaf
1 pound cabbage, shredded
1 cup Jerusalem artichoke, cut in chunks (optional)
1/2 cup parsnip, diced
1 cup turnip, cut in chunks
14-ounce can peeled and seeded tomatoes, coarsely chopped
4 cups Basic Vegetable Stock (page 94) or water
2 tablespoons apple cider vinegar
sea salt and freshly ground white pepper, to taste

Heat oil in a stockpot. Add onion, garlic, carrots, celery, bouquet garni, caraway and bay leaf, and sauté for 5 minutes. Add the rest of the ingredients and bring soup to a boil. Lower heat and simmer 30 minutes. Season to taste. Remove bay leaf.

[serves 8]

Nutrition Per Serving: Calories 95, Total Fat 2g, Saturated Fat trace, Cholesterol 0mg, Sodium 129mg, Potassium 556mg, Total Carbohydrate 20g, Dietary Fiber 4g, Protein 3g, Calcium 72mg, Iron 2mg, Vitamin C 36mg, Vitamin A 4916 IU, Vitamin B6 .2mg, Thiamin B1 .1mg, Riboflavin B2 .1mg, Folacin 53mcg, Niacin 1mg

Gentle Cauliflower Soup

The Diet Doctor's Wife: This is a simple soup that is terrific for times when you have the sniffles.

5 cups water or Basic Vegetable Stock (page 94)
2 carrots, thinly sliced
1 head cauliflower, cut in florets
4 cabbage leaves, shredded
1 Jerusalem artichoke, parsnip or turnip, peeled and thinly sliced
1 leek, white and pale green part only, thinly sliced
sea salt, to taste

Boil water. Add vegetables. Reduce heat to simmer for 20 minutes. Puree. Season to taste.

[serves 6]

Nutrition Per Serving: Calories 46, Total Fat trace, Saturated Fat trace, Cholesterol 0mg, Sodium 26mg, Potassium 300mg, Total Carbohydrate 11g, Dietary Fiber 2g, Protein 2g, Calcium 34mg, Iron 1mg, Vitamin C 18mg, Vitamin A 6794 IU, Vitamin B6 .1mg, Thiamin B1 .1mg, Folacin 32mcg, Niacin 1mg

Hungarian Cauliflower Soup

The Diet Doctor's Wife: This recipe is inspired by Gladys Bauer's cauliflower soup with dumplings. Gladys used to help my mother with the housework as well as care for my brothers and me. She was quite a personality and a superb Hungarian cook. Her wonderfully hearty soup was the standard starter that warmed us during the cold winter months. My version is vegetarian, sans dumplings and considerably less fatty, but still true to my childhood memory.

The Diet Doctor: Don't let the simplicity of the ingredients fool you. This is one of my favorite soups in the book. The black pepper creates an unexpected yet welcomed zing - just enough of a push, to send your taste buds off into the stratosphere. And the calorie count is suspiciously low.

1 onion, chopped
1 head of cauliflower, chopped
1 carrot, chopped
4 cups water or Basic Vegetable Stock (page 94)
sea salt, to taste
1/4-1/2 teaspoon freshly ground black pepper

Place first 4 ingredients in a pressure cooker. Secure lid and bring up to pressure over medium heat. Reduce heat to medium low and cook for 10 minutes. When pressure comes down, remove lid, puree the soup and season to taste. (If you don't have a pressure cooker, bring the ingredients to a boil, lower heat and simmer 30-45 minutes. Puree and season to taste.)

[serves 6]

Nutrition Per Serving: Calories 17, Total Fat trace, Saturated Fat trace, Cholesterol 0mg, Sodium 15mg, Potassium 119mg, Total Carbohydrate 4g, Dietary Fiber 1g, Protein 1g, Calcium 14mg, Vitamin C 10mg, Vitamin A 3379 IU, Vitamin B6 .1mg, Folacin 15mcg

Red Squash Soup

The Diet Doctor's Wife: This soup is simple and hearty. I like it best made with buttercup squash, although butternut and other varieties of winter squash are more readily available.

2 pounds winter squash (buttercup, butternut, acorn, red kuri)
2 teaspoons extra virgin olive oil
1 carrot, chopped
1 stalk celery, chopped
1 small onion, chopped
bouquet garni (1 sprig thyme, 6 sprigs parsley and 1 bay leaf, tied together with string)
4 cups Basic Vegetable Stock (page 94) or water
sea salt and freshly ground black pepper, to taste
1 teaspoon fresh thyme leaves

Preheat oven to 450 degrees F.

Cut squash in half, and scoop out seeds and fibers. Place squash halves on a baking sheet, cut side down, and bake for 30-45 minutes until tender. Scoop out cooked flesh and set aside.

In a soup pot, heat oil on medium and add carrot, celery, onion and bouquet garni. Sauté until vegetables start to release their juices, about 2-3 minutes. Add squash flesh and stock. Bring to a boil and then reduce heat to a gentle simmer for 30 minutes with lid partially off. Remove bouquet garni. Puree and season to taste. Add fresh thyme leaves and allow soup to rest for 5 minutes. Ladle soup into serving bowls.

[serves 6]

Nutrition Per Serving: Calories 97, Total Fat 1g, Saturated Fat trace, Cholesterol 0mg, Sodium 32mg, Potassium 535mg, Total Carbohydrate 21g, Dietary Fiber 3g, Protein 2g, Calcium 71mg, Iron 1mg, Vitamin C 30mg, Vitamin A 13,306 IU, Vitamin B6 .2mg, Thiamin B1 .1mg, Folacin 41mcg, Niacin 2mg

Curried Red Squash Soup

The Diet Doctor: I'm not a big fan of curry, but in this soup, it works. There's just the right amount to create interest without going too far.

2 pounds winter squash (butternut, buttercup, kabocha, red kuri, etc.)
2 teaspoons extra virgin olive oil
1 carrot, diced
1 small onion, chopped
bouquet garni (1 sprig thyme, 6 sprigs parsley and 1 bay leaf, tied together with string)
1 tablespoon curry
4 cups Basic Vegetable Stock (page 94) or water
sea salt and freshly ground black pepper, to taste

Preheat oven to 450 degrees F. Cut squash in half, and scoop out seeds and fibers. Place squash halves on a baking sheet, cut side down, and bake for 30-45 minutes, until tender. Scoop out cooked flesh and set aside.

In a soup pot, heat oil on medium and add carrot, onion, bouquet garni and curry. Sauté until vegetables start to release their juices, about 2-3 minutes. Add squash flesh and stock. Bring to a boil and then reduce heat to a gentle simmer for 30 minutes with lid partially off. Remove bouquet garni. Puree and season to taste. Allow soup to rest for 5 minutes. Ladle soup into serving bowls.

[serves 8]

Nutrition Per Serving: Calories 75, Total Fat 1g, Saturated Fat trace, Cholesterol 0mg, Sodium 20mg, Potassium 398mg, Total Carbohydrate 16g, Dietary Fiber 2g, Protein 1g, Calcium 55mg, Iron 1mg, Vitamin C 22mg, Vitamin A 9976 IU, Vitamin B6 .2mg, Thiamin B1 .1mg, Folacin 31mcg, Niacin 1mg

Pot Au Feu I

The Diet Doctor: Pot au Feu is very simple fare - an extremely low fat, one-pot wonder.

3 cups Basic Vegetable Stock (page 94)
8 whole black peppercorns

bouquet garni (1 bay leaf, 6 sprigs parsley and 6 chives, tied together with string)
4 carrots, peeled and cut in large chunks
4 leeks, white and pale green parts only, cut in 2-inch chunks
2 onions, peeled and halved
2 small turnips, peeled and halved
2 small parsnips, peeled and halved
2 celery hearts, each 6 inches long, halved lengthwise or 4 celery ribs, halved
sea salt and freshly ground black pepper, to taste
fresh chopped parsley, for garnish

Place all ingredients (except for garnish) in a pressure cooker. Pressure cook for 10 minutes. Remove bouquet garni. Season to taste.

To serve, arrange vegetables in serving bowls and spoon broth on top. Garnish with chopped parsley.

[serves 4]

Nutrition Per Serving: Calories 230, Total Fat 1g, Saturated Fat trace, Cholesterol 0mg, Sodium 150mg, Potassium 1138mg, Total Carbohydrate 54g, Dietary Fiber 12g, Protein 5g, Calcium 159mg, Iron 3mg, Zinc 1mg, Vitamin C 56mg, Vitamin A 20,394 IU, Vitamin B6 .5mg, Thiamin B1 .3mg, Riboflavin B2 .2mg, Folacin 174mcg, Niacin 2mg

Pot Au Feu II

2 teaspoons extra virgin olive oil
1 cup pearl onions, peeled
3 cloves garlic, peeled
1/4 cup dry white wine
3 cups Basic Vegetable Stock (page 94) or water
8 whole black peppercorns
bouquet garni (2 bay leaves, 6 sprigs parsley and 5 chives, tied together with string)
4 carrots, peeled and cut in large chunks
4 leeks, white and pale green parts only, cut in 2-inch chunks

2 small turnips, peeled and halved
2 parsnips, peeled and cut in large chunks
2 celery hearts, each 6 inches long, cut in half lengthwise or 4 celery ribs, halved
sea salt and freshly ground black pepper, to taste

In a pressure cooker, heat olive oil and sauté onions and garlic until golden. Add wine and cook until mostly evaporated. Add the rest of ingredients. Pressure cook for 10 minutes.

Remove bouquet garni. Season to taste.

To serve, arrange vegetables in serving bowls and spoon broth on top.

[serves 4]

Nutrition Per Serving: Calories 254, Total Fat 3g, Saturated Fat trace, Cholesterol 0mg, Sodium 250mg, Potassium 1136mg, Total Carbohydrate 53g, Dietary Fiber 12g, Protein 5g, Calcium 165mg, Iron 3mg, Zinc 1mg, Vitamin C 55mg, Vitamin A 20,394 IU, Vitamin B6 .6mg, Thiamin B1 .3mg, Riboflavin B2 .1mg, Folacin 168mcg, Niacin 2mg

Matzoh Ball Soup

The Diet Doctor's Wife: My mother used to serve chicken soup with big chunks of carrots and herb-flecked matzoh balls. This is a lower fat, vegetarian version of that old familiar treat.

The Diet Doctor: This really does taste like matzoh ball soup. I didn't think it possible without the chicken.

Matzoh Balls

1 tablespoon olive oil
1 free-range egg
1/4 cup water or Basic Vegetable Stock (page 94)
1/2 cup matzoh meal
1/2 teaspoon sea salt
2 tablespoons fresh dill and/or parsley, finely minced

Beat together oil and egg until light and foamy. Add water or stock and beat until incorporated. In a separate bowl, combine matzoh meal, salt and herbs. Add dry ingredients to egg mixture and stir with a wooden spoon just until a batter is formed. Batter should be soft. If it is too dry, add 1-2 tablespoons of water or stock and mix to combine. Cover and refrigerate for at least 1 hour, up to 24 hours. Form 6-8 balls.

Soup

5 cups Basic Vegetable Stock (page 94)
1 teaspoon sea salt
bouquet garni (6 chives, 6 sprigs parsley, a handful of celery leaves and 1 bay leaf, tied together with string)
2 carrots, peeled and cut in large chunks
4 leeks, white and pale green parts only, halved lengthwise
2 small turnips, peeled and quartered
1 parsnip, peeled and cut in large chunks
2 celery hearts, each 6 inches long or 4 celery ribs, halved
6-8 matzoh balls
1/4 cup fresh dill and/or parsley, finely chopped
sea salt and freshly ground black pepper, to taste
fresh chopped dill and/or parsley, for garnish

Place first 9 ingredients in a pressure cooker. Pressure cook for 10 minutes.

Remove bouquet garni. With a slotted spoon, remove all vegetables and set aside. Add chopped dill to broth and check for seasoning.

If using celery hearts, cut in 6-8 portions.

To serve, distribute vegetables among 6-8 serving bowls. Add a matzoh ball to each bowl. Ladle broth on top. Garnish with fresh chopped dill and/or parsley, if desired.

[serves 6-8]

Nutrition Per Serving: Calories 195, Total Fat 4g, Saturated Fat 1g, Cholesterol 31mg, Sodium 800mg, Potassium 681mg, Total Carbohydrate 37g, Dietary Fiber 6g, Protein 5g, Calcium 157mg, Iron 4mg, Zinc 1mg, Vitamin C 30mg, Vitamin A 7018 IU, Vitamin B6 .3mg, Vitamin B12 .1mcg, Thiamin B1 .2mg, Riboflavin B2 .1mg, Folacin 93mcg, Niacin 1mg

Whole Turnip Soup

The Diet Doctor's Wife: This soup is inspired by an Alice Waters recipe. I have created a lower fat, vegetarian version that works quite well. I have replaced the pancetta with chipotle pepper, which gives the soup a subtle smoky flavor. And naturally, I use vegetable stock instead of chicken stock.

1 medium yellow onion
2 cloves garlic
2 teaspoons extra virgin olive oil
1 teaspoon Clarified Butter (page 346) or ghee (optional)
*2 pounds young turnips with leaves
1 bay leaf
1 sprig fresh thyme
1 dried chipotle pepper
8 cups Basic Vegetable Stock (page 94)
sea salt and freshly ground black pepper, to taste

Thinly slice the onion and garlic. In a soup pot, heat olive oil and clarified butter over medium heat. Add onion, garlic and a splash of water and cook, covered, for 5 minutes until onion becomes soft and translucent.

Remove leaves from turnips and set aside. Trim off roots and discard. Slice turnips thinly (young turnips do not need to be peeled), and add to the pot. Cook for 3-5 minutes until turnips begin to release their juices. Add bay leaf, thyme, chipotle, vegetable stock, salt and pepper. Bring to a boil. Reduce heat to low, cover, and simmer for 15 minutes.

Remove and discard stems from turnip leaves. Cut leaves into thin strips and add them to the soup. Simmer soup for another 10-15 minutes until turnip leaves become soft and tender. Remove chipotle pepper, bay leaf and thyme sprig. Taste for seasoning.

[serves 10]

Nutrition Per Serving: Calories 38, Total Fat 1g, Saturated Fat trace, Cholesterol 1mg, Sodium 37mg, Potassium 176mg, Total Carbohydrate 5g, Dietary Fiber 2g, Protein 1g, Calcium 66mg, Iron 1mg, Vitamin C 33mg, Vitamin A 1793 IU, Vitamin B6 .1mg, Folacin 54mcg

*Note: It is important to use young turnips. Older turnips give the soup a bitter taste.

Thai Tofu and Coconut Soup

The Diet Doctor's Wife: The only way Bill will eat Thai food is if I prepare it at home. He can't bring himself to indulge in the full fat coconut milk used in Thai restaurants. Plus he prefers more subtle seasoning.

10 ounces tofu, cut in 1-inch cubes

Marinade

1/4 teaspoon fresh hot chili pepper, finely chopped
2 scallions, thinly sliced
1 clove garlic, crushed
1 teaspoon fresh ginger root, grated
1 tablespoon fresh lemongrass, thinly sliced
2 tablespoons water
1 tablespoon Thai fish sauce
juice of 1 lime

Place tofu in a shallow bowl. Combine ingredients of marinade and pour over tofu. Marinate the tofu for at least 1 hour, preferably overnight. Drain tofu.

Soup

2 teaspoons grapeseed oil
2-inch piece fresh ginger root, peeled and grated
3 cloves garlic, crushed
1 small fresh red chili pepper, finely chopped or 1 whole dried red chili pepper
4 cilantro roots, finely chopped (optional)
5 scallions, finely chopped
5 button mushrooms, trimmed and halved
1 stalk lemongrass, bottom 3 inches only, bruised with a meat-tenderizing mallet
3 tablespoons freshly squeezed lime juice
1 tablespoon Thai fish sauce or 2 tablespoons soy sauce
3 cups Basic Vegetable Stock (page 94)
1 cup reduced fat coconut milk
2 tablespoons maple syrup
4 fresh or dried kaffir lime leaves
1/2 cup fresh cilantro leaves, chopped

Heat oil in a soup pot over medium heat. Add ginger, garlic, chili pepper, cilantro roots and scallions. Sauté 1 minute. Add mushrooms and lemongrass and cook for another minute or so. Add lime juice, Thai fish sauce, stock, coconut milk, maple syrup, lime leaves and tofu. Bring to a boil and then reduce heat to simmer for 15 minutes. Taste for seasoning. Remove lime leaves and lemongrass. Serve in individual bowls and garnish with chopped cilantro leaves.

[serves 6]

Nutrition Per Serving: Calories 163, Total Fat 8g, Saturated Fat 2g, Cholesterol trace, *Sodium 635mg, Potassium 425mg, Total Carbohydrate 21g, Dietary Fiber 2g, Protein 8g, Calcium 115mg, Iron 12mg, Zinc 1mg, Vitamin C 12mg, Vitamin A 136 IU, Vitamin B6 .1mg, Thiamin B1 .1mg, Riboflavin B2 .3mg, Folacin 38mcg, Niacin 3mg

*Note: This is a relatively high sodium dish. Make sure to watch your sodium intake for the rest of the day and drink plenty of water.

Chinese Vegetable Soup

4 cups Chinese Stock (page 95)
6 ounces Chinese greens, coarsely chopped
1 carrot, sliced in thin rounds
3 scallions, cut in 2-inch lengths
1 tablespoon soy sauce
sea salt and freshly ground white pepper, to taste

Bring stock to a boil over medium heat. Lower temperature to medium low and add vegetables. Simmer 1-2 minutes. Season with soy sauce, salt and pepper. Simmer for 1 minute more and serve.

[serves 4]

Nutrition Per Serving: Calories 35, Total Fat trace, Saturated Fat trace, Cholesterol 0mg, Sodium 276mg, Potassium 248mg, Total Carbohydrate 5g, Dietary Fiber 2g, Protein 2g, Calcium 58mg, Iron 1mg, Vitamin C 34mg, Vitamin A 7360 IU, Vitamin B6 .1mg, Riboflavin B2 .1mg, Folacin 90mcg, Niacin 1mg

Chinese Mushroom Soup

4 dried shitake mushrooms, soaked in hot water for 20 minutes
3 ounces assorted fresh mushrooms, trimmed
4 cups Chinese Stock (page 95)
1/2-inch piece fresh ginger root, peeled and minced
1 clove garlic, peeled and minced
2 tablespoons dry sherry
2 tablespoons low sodium tamari
3 ounces fresh tofu, cut in 1/2-inch cubes
6 ounces bok choy leaves and stems, chopped
1 tablespoon arrowroot or kuzu, mixed with 2 tablespoons cold water
sea salt and freshly ground white pepper, to taste
3 tablespoons scallions, chopped

Drain soaked mushrooms and squeeze out any excess water. Cut away stems and discard. Slice caps and set aside. Slice the fresh mushrooms. If using button mushrooms, you may want to cut them in halves or quarters.

Pour stock in a soup pot and add ginger, garlic, sherry and tamari. Bring to a boil and reduce heat to simmer. Stir in mushrooms, tofu and greens. Simmer 5 minutes and then add arrowroot mixture and stir until thickened. Season to taste. Ladle into soup bowls and garnish with chopped scallions.

[serves 6]

Nutrition Per Serving: Calories 48, Total Fat 1g, Saturated Fat trace, Cholesterol 0mg, Sodium 241mg, Potassium 204mg, Total Carbohydrate 6g, Dietary Fiber 1g, Protein 3g, Calcium 51mg, Iron 1mg, Vitamin C 14mg, Vitamin A 874 IU, Vitamin B6 .1mg, Riboflavin B2 .1mg, Folacin 31mcg, Niacin 1mg

Hot-and-Sour Soup

The Diet Doctor's Wife: I prefer this vegetarian version of hot-and-sour soup to the Chinese classic. It is lighter and more delicate, yet still has a wonderful spicy flavor.

1/4 ounce dried tree ear fungus
8 fresh shitake mushrooms, stalks removed
3 ounces tofu
1/2 cup canned bamboo shoots, artichoke hearts or hearts of palm
1/3 cup Pressed Salad (page 285), drained
4 cups Chinese Stock (page 95)
1/4 cup brown rice syrup or 2 tablespoons maple syrup
1-2 tablespoons brown rice vinegar
1 tablespoon low sodium tamari
1/2 teaspoon hot chili oil
sea salt, to taste
1/8 teaspoon freshly ground white pepper, or more to taste

*1 tablespoon arrowroot or kuzu, mixed with 2 tablespoons cold water
1/4 teaspoon toasted sesame oil
2 scallions, cut in fine rounds

Reconstitute tree ear fungus in hot water for 30 minutes. Drain and squeeze out excess water. Trim away hard section and discard. Cut fungus into 1/4-inch strips.

Slice shitake mushroom caps into thin strips. Cut tofu into 1/2-inch cubes. Rinse and drain bamboo shoots, and cut into thin julienne strips. Rinse and drain Pressed Salad.

In a large saucepan, bring stock, mushrooms, tofu, bamboo shoots, Pressed Salad, and tree ear fungus to a boil. Reduce heat and simmer for 5 minutes. Add rice syrup, vinegar, tamari, chili oil, salt, pepper and arrowroot mixture. Stir continually until broth thickens a bit. Just before serving, add sesame oil. Garnish each serving with scallion rounds.

[serves 6]

Nutrition Per Serving: Calories 83, Total Fat 1g, Saturated Fat trace, Cholesterol 0mg, Sodium 282mg, Potassium 151mg, Total Carbohydrate 14g, Dietary Fiber 1g, Protein 2g, Calcium 26mg, Iron 1mg, Zinc 1mg, Vitamin C 4mg, Vitamin A 1174 IU, Vitamin B6 .1mg, Riboflavin B2 .1mg, Folacin 18mcg, Niacin 1mg

*Note: Cornstarch is usually used to thicken Chinese dishes. I use arrowroot or kuzu instead, since cornstarch is a highly refined product made with bleaches and extractive chemicals.

Cool Weather Miso Soup

The Diet Doctor: This is a hearty and satisfying winter soup that according to Gabrielle takes practically no time to prepare.

1 tablespoon instant wakame flakes or arame (optional)
1/4 cup daikon, sliced in thin rounds cut in half
1/4 cup carrot, sliced in thin rounds cut in half
4 fresh shitake mushroom caps, thinly sliced

2 tablespoons scallions, chopped
1 handful chopped seasonal greens (kale, collards, mustard)
1 quarter-size slice fresh ginger root, julienned
2 cups water, Basic Vegetable Stock (page 94) or Japanese Stock (page 95)
2 tablespoons red or barley miso
1-2 drops toasted sesame oil
1-2 drops sake
1-2 drops tamari

Place first 8 ingredients in a pot. Bring to a boil. Reduce heat and gently simmer for 5 minutes.

Remove 1/4 cup of broth from the pot and whisk together with miso until a liquid puree is formed. Pour miso mixture back into the pot. Season with sesame oil, sake and tamari. Allow to simmer 1 minute and serve.

[serves 4]

Nutrition Per Serving: Calories 43, Total Fat 1g, Saturated Fat trace, Cholesterol 0mg, Sodium 331mg, Potassium 193mg, Total Carbohydrate 8g, Dietary Fiber 2g, Protein 2g, Calcium 37mg, Iron 1mg, Zinc 1mg, Vitamin C 23mg, Vitamin A 3770 IU, Vitamin B6 .1mg, Riboflavin B2 .1mg, Folacin 18mcg, Niacin 1mg

Warm Weather Miso Soup

The Diet Doctor's Wife: You will enjoy this light and refreshing miso soup in the warm weather months. Best of all, it takes only minutes to prepare.

2 scallions, thinly sliced or 6 chives, chopped
1/2 carrot, thinly sliced
1 quarter-size slice fresh ginger root, julienned
pinch of wakame flakes or arame (optional)
2 handfuls tat soi or watercress
3 ounces silken tofu, cut in small cubes
2 cups water, Basic Vegetable Stock (page 94) or Japanese Stock (page 95)

2 tablespoons yellow miso
1/2 teaspoon sake
2-3 drops tamari
1 tablespoon fresh dill, minced

Place first 7 ingredients in a pot. Bring to a boil. Reduce heat and gently simmer for 3-5 minutes. Remove 1/4 cup of broth from the pot and whisk together with miso until a liquid puree is formed. Pour miso mixture back into the pot. Add sake, tamari and dill. Allow to simmer 1 minute and serve.

[serves 4]

Nutrition Per Serving: Calories 43, Total Fat 2g, Saturated Fat trace, Cholesterol 0mg, Sodium 334mg, Potassium 149mg, Total Carbohydrate 5g, Dietary Fiber 2g, Protein 3g, Calcium 59mg, Iron 2mg, Zinc 1mg, Vitamin C 10mg, Vitamin A 3396 IU, Vitamin B6 .1mg, Riboflavin B2 .1mg, Folacin 14mcg

Bonito Miso

The Diet Doctor: This miso tastes exactly like what you get in Japanese restaurants, except without the chemicals or preservatives.

2 cups Bonito Dashi (page 96)
1 1/2 tablespoons yellow miso
1 tablespoon instant wakame flakes, soaked 1 minute and drained
4 ounces silken tofu, cut in small cubes
1 tablespoon scallions, sliced in thin rounds

Bring Bonito Dashi to a boil. Reduce heat to simmer. Remove 1/4 cup of broth and whisk together with miso until a liquid puree is formed. Add miso mixture to soup and give it a stir. Simmer for 30 seconds to 1 minute longer. Divide wakame, tofu and scallions among 4 serving bowls. Add broth to each bowl. Serve immediately.

[serves 4]

Nutrition Per Serving: Calories 19, Total Fat trace, Saturated Fat trace, Cholesterol 0mg, Sodium 273mg, Potassium 15mg, Total Carbohydrate 2g, Protein 1g, Calcium 7mg, Vitamin A 16 IU, Folacin 6mcg

Japanese Tofu Nabe

The Diet Doctor's Wife: Japanese noodle soups are so easy to prepare at home and taste far better than the ones you get in fast food noodle shops. And if you follow this recipe, there is no fear of ingesting mystery chemicals and preservatives.

8 ounces dried somen noodles
12 dried shitake mushrooms, soaked in hot water for 1/2 hour
4 cups Japanese Stock (page 95)
1 tablespoon low sodium tamari
2 tablespoons mirin
6 ounces Chinese cabbage (boy choy, Napa, etc.)
1 medium carrot, sliced on the diagonal
1/2 cup daikon, sliced in half-rounds
12 snow peas, de-stringed
1 pound firm tofu, cut in 1-inch cubes
sea salt, to taste

Condiments

1/2 cup scallions, finely chopped, liquid squeezed out
2 tablespoons fresh ginger root, grated

To prepare noodles, bring 3 quarts of water to a rolling boil. Add noodles and cook until al dente (tender but still firm to the bite). Stir occasionally to prevent noodles from sticking. Two or three times throughout cooking, shock the noodles with 1/2 cup of cold water to allow them to firm up slightly, and then allow cooking water to come back to a rolling boil. When the noodles are done, drain and allow to cool. Reserve cooking water.

Drain mushrooms, reserving the soaking liquid. Remove mushroom stems and discard. Set mushroom caps aside. Strain mushroom soaking liquid through a cheesecloth-lined wire-mesh strainer, and set aside.

Place Japanese Stock, mushroom caps and strained mushroom liquid in a large pot. Bring to a boil and then reduce heat to low. Add tamari and mirin. Simmer gently until ready to serve.

In a separate pot, reheat the water used to cook the noodles and bring to a boil. Parboil cabbage leaves. Drain and allow to cool. Reserve the cooking liquid. Boil the carrots in the reserved cooking liquid until tender. Drain and allow to cool. Reserve the cooking liquid. Boil the daikon rounds in the reserved cooking liquid until tender. Drain and allow to cool, reserving the cooking liquid once more. Blanch the snow peas in the reserved cooking liquid. Drain and refresh in cold water. Drain again.

Distribute the noodles, vegetables and tofu among 6 serving bowls. Ladle some of the simmering broth on top. Serve with the condiments.

[serves 6]

Nutrition Per Serving: Calories 292, Total Fat 5g, Saturated Fat 1g, Cholesterol 0mg, Sodium 193mg, Potassium 739mg, Total Carbohydrate 47g, Dietary Fiber 7g, Protein 17g, Calcium 233mg, Iron 6mg, Zinc 2mg, Vitamin C 93mg, Vitamin A 4446 IU, Vitamin B6 .4mg, Thiamin B1 .4mg, Riboflavin B2 1mg, Folacin 117mcg, Niacin 3mg

Japanese Fish Nabe

The Diet Doctor's Wife: This is a soup that can be served as a meal. It is nutritionally balanced, filling, yet not at all heavy.

The Diet Doctor: I used to love ordering cook-it-yourself dishes in Japanese restaurants, but unfortunately, I'd wake up the next morning feeling so groggy. I imagine the feeling came from an allergic reaction to the chemicals and "mystery" ingredients in the bottled stocks and sauces.

But at home, I don't have to worry about that. Gabrielle just heats up some of her Japanese stock, adds some fish and vegetables, and 10 minutes later we're feasting. The next day I feel just fine.

1/2 bok choy, leaves shredded, stalks cut in diagonal strips
2 carrots, cut in 1/2–inch diagonals
5 cups Bonito Dashi (page 96) or Japanese Stock (page 95)
1 tablespoon low sodium tamari, plus extra if desired
2 tablespoons mirin
1 pound salmon, skin removed, cut in 4 pieces
1/2 pound tofu, cut in 1-inch cubes
1 package okonomi mushrooms, separated or 3 ounces button mushrooms, sliced

Condiments

2 tablespoons fresh ginger root, peeled and grated
1/2 cup daikon radish, peeled and grated, liquid squeezed out
4 scallions, finely chopped, liquid squeezed out
1 small fresh red chili pepper, sliced in thin rounds or wasabi paste
tamari

In a pot of salted boiling water, parboil bok choy stalks. Remove stalks with a slotted spoon. Reheat water and boil the carrots until tender. Drain carrots and allow to cool.

In a large pot, bring Bonito Dashi, tamari and mirin to a boil. Add fish and allow to come back to a boil. Lower heat and simmer until fish is cooked through. Add bok choy stems and leaves, carrots and tofu. Simmer until all ingredients are warmed through.

Evenly distribute the fish and vegetables among 4 serving bowls. Top with okonomi mushrooms. Ladle broth on top.

Pass around condiments for seasoning according to individual taste.

[serves 4]

Nutrition Per Serving: Calories 237, Total Fat 7g, Saturated Fat 1g, Cholesterol 59mg, Sodium 325mg, Potassium 816mg, Total Carbohydrate 10g, Dietary Fiber 3g, Protein 29g, Calcium 116mg, Iron 5mg, Zinc 1mg, Vitamin C 45mg, Vitamin A 10,715 IU, Vitamin B6 .4mg, Vitamin B12 3.4mcg, Thiamin B1 .3mg, Riboflavin B2 .3mg, Folacin 49mcg,, Niacin 7mg

Caldo Verde with Fresh Cod

The Diet Doctor's Wife: I consider this soup to be medicinal. It is packed with nutrients, yet light and easy to digest. And it tastes good too. Caldo Verde with Cod was the first real meal I served to Bill after his appendectomy and to my mother after her hip surgery.

2 teaspoons extra virgin olive oil
6 large cloves garlic, finely minced
1 carrot, cubed
1/8-1/4 teaspoon red pepper flakes
1/2 pound turnips or daikon, peeled and cubed
1/2 pound cauliflower florets
1 quart Basic Vegetable Stock (page 94)
1 cup white wine
1 cup water
6 ounces kale leaves with stems removed, shredded
1 pound cod fillets with skin removed, cut in chunks
sea salt, to taste

Heat extra virgin olive oil in a large heavy soup pot on medium heat. Add garlic, carrot and pepper flakes, and sauté for 1 minute. Add turnips, cauliflower, stock, white wine and water. Bring to a boil and then reduce heat to simmer for 15 minutes.

With a potato masher, lightly break up carrots, cauliflower and turnips directly in the soup pot. Add kale leaves. Simmer another 10 minutes. Add cod and salt. Simmer another 5 minutes until fish is cooked through. Taste for seasoning.

[serves 6-8]

Nutrition Per Serving: Calories 157, Total Fat 2g, Saturated Fat trace, Cholesterol 33mg, Sodium 109mg, Potassium 695mg, Total Carbohydrate 13g, Dietary Fiber 2g, Protein 16g, Calcium 81mg, Iron 1mg, Zinc 1mg, Vitamin C 61mg, Vitamin A 5938 IU, Vitamin B6 .4mg, Vitamin B12 .7mcg, Thiamin B1 .1mg, Riboflavin B2 .1mg, Folacin 41mcg, Niacin 2mg

Provencal Fish Stew

The Diet Doctor's Wife: This soup is heavenly. It's aromatic, delicate, yet truly satisfying. I often serve Provencal Fish Stew at lunch for special occasions. It is basically a bouillabaisse without the shellfish.

3 pounds white-fleshed fish fillets (red snapper, grouper, cod), skin removed
4 teaspoons extra virgin olive oil
5 plump cloves garlic, chopped
2 large onions, coarsely chopped
1-2 tablespoons tomato paste or 3 large tomatoes, peeled, cored, seeded and chopped
1/8 teaspoon grated orange peel
1/8 teaspoon fennel seeds, crushed with a mortar and pestle
pinch each of dried thyme, dried basil and dried oregano
bouquet garni (1 sprig thyme, 6 sprigs parsley and 2 bay leaves, tied together with string)
2 carrots, chopped
2 leeks, chopped
sea salt and freshly ground black pepper, to taste
6 cups Basic Vegetable Stock (page 94)
1 cup dry white wine
1 teaspoon saffron threads
2-3 teaspoons Pernod® or licorice flavored liqueur

Cut fish fillets in 2-inch cubes. Place in a shallow pan.

Marinate fish in 2 teaspoons olive oil and 1/2 teaspoon chopped garlic. Refrigerate for 1-3 hours.

In a large saucepan, heat 2 teaspoons of oil over medium low heat. Add the onions and remaining chopped garlic, and sauté for 4-5 minutes. If the pan gets too dry, add a splash of water.

Add tomato paste, orange peel, crushed fennel seeds, dried thyme, dried basil, dried oregano, bouquet garni, carrots, leeks, salt and pepper. Cook, covered, for 10 minutes. Add stock and wine. Bring to a boil. Lower heat and simmer, uncovered, for 30 minutes. Remove from the heat.

Pour mixture into the bowl of a food processor and pulse to blend. Strain, if desired.

Return soup to the saucepan. Add fish and cook at a gentle boil for 10 minutes. Add saffron and simmer for 5 minutes. Add Pernod®. Taste for seasoning.

Pour soup into bowls. Serve with Eggless Rouille (page 339).

[serves 8]

Nutrition Per Serving: Calories 255, Total Fat 5g, Saturated Fat 1g, Cholesterol 69mg, Sodium 154mg, Potassium 816mg, Total Carbohydrate 12g, Dietary Fiber 2g, Protein 33g, Calcium 65mg, Iron 1mg, Zinc 1mg, Vitamin C 9mg, Vitamin A 5321 IU, Vitamin B6 .7mg, Vitamin B12 2.4mcg, Thiamin B1 .2mg, Riboflavin B2 .1mg, Folacin 32mcg, Niacin 3mg

Note: Traditionally this soup is served with toasted baguette slices, which are rubbed with whole garlic cloves. Each baguette slice is placed in a soup bowl with a dollop of rouille. Our feeling is that the addition of bread adds nothing more than calories.

Fish Chowder

The Diet Doctor's Wife: This fish chowder is one of the first dishes I prepared for Bill, months before we embarked on our quasi-macrobiotic journey. Bill still requests it, especially when the weather starts to get a bit chilly.

The Diet Doctor: This dish is really simple. That's why it's so good.

2 teaspoons extra virgin olive oil
1 medium onion, diced
2 leeks, white and pale green parts only, chopped
5 stalks celery, diced
1 large carrot, chopped
1/4 cup garlic, finely chopped
14-ounce can tomatoes, drained with liquid reserved
1 medium turnip, peeled and diced in 1-inch cubes or 1/2 head cauliflower, cut in small florets
1 teaspoon saffron threads
2 bay leaves
1 teaspoon dried thyme
sea salt and freshly ground black pepper, to taste
1/2 cup dry white wine
4 cups Basic Vegetable Stock (page 94)
1 pound cod fillet, skin removed and cubed

Heat olive oil in a heavy-bottomed soup pot over medium heat. Add onion, leeks, celery and carrot, and sauté until vegetables release their juices, about 5 minutes. Add garlic, tomatoes, turnip, saffron, bay leaves, thyme, salt and pepper. Sauté 2 minutes. Add white wine and cook 5 minutes until most of the liquid has been absorbed.

Add stock and reserved tomato liquid, and bring to a boil. Reduce heat and gently simmer for 30 minutes.

Add fish. Cook at a strong simmer for 5 minutes. Remove bay leaves. Taste for seasoning.

[serves 4]

Nutrition Per Serving: Calories 235, Total Fat 4g, Saturated Fat 1g, Cholesterol 49mg, Sodium 295mg, Potassium 1154mg, Total Carbohydrate 23g, Dietary Fiber 5g, Protein 24g, Calcium 141mg, Iron 3mg, Zinc 1mg, Vitamin C 38mg, Vitamin A 5826 IU, Vitamin B6 .7mg, Vitamin B12 1mcg, Thiamin B1 .2mg, Riboflavin B2 .1mg, Folacin 74mcg, Niacin 4mg

Grains

WHOLE GRAINS

Whole grains (brown rice, whole barley, millet) should be eaten daily. They are a good source of B complex vitamins, vitamin E, calcium, iron, magnesium, phosphorous, potassium, essential fatty acids and dietary fiber. Processed whole grains (whole wheat flour, rolled oats, rye flakes) can be eaten in moderation. Although rich in essential vitamins and minerals, they are lower in dietary fiber and can become rancid over a 3-month period. Eating a lot of processed whole grains and their products can also lead to weight gain. Refined grains and their products (white rice, white flour, cornstarch) should be eaten rarely or avoided whenever possible. The reason is that much of the nutrition is lost in the refining process. Chemical additives may also be present.

Below is a list of whole grains and whole grain products (whole grain products are indicated in italics):

Rice - brown rice (short, medium and long grain), sweet brown rice, wild rice, *puffed brown rice crackers, mochi, brown rice flour, brown rice pasta*

Barley - whole barley, pearl barley, *barley tea, barley flour, barley flour baked goods*

Buckwheat - buckwheat groats, *buckwheat flour, buckwheat pasta, buckwheat flour baked goods*

Corn - fresh corn, popped corn, *cornmeal, corn flour, tortilla chips*

Millet - millet, *millet flour, millet flour baked goods*

Oats - whole oats, *steel-cut oats, rolled oats, oat flakes, oat flour, oat flour baked goods*

Rye - rye berries, *rye flakes, rye flour, rye flour pasta, rye bread*

Spelt - spelt berries, *spelt flour, spelt flour baked goods*

Whole Wheat - wheat berries, *bulgur, whole wheat flour, whole wheat pasta, whole wheat couscous, seitan, fu, whole wheat bread, whole wheat crackers, whole wheat flour baked goods*

WASHING GRAINS

Whole grains must be washed thoroughly before you cook them. To wash whole grains just place them in a large pot and cover with water. Swish the grains around. The water will likely be cloudy. Drain through a mesh colander. Continue the washing procedure until the water runs clear. Drain.

SOAKING GRAINS

In addition to being washed thoroughly, some whole grains need to be soaked in cold water before you cook them. Soaking allows the grains to swell, which creates a sweeter taste and softer texture. Soaking also decreases cooking time. Soaking time depends on the type of grain, how long the grain has been stored and the season. In general, hard-kernelled whole grains (barley, rye berries and wheat berries) should be soaked for 4-8 hours. Brown rice can be soaked, if desired, anywhere from 1-8 hours. Grains with thin kernel walls (millet and buckwheat groats) do not require soaking at all.

Grains require shorter soaking time in the warmer months. If you do not have time to soak a hard-kernelled grain, cook a bit longer and with a bit more water than the recipe calls for.

COOKING METHODS

The grain recipes in this cookbook call for boiling or pressure-cooking. My preference is pressure-cooking since it creates a richer flavor and softer texture. Cooking times vary according to the type of grain and method of cooking.

You may want to slip a flame deflector under your pot while your grains are cooking. This lowers the temperature slightly so that the grains do not stick to the bottom of the pot.

1. Pressure Cooking

Wash and drain whole grains. Put washed and drained grains in a pressure cooker. Add the indicated quantity of water. Add sea salt. Lock cover and place cooker over medium heat. Bring up to pressure and then slip a flame deflector under the cooker. Turn the heat to medium low. Cook for the required time.

In general, for every cup of grain, use 1 1/2 cups of water. Note that hard-kernelled grains need to be soaked before cooking. If desired, you may also choose to soak brown rice. The soaking water can be used for cooking. Add sea salt and any other seasoning after grains have been soaked.

2. Boiling

Wash and drain whole grains. Put washed and drained grains in a heavy pot. Add the indicated quantity of water. Add sea salt. Cover and bring to a boil. Simmer over low heat for the required cooking time.

In general, for every cup of grain, use 2 cups of water. Note that hard-kernelled grains need to be soaked before cooking. The soaking water can be used for cooking. Add sea salt or any other seasoning after the grains have been soaked.

Boiling is an ideal way to cook brown rice, basmati rice, Arborio rice, grains with a thin kernel wall (millet and buckwheat groats), and grains that are rolled or cut (rolled oats, steel-cut oats, barley flakes, rye flakes, polenta and cornmeal).

3. Baking

Grains can also be baked. There are no baked grain recipes in this cookbook.

Pressure Cooked Brown Rice

The Diet Doctor's Wife: I make Pressure Cooked Brown Rice several times a week. The pressure cooking creates richness without the use of fat. And the texture is wonderful.

2 cups brown rice, preferably short grain
3 cups water
1/4 teaspoon sea salt

Place rice, water and salt in a pressure cooker. Cover and bring up to pressure over high heat. Reduce heat to medium low and place a flame deflector under the cooker. Cook for 45 minutes.

Remove cooker from the heat and let pressure come down naturally. Remove lid and let sit for 5 minutes.

[serves 8]

Nutrition Per Serving: Calories 172, Total Fat 1g, Saturated Fat trace, Cholesterol 0mg, Sodium 63mg, Potassium 127mg, Total Carbohydrate 36g, Dietary Fiber 1g, Protein 4g, Calcium 17mg, Iron 1mg, Zinc 1mg, Vitamin B6 .2mg, Thiamin B1 .2mg, Folacin 10mcg, Niacin 2mg

Note: For a softer texture and sweeter flavor, soak the rice in the 3 cups of water for 1-8 hours before cooking. Then place the rice, soaking water, and salt in a pressure cooker. Cook according to the directions in the recipe above.

Boiled Brown Rice

2 cups brown rice
4 cups water
1/4 teaspoon sea salt

Place rice, water and salt in a heavy pot. Cover and bring to a boil. Reduce heat to medium low and place a flame deflector under the pot. Simmer for 1 hour.

Remove pot from the heat. Take off lid. Let sit for 5 minutes.

[serves 8]

Nutrition Per Serving: Calories 172, Total Fat 1g, Saturated Fat trace, Cholesterol 0mg, Sodium 63mg, Potassium 127mg, Total Carbohydrate 36g, Dietary Fiber 1g, Protein 4g, Calcium 17mg, Iron 1mg, Zinc 1mg, Vitamin B6 .2mg, Thiamin B1 .2mg, Folacin 10mcg, Niacin 2mg

Brown Basmati Rice

1 cup brown basmati rice
1 1/2 cups water
1/4 teaspoon sea salt

Add rice and water to a heavy pot and allow to sit for 1 hour. Add sea salt. Cover the pot and bring to a boil over medium heat. Reduce heat to low and place a flame deflector under the pot. Simmer for 20-25 minutes. Remove from heat and let sit, covered, for 10 minutes.

[4 servings]

Nutrition Per Serving: Calories 172, Total Fat 1g, Saturated Fat trace, Cholesterol 0mg, Sodium 63mg, Potassium 127mg, Total Carbohydrate 36g, Dietary Fiber 1g, Protein 4g, Calcium 17mg, Iron 1mg, Zinc 1mg, Vitamin B6 .2mg, Thiamin B1 .2mg, Folacin 10mcg, Niacin 2mg

Sushi Rice

*2 cups short grain brown rice or sweet brown rice
3 cups water
1/4–1/2 teaspoon sea salt
4 tablespoons brown rice vinegar
3 tablespoons brown rice syrup

Place the rice, water and sea salt in a pressure cooker. Cover and bring up to pressure. Reduce heat to medium low and place a flame deflector under the pressure cooker. Cook for 45 minutes. Remove from heat and allow pressure to come down naturally. Remove cover and allow rice to rest for 5 minutes. Place rice in a shallow bowl.

In a saucepan, heat vinegar and rice syrup until syrup liquefies. Stir and allow to cool.

Add vinegar and rice syrup mixture to the cooked rice. Mix together. Fan the rice with one hand, to cool.

[serves 8]

Nutrition Per Serving: Calories 189, Total Fat 1g, Saturated Fat trace, Cholesterol 0mg, Sodium 64mg, Potassium 135mg, Total Carbohydrate 41g, Dietary Fiber 1g, Protein 4g, Calcium 18mg, Iron 1mg, Zinc 1mg, Vitamin B6 .2mg, Thiamin B1 .2mg, Folacin 10mcg, Niacin 2mg

*Note: You can make this dish with half white sushi rice and half short grain brown rice. Use 2 1/2 to 2 3/4 cups of water for 2 cups of the combined raw rice.

Inside-Out Sushi

4 sushi nori sheets
3 cups Sushi Rice (page 133)
2 tablespoons tan sesame seeds, toasted and lightly crushed
*1-2 pickling cucumbers or 1/2 Japanese cucumber, cut in thin sticks
1/3 avocado, peeled, pitted and sliced in thin wedges
1-2 carrots, cut in thin sticks

Condiments

Wasabi paste
soy sauce or tamari
ginger pickles

Cover a sushi mat with a sheet of plastic wrap. Fold the wrap over the edges of the mat. The smooth plastic side should be facing up. Place 1 nori sheet on the mat. Take 3/4 cup of rice and form into a ball. Place ball of rice at the bottom of the nori sheet. Spread the rice to the edges of the nori sheet. Sprinkle sesame seeds evenly over the top of the rice.

Taking the top 2 corners, pick up the rice-covered nori sheet and quickly turn it over, rice side down, and rest it on the mat. Place one quarter of the cucumber, avocado and carrots across the center of the nori. Roll the mat over the vegetables, pressing them with your fingers as you roll. This will keep the vegetables in place. Continue to roll, leaving a 3/4-inch strip of nori free at the end. Press gently to keep the roll firm. Use the mat to gently move the roll back and forth in order to seal the seam. Press gently once again to keep the roll firm and to maintain its shape.

Cut the roll in half. Cut each half in half, and in half again. You should have 8 equal-size slices. Repeat the whole process with the 3 remaining nori sheets. Serve with wasabi paste, soy sauce and ginger pickles.

[serves 4 (4 rolls, 32 pieces)]

Nutrition Per Serving: Calories 270, Total Fat 6g, Saturated Fat 1g, Cholesterol 0mg, Sodium 135mg, Potassium 396mg, Total Carbohydrate 49g, Dietary Fiber 5g, Protein 6g, Calcium 83mg, Iron 2mg, Zinc 2mg, Vitamin C 11mg, Vitamin A 5856 IU, Vitamin B6 .4mg, Thiamin B1 .2mg, Riboflavin B2 .1mg, Folacin 48mcg, Niacin 3mg

*Note: Pickling and Japanese cucumbers are used because of their thin skin and small seeds. If a thicker, larger seeded cucumber is used, peel the skin and remove the seeds before cutting into thin strips.

California Sushi Bowl

The Diet Doctor's Wife: This is a no-fuss way to enjoy sushi. No complicated rolling techniques are required.

The Diet Doctor: If you have high cholesterol, you may want to substitute the shrimp in this dish with smoked salmon or bonito flakes. For those of

you who are losing weight, the relatively high cholesterol in the shrimp is not that significant. Shrimp is low in calories, which makes it a good diet food. As you lose weight, your body fat decreases; this helps to lower your cholesterol.

3 cups Sushi Rice (page 133)
1/2 cup cucumber, sliced in 1/8-inch rounds
1/3 cup carrot, thinly sliced
2 tablespoons pickled ginger slices, chopped
1 cup cooked baby shrimp or smoked salmon pieces (nitrite-free), or 3 tablespoons bonito flakes (optional)
1/3 cup avocado, cubed (optional)
1 sheet sushi nori, cut in thin strips
*2 tablespoons tan sesame seeds, toasted

Condiments

wasabi paste
soy sauce or tamari

Place cucumber slices in a colander. Lightly sprinkle with sea salt and allow to sit and drain for 1/2 hour. Pat dry with a paper towel.

Distribute rice among 4 serving bowls. Scatter cucumber, carrot, ginger pickle, shrimp and avocado on top. Garnish with nori strips and sesame seeds. Serve with a dipping sauce made of wasabi mixed with soy sauce.

[serves 4]

Nutrition Per Serving: Calories 264, Total Fat 4g, Saturated Fat 1g, Cholesterol 111mg, Sodium 135mg, Potassium 253mg, Total Carbohydrate 40g, Dietary Fiber 3g, Protein 16g, Calcium 87mg, Iron 3mg, Zinc 2mg, Vitamin C 4mg, Vitamin A 3296 IU, Vitamin B6 .3mg, Vitamin B12 .8mcg, Thiamin B1 .2mg, Folacin 19mcg, Niacin 4mg

*Note: To toast sesame seeds, refer to recipe for Sesame Salt on page 327.

Thin Cucumber Rolls

5 sheets sushi nori
2 cups Sushi Rice (page 133)

*3 pickling cucumbers or 1 Japanese cucumber, cut into 1/4-inch thick strips
**1 tablespoon sesame seeds, toasted
wasabi paste

Cut nori sheets in half lengthwise. Cut 3/4-inch off the bottom of each 1/2-sheet. Place one trimmed nori sheet lengthwise, shiny side down, on a bamboo sushi mat. The nori sheet should be placed 1 inch from the bottom edge of the mat.

Wet hands and take a handful of rice and form into a ball. Place the rice ball just below the center of the nori sheet. Spread rice to evenly cover the surface of the nori, leaving a 3/4-inch strip uncovered at the top edge.

To keep the filling in place, build up the rice a bit at the bottom edge of the nori sheet to create a low ridge. Dab some wasabi across the center of the rice. Sprinkle some sesame seeds on top of the wasabi. Place the cucumber strips on top of the sesame seeds in a horizontal line along the center of the rice.

Hold the cucumber strips in place with flat fingers, as you lift the edge of the bamboo mat that is closest to you. Roll the mat away from you to form the cucumber roll, pressing gently to keep the roll firm. When both rice edges meet, there will be a 3/4-inch strip of bare nori left over. Using the mat, gently move the roll back and forth to seal the nori edge. Press gently to keep the roll firm and to maintain its shape.

Slice the roll in half, and then each half-slice in thirds. Continue the whole process with the remaining nori sheets.

[serves 10 (10 rolls, 60 pieces)]

Nutrition Per Serving: Calories 59, Total Fat 1g, Saturated Fat trace, Cholesterol 0mg, Sodium 4mg, Potassium 106mg, Total Carbohydrate 12g, Dietary Fiber 1g, Protein 2g, Calcium 15mg, Vitamin C 4mg, Vitamin A 362 IU, Vitamin B6 .1mg, Thiamin B1 .1mg, Folacin 16mcg, Niacin 1mg

*Note 1: Pickling and Japanese cucumbers are used because of their thin skin and small seeds. If a thicker, larger seeded cucumber is used, peel the skin and remove the seeds before cutting into thin strips.

**Note 2: To toast sesame seeds, refer to recipe for Sesame Salt on page 327.

Wappa for Two

The Diet Doctor's Wife: In Japan Town in San Francisco, there is a tiny restaurant called Maki that is out of this world. Their signature Wappa dishes are delicious rice preparations served in small bamboo steamers. The esthetic is simple and refined. I have created my own version below.

1/2 cup Japanese Stock (page 95)
1 tablespoon tamari
1 tablespoon mirin
1 tablespoon sake
1 tablespoon maple syrup
2 teaspoons fresh ginger root, grated
1/8 teaspoon toasted sesame oil
1 cup Chinese greens (tat soi, Napa cabbage, bok choy), chopped
2 fresh shitake mushroom caps, sliced
1/4 cup carrots, julienned
1/4 cup daikon radish, julienned
6 fresh snow peas
2 ounces tofu strips, julienned
2 cups cooked short grain brown rice
2 Napa cabbage leaves, to line bamboo steamers

Take out 2 individual-serving-size bamboo steamers.

To prepare marinade, combine Japanese Stock, tamari, mirin, sake and maple syrup in a small saucepan. Heat mixture on medium low until warmed through. Squeeze the juice out of the grated ginger into the marinade mixture. Discard ginger pulp. Stir in sesame oil. Remove from heat. Allow to cool.

Pour marinade over vegetables and tofu. Marinate for at least 1 hour. Drain and reserve marinade liquid.

In a bowl, combine marinated vegetables and tofu with rice. To best integrate, alternately layer rice and marinated ingredients. Then lightly mix with a wooden spoon.

Place a Napa cabbage leaf on the bottom of each steamer to completely cover slats. Top each Napa leaf with 1/2 the rice mixture. Spoon 1-2 tablespoons of marinade liquid over each of the rice mixtures. Stack steamers and cover with bamboo lid. To begin steaming, add cold water to a wok to a level of 1-2 inches. Bring to a simmer. Place stacked steamers inside the wok over the simmering water. Cover wok and steam for 10 minutes. Serve in the bamboo steamers.

[serves 2]

Nutrition Per Serving: Calories 322, Total Fat 3g, Saturated Fat 1g, Cholesterol 0mg, Sodium 337mg, Potassium 405mg, Total Carbohydrate 61g, Dietary Fiber 5g, Protein 9g, Calcium 111mg, Iron 4mg, Zinc 2mg, Vitamin C 26mg, Vitamin A 5379 IU, Vitamin B6 .5mg, Thiamin B1 .3mg, Riboflavin B2 .1mg, Folacin 52mcg, Niacin 4mg

Mah Zeh Rice

The Diet Doctor's Wife: This is my rendition of Bill's favorite rice dish from Souen, a wonderful macrobiotic restaurant in New York City. Mah Zeh is a mispronunciation of the original name and also means "what's that?" in Hebrew.

8 dried shitake mushrooms, soaked in hot water for 15 minutes
1 medium carrot, julienned
1 small burdock root, julienned
1/3 cup green beans or asparagus, cut in 1/4-inch pieces
3 tablespoons reconstituted kombu, julienned
1 cup Japanese Stock (page 95), plus more if needed
1 tablespoon tamari
1 tablespoon mirin
1 tablespoon sake
4 cups cooked short grain brown rice
finely cut strips of nori, for garnish

Squeeze liquid out of reconstituted shitake mushrooms. Remove and discard stems. Slice caps thinly.

Combine shitake mushroom cap slices, carrots, burdock, green beans and kombu in a small bowl. Add Japanese stock, tamari, mirin and sake. Allow to marinate overnight. (For a quicker version, combine stock and burdock in a small saucepan. Bring to a boil and reduce heat to simmer, covered, for 5 minutes. Add carrots and green beans. Simmer another minute. Remove from the heat and add tamari, mirin and sake. Allow vegetables to marinate for at least 1/2 hour.)

Heat a wok on medium. Add rice, vegetables and any leftover marinade. Add a splash of stock or water. Stir to combine and cook until mixture is heated through and liquid has evaporated.

Place in serving bowls and garnish with nori strips, if desired.

[serves 4]

Nutrition Per Serving: Calories 293, Total Fat 2g, Saturated Fat trace, Cholesterol 0mg, Sodium 272mg, Potassium 406mg, Total Carbohydrate 61g, Dietary Fiber 6g, Protein 7g, Calcium 52mg, Iron 2mg, Zinc 2mg, Vitamin C 5mg, Vitamin A 5129 IU, Vitamin B6 .5mg, Thiamin B1 .2mg, Riboflavin B2 .1mg, Folacin 42mcg, Niacin 4mg

Variation: Add Roasted Salmon Japanese Style (page 242) to this dish, either whole or flaked.

Outback Rice Dinner

The Diet Doctor: Gabrielle and I often order take-out salmon dinner (no butter on the fish or vegetables) from the Outback Steakhouse near the office. It's plain, good food for times when we are too tired or too lazy to cook. We like it so much that we have created a home version with a quasi-macrobiotic twist. As far as we're concerned, this dish qualifies as comfort food – the kind that won't kill you.

2 tablespoons low sodium tamari
2 tablespoons sake
2 tablespoons mirin
1 cup cauliflower florets
1 cup broccoli florets
1 medium carrot, cut in 1/4-inch thick slices
6-ounce salmon fillet
2 cups cooked brown rice
water or Basic Vegetable Stock (page 94)

Combine tamari, sake and mirin in a small bowl. Place vegetables in a separate bowl and marinate in 4 tablespoons of the tamari mixture. Marinate the salmon in the remaining 2 tablespoons of the tamari mixture. Allow to rest for 15-30 minutes.

Steam the vegetables until tender. Set aside. Steam the salmon until cooked through. Remove and discard the salmon skin.

Heat a wok on medium. Add rice, steamed vegetables and fish. Cook to heat through. If the pan gets too dry, add a dash of water or stock. Season to taste.

[serves 2]

Nutrition Per Serving: Calories 405, Total Fat 5g, Saturated Fat 1g, Cholesterol 44mg, Sodium 697mg, Potassium 784mg, Total Carbohydrate 57g, Dietary Fiber 7g, Protein 25g, Calcium 73mg, Iron 3mg, Zinc 2mg, Vitamin 60mg, Vitamin A 11336 IU, Vitamin B6 .6mg, Vitamin B12 2.5mcg, Thiamin B1 .4mg, Riboflavin B2 .2mg, Folacin 73mcg, Niacin 8mg

Garlic and Mushroom Rice

1 clove garlic, minced
1 teaspoon toasted sesame oil
5 fresh button or shitake mushrooms, trimmed and sliced
1 cup short grain brown rice, washed and drained
2 cups cold water
1/4 teaspoon sea salt

In a heavy saucepan, sauté garlic in sesame oil over medium heat for 1 minute. Add mushrooms and sauté for 2-3 minutes. If the pan gets too dry, add a splash of water or stock. Add rice and sauté another 2-3 minutes. Add water and salt. Cover and bring to a boil. Reduce heat to low and place a flame deflector under the pan. Cook for 50 minutes.

[serves 4]

Nutrition Per Serving: Calories 189, Total Fat 2g, Saturated Fat trace, Cholesterol 0mg, Sodium 124mg, Potassium 214mg, Total Carbohydrate 37g, Dietary Fiber 1g, Protein 4g, Calcium 21mg, Iron 1mg, Zinc 1mg, Vitamin C 1mg, Vitamin B6 .3mg, Thiamin B1 .2mg, Riboflavin B2 .1mg, Folacin 14mcg, Niacin 3mg

Brown and Wild Rice with Vegetables

1 teaspoon toasted sesame oil
1/4 cup shallots or onions, finely chopped
1 1/2 cups fresh shitake mushroom caps, sliced
tamari
1/2 cup burdock, cubed
1/2 cup carrots, cubed
1 cup brown basmati rice
1 cup wild rice
1/4 teaspoon sea salt
3 1/2 cups water

In a pressure cooker, heat oil and sauté shallots for 1 minute. Add mushrooms and sauté for another minute. Add a few drops of tamari and continue cooking for another minute. Add burdock and carrots. Cook for another minute, adding a few more drops of tamari, if desired. Add rices, salt and water.

Cover and bring up to pressure. When pressure is up, reduce heat to medium low and place a flame deflector under the cooker. Cook 45-50 minutes. Remove cooker from heat and allow pressure to come down naturally. Remove cover and allow rice to sit for 5-10 minutes.

[serves 8-10]

Nutrition Per Serving: Calories 306, Total Fat 2g, Saturated Fat trace, Cholesterol 0mg, Sodium 76mg, Potassium 883mg, Total Carbohydrate 69g, Dietary Fiber 8g, Protein 9g, Calcium 23mg, Iron 2mg, Zinc 5mg, Vitamin C 3mg, Vitamin A 2888 IU, Vitamin B6 .6mg, Thiamin B1 .2mg, Riboflavin B2 .6mg, Folacin 100mcg, Niacin 9mg

Vegetable Fried Rice

1 1/2 teaspoons grapeseed oil
2 scallions, thinly sliced
1 tablespoon fresh ginger root, grated
1/2 cup celery, minced
1/2 cup carrot, minced
1/4 cup daikon, minced
6 fresh shitake mushroom caps, thinly sliced
tamari or soy sauce
4 cups cooked brown rice
1-2 drops toasted sesame oil
sea salt, to taste
chopped fresh scallions, chives or dill, for garnish

Heat grapeseed oil in a wok over medium heat. Warm scallions and ginger for about 1 minute. Add the rest of the vegetables and sauté. If the pan gets too dry, add a couple of tablespoons of water or stock, and cook for 1 minute. Add a few drops of tamari and stir to incorporate. Add rice and a few more drops of tamari and a drop of toasted sesame oil. Sauté until rice is heated through. If the wok gets too dry, add a bit more water or stock. Sauté until liquid is evaporated. Season to taste. Garnish with finely chopped scallions, chives or dill.

[serves 6]

Nutrition Per Serving: Calories 176, Total Fat 2g, Saturated Fat trace, Cholesterol 0mg, Sodium 18mg, Potassium 204mg, Total Carbohydrate 35g, Dietary Fiber 3g, Protein 4g, Calcium 25mg, Iron 1mg, Zinc 1mg, Vitamin C 4mg, Vitamin A 3046 IU, Vitamin B6 .2mg, Thiamin B1 .1mg, Riboflavin B2 .1mg, Folacin 20mcg, Niacin 2mg

Fried Rice A La Om Cafe

The Diet Doctor's Wife: This is a lower fat version of a dish that Bill and I often order at the Om Cafe in Ferndale, Michigan. It's simple and satisfying.

1 1/2 teaspoons grapeseed oil
2 carrots, sliced on the diagonal and then halved
3 cups broccoli florets, stems no more than 2 inches long
1 cup red onion, sliced in 1/8-inch thick half-moons
1/2 teaspoon dried basil
4 cups cooked short grain brown rice
1 teaspoon soy sauce
sea salt, to taste

Heat oil in a wok on medium. Sauté carrots, broccoli and red onion for 5 minutes. If the wok gets too dry, reduce heat or add a splash of water.

Add 1/2 cup water, cover and cook another 3 minutes on medium heat. Add basil and brown rice. Stir to incorporate. Cook away liquid. Stir in soy sauce. (If rice mixture is too dry, add 1-2 tablespoons of water.) Cook 1 minute longer. Season to taste.

[serves 6]

Nutrition Per Serving: Calories 188, Total Fat 2g, Saturated Fat trace, Cholesterol 0mg, Sodium 76mg, Potassium 301mg, Total Carbohydrate 37g, Dietary Fiber 5g, Protein 5g, Calcium 45mg, Iron 1mg, Zinc 1mg, Vitamin C 38mg, Vitamin A 7863 IU, Vitamin B6 .3mg, Thiamin B1 .2mg, Riboflavin B2 .1mg, Folacin 40mcg, Niacin 2mg

Mexican Rice

2 cups short grain brown rice
1 1/2 teaspoons extra virgin olive oil
2 cloves garlic, minced
1 medium onion, chopped
2 tomatoes, peeled, seeded and chopped (optional)

1 teaspoon fresh chili pepper, minced (optional)
1/4 teaspoon ground cumin
4 cups water
1/4 teaspoon sea salt
3 tablespoons fresh coriander leaves, chopped

Soak rice for 1 hour. Drain.

Heat oil in a medium-size heavy pot. Add garlic and onion, and sauté 2-3 minutes. Add tomato, chili pepper, cumin, rice, water and salt. Cover pot. Bring to a boil, reduce to low and place a flame deflector under the pot. Cook for 1 hour. Remove from heat and let sit, covered, for 15 minutes. Mix in fresh coriander leaves and serve.

[serves 8]

Nutrition Per Serving: Calories 194, Total Fat 2g, Saturated Fat trace, Cholesterol 0mg, Sodium 69mg, Potassium 253mg, Total Carbohydrate 39g, Dietary Fiber 1g, Protein 4g, Calcium 33mg, Iron 1mg, Zinc 1mg, Vitamin C 12mg, Vitamin A 235 IU, Vitamin B6 .3mg, Thiamin B1 .2mg, Folacin 19mcg, Niacin 2mg

Herbed Basmati Rice

1 teaspoon extra virgin olive oil
1 cup brown basmati rice
1/4 teaspoon sea salt
bouquet garni (6 sprigs parsley, 6 basil leaves, 1 sprig rosemary, 1 sprig thyme and 1 bay leaf, tied together with string)
1 1/2 cups water or Basic Vegetable Stock (page 94)

In a medium heavy saucepan, combine oil and rice, and toss to coat. Cook over low heat, stirring occasionally until there is a light toasted aroma, about 2-3 minutes. Add salt, bouquet garni and water. Stir and bring to a boil over high heat. Cover and simmer on low for 20-25 minutes. Remove from heat and let sit, covered, for 10 minutes. Discard bouquet garni.

[4 servings]

Nutrition Per Serving: Calories 182, Total Fat 2g, Saturated Fat trace, Cholesterol 0mg, Sodium 122mg, Potassium 133mg, Total Carbohydrate 36g, Dietary Fiber 1g, Protein 4g, Calcium 19mg, Iron 1mg, Zinc 1mg, Vitamin C 1mg, Vitamin A 52 IU, Vitamin B6 .2mg, Thiamin B1 .2mg, Folacin 11mcg, Niacin 2mg

Brown Rice with Kale

The Diet Doctor's Wife: This recipe is not only very tasty, but also incredibly nutritious. A great dish to take to a potluck dinner.

1 1/2 cups brown basmati rice
1 1/2 pounds fresh kale or collards, stems removed
1 1/2 teaspoons grapeseed oil
1 medium onion, chopped
3/4 teaspoon ground cumin
3/4 teaspoon ground coriander
1/4 teaspoon mace or nutmeg
1/2 teaspoon sea salt

Soak rice in 3 cups water for 1 hour.

Blanch kale in boiling water for 2 minutes. Drain and allow to cool. Chop kale leaves.

In a large heavy saucepan, heat oil on medium low. Add onion and sauté until translucent. Add kale and sauté for 1 minute. Reduce heat to low and cook for another 15 minutes. Add rice, soaking liquid and spices. Bring to a boil over medium heat. Cover and reduce heat to low and cook for 1 hour. Remove from heat and leave covered for 15 minutes.

[serves 6-8]

Nutrition Per Serving: Calories 248, Total Fat 3g, Saturated Fat trace, Cholesterol 0mg, Sodium 208mg, Potassium 671mg, Total Carbohydrate 49g, Dietary Fiber 3g, Protein 8g, Calcium 177mg, Iron 3mg, Zinc 2mg, Vitamin C 137mg, Vitamin A 10105 IU, Vitamin B6 .6mg, Thiamin B1 .3mg, Riboflavin B2 .2mg, Folacin 46mcg, Niacin 3mg

Risotto with Mushrooms

.35 ounces dried porcini mushrooms
8 ounces fresh mixed mushrooms, sliced
1/4 cup dry sherry or red wine
2-3 cups Basic Vegetable Stock (page 94)
2 teaspoons extra virgin olive oil
1/4 cup onion, finely chopped
2 cloves garlic, minced
1 sprig fresh thyme
sea salt, to taste
1 cup Arborio rice

Soak dried mushrooms in 1 cup of hot water and allow to sit for 30 minutes. Remove mushrooms with a slotted spoon and squeeze out extra liquid. Finely chop the reconstituted mushrooms and set aside.

Strain soaking liquid through a fine meshed strainer lined with cheesecloth. Reserve strained liquid.

While the dried mushrooms are soaking, marinate fresh mushrooms in sherry for 30 minutes. Strain fresh mushrooms and reserve sherry.

Heat stock to a gentle simmer. Add reserved mushroom soaking liquid to the simmering stock.

In a heavy sauté pan, heat oil over medium heat. Add onions, garlic, the sprig of thyme and a pinch of salt. Cook until onions become translucent. Add fresh mushrooms and cook until softened, about 5 minutes. If mushrooms begin to stick, reduce heat to medium low. If sticking continues, add a splash of water. Stir in the rice and coat with mushroom mixture. Cook about 1 minute. Add the strained off sherry and sauté until liquid evaporates. Stir in the reconstituted mushrooms. Add 1/2 cup of simmering stock and stir until liquid is absorbed. Continue adding stock, 1/2 cup at a time, stirring constantly until liquid is absorbed before adding the next 1/2 cup. This process should take between 20 and 25 minutes. Cook until the rice is al dente. Season to taste.

[serves 4]

Nutrition Per Serving: Calories 241, Total Fat 3g, Saturated Fat trace, Cholesterol 0mg, Sodium 55mg, Potassium 275mg, Total Carbohydrate 45g, Dietary Fiber 1g, Protein 5g, Calcium 11mg, Iron 1mg, Zinc 1mg, Vitamin C 4mg, Vitamin A 29 IU, Vitamin B6 .1mg, Riboflavin B2 .3mg, Folacin 18mcg, Niacin 3mg

Fish Porridge

The Diet Doctor's Wife: When I was living in Singapore, my friend and colleague, Mark Stevens, used to rave about fish congee. Fish congee is a rice porridge flecked with thin pieces of steamed fish. The idea of fish porridge didn't really appeal to me, but Mark was so enthusiastic that I agreed to try it. So one morning we met for an early breakfast at a restaurant known to have the best fish congee in town. It was quite a trek but well worth it. I found the congee simple and satisfying, and a welcomed change from the heavy-handed hot and spicy seasoning that Singaporean cuisine is known for. My version is made with brown rice, which adds heartiness and fiber.

1/2 cup sweet brown rice
1/2 teaspoon sea salt
4 cups water
4 cups Basic Vegetable Stock (page 94)
1/4 pound white-fleshed fish fillet, skin removed
1 tablespoon slivered ginger root
2 teaspoons soy sauce
pinch of white pepper
1/4 teaspoon toasted sesame oil
1 tablespoon scallion, chopped
2 tablespoons fresh coriander leaves, chopped

Condiments

fresh hot chili peppers, chopped
soy sauce

Put washed rice in a pressure cooker with sea salt. Add water and broth. Bring to a boil, secure lid and pressure cook on low for 1 hour.

Meanwhile, wrap fish in plastic wrap and freeze for 1 hour. Remove from the freezer. With a sharp knife, slice fish very thinly. Combine ginger, soy, white pepper, and oil. Pour over fish. Sprinkle scallion and fresh coriander on top.

Ladle piping hot porridge into 6 serving bowls. Divide fish mixture among the bowls and stir into the porridge. The fish steams instantly. Serve with condiments, if desired. (Place a pinch of chopped chili pepper in each of 6 condiment-size bowls. Add some soy sauce. Add soy-soaked chili pepper to the porridge, according to taste.)

[serves 6]

Nutrition Per Serving: Calories 79, Total Fat 1g, Saturated Fat trace, Cholesterol 8mg, Sodium 286mg, Potassium 159mg, Total Carbohydrate 13g, Protein 5g, Calcium 20mg, Iron 1mg, Vitamin C 4mg, Vitamin A 47 IU, Vitamin B6 .1mg, Vitamin B12 .2mcg, Thiamin B1 .1mg, Folacin 7mcg, Niacin 1mg

Tabouleh

The Diet Doctor's Wife: The first time I had Tabouleh was at my cousin Michele's. It was my 18th birthday, which fell on Canadian Thanksgiving and the beginning of the Kitchener Oktoberfest. Michele, who was living in Kitchener at the time, invited my parents and me to spend the weekend at her home for a family celebration. It was a magical time. The fall color was at its peak, the air was crisp and clean, and most important, I was with the people I loved most. We toasted my coming of age with champagne accompanied by a fabulous German Black Forest cake from the renowned Café Mozart. And somewhere in between, we feasted on delightful hors d'oeuvres. The one that stood out most for me was the Tabouleh, which Michele served with potato chips – an inspired combination, although lower fat accompaniments are just as tasty.

1/2 cup bulgur wheat
1/4 teaspoon sea salt
freshly ground black pepper, to taste

1 1/2 tablespoons freshly squeezed lemon juice, plus more to taste
1 1/2 tablespoons extra virgin olive oil
3/4 cup fresh flat-leafed parsley leaves, chopped
1/4 cup fresh mint leaves, chopped
3 scallions, chopped
3 tomatoes, seeded and diced

Soak the bulgur wheat in cold water for 10 minutes. Drain through a cheesecloth-lined mesh strainer. Squeeze out excess water. Put bulgur in a bowl and add salt, pepper, lemon juice and olive oil. Let stand for 1/2 hour. Add parsley, mint, scallions and tomatoes. Stir to integrate. Sprinkle with extra lemon juice, if desired.

[serves 4]

Nutrition Per Serving: Calories 136, Total Fat 6g, Saturated Fat 1g, Cholesterol 0mg, Sodium 139mg, Potassium 403mg, Total Carbohydrate 20g, Dietary Fiber 5g, Protein 4g, Calcium 46mg, Iron 2mg, Zinc 1mg, Vitamin C 38mg, Vitamin A 1434 IU, Vitamin B6 .1mg, Thiamin B1 .1mg, Riboflavin B2 .1mg, Folacin 50mcg, Niacin 2mg

Bulgur, Chickpea and Tomato Pilaf

The Diet Doctor's Wife: There is a company in Toledo, Ohio that packages this pilaf for the prepared food sections of our local food markets. I just love it, especially on days when I don't feel like cooking. Of course I had to create my own version and make a few minor adjustments. Mine is considerably less fatty with more subtle seasoning.

2 teaspoons extra virgin olive oil
1 onion, chopped
1/2 green pepper, chopped (optional)
1 1/2 cups fresh tomatoes, peeled, seeded and chopped
1 cup cooked chickpeas
1/2 teaspoon ground allspice
1/4 cup fresh parsley, chopped
1 cup bulgur

1 cup water
3/4 teaspoon sea salt
freshly ground black pepper, to taste

Heat oil in a heavy saucepan on medium. Add onion and pepper, and sauté for 2 minutes. Add the tomatoes and cook for 2 minutes longer. Add the chickpeas, allspice and parsley. Cook another 2 minutes. Add bulgur, water and salt. Cover and bring to a boil. Reduce heat to low to gently simmer for 30 minutes. Remove from the heat. Remove the lid and cover the saucepan with a dishtowel. Cover the dishtowel with the lid. Let the bulgur mixture sit for 20 minutes. Add freshly ground black pepper to taste and stir to combine.

[serves 6]

Nutrition Per Serving: Calories 156, Total Fat 3g, Saturated Fat trace, Cholesterol 0mg, Sodium 248mg, Potassium 320mg, Total Carbohydrate 29g, Dietary Fiber 6g, Protein 6g, Calcium 33mg, Iron 2mg, Zinc 1mg, Vitamin C 14mg, Vitamin A 420 IU, Vitamin B6 .2mg, Thiamin B1 .1mg, Riboflavin .1mg, Folacin 67 mcg, Niacin 2mg

Boiled Barley

1 cup barley, soaked in water for 4-8 hours
2 cups water or Basic Vegetable Stock (page 94)
1/4 teaspoon sea salt

Drain barley. Place drained barley in a pot with 2 cups water and 1/4 teaspoon sea salt. Cover, bring to a boil and then reduce heat to low. Place a flame deflector under the pot and simmer for 1 1/4 hours. The barley will have a soft texture, each grain still retaining its shape. For a firmer texture, soak the barley for less time or not at all.

[serves 4]

Nutrition Per Serving: Calories 163, Total Fat 1g, Saturated Fat trace, Cholesterol 0mg, Sodium 127mg, Potassium 208mg, Total Carbohydrate 34g, Dietary Fiber 7g, Protein 6g, Calcium 18mg, Iron 2mg, Zinc 1mg, Vitamin A 10 IU, Vitamin B6 .1mg, Thiamin B1 .3mg, Riboflavin B2 .1mg, Folacin 9mcg, Niacin 2mg

Northern Grains

1 cup brown rice, soaked 1-8 hours
1/2 cup barley, soaked 4-8 hours
1/2 cup buckwheat groats
1/2 teaspoon caraway seeds
1/2 teaspoon sea salt
3 cups water

Drain rice and barley. Place all ingredients in a pressure cooker. Secure lid and bring up to pressure over medium heat. Reduce heat to medium low and slip a flame deflector under the cooker. Cook for 45 minutes. Remove from the heat and allow pressure to release naturally. Allow grains to rest for 5 minutes before serving.

[serves 8]

Nutrition Per Serving: Calories 166, Total Fat 1g, Saturated Fat trace, Cholesterol 0mg, Sodium 123mg, Potassium 133mg, Total Carbohydrate 36g, Dietary Fiber 3g, Protein 4g, Calcium 16mg, Iron 1mg, Zinc 1mg, Vitamin A 3 IU, Vitamin B6 .2mg, Thiamin B1 .1mg, Riboflavin B2 .1mg, Folacin 12mcg, Niacin 2mg

Japanese Style Mixed Grains

The Diet Doctor's Wife: This is an easy, satisfying dish that is great to make in large quantities. On it's own or added to a stir-fry, it is nutritious and delicious.

1/3 cup barley, soaked 4-8 hours
1/3 cup adzuki beans, soaked 6-8 hours
1 cup short grain brown rice
1/3 cup millet
1/2 teaspoon sea salt
3 cups water

Drain soaked barley and adzuki beans. The soaking water can be used as part of the cooking water. Put all ingredients in a pressure cooker. Secure lid and bring up to pressure over medium heat. Reduce heat to medium low. Put a flame deflector under the cooker and cook for 45 minutes. Remove from heat and allow pressure to come down naturally. Remove lid and let rice mixture sit for 5 minutes before serving.

Serve with Sesame Salt (page 327), chopped scallions, chopped pickle, etc.

[serves 8]

Nutrition Per Serving: Calories 172, Total Fat 1g, Saturated Fat trace, Cholesterol 0mg, Sodium 120mg, Potassium 217mg, Total Carbohydrate 35g, Dietary Fiber 3g, Protein 5g, Calcium 16mg, Iron 1mg, Zinc 1mg, Vitamin A 3 IU, Vitamin B6 .2mg, Thiamin B1 .2mg, Riboflavin B2 .1mg, Folacin 64mcg, Niacin 2mg

Cabbage Stuffed with Mixed Grains

Mixed Grains

1/2 cup long grain brown rice, soaked 1 hour
1/4 cup wild rice, soaked 1 hour
1/4 cup buckwheat groats
1/3 cup onion, chopped
1/3 cup burdock root, peeled and diced
1/3 cup carrot, peeled and diced
1/3 cup celery, diced or celery root, peeled and diced
1 bay leaf
1 tablespoon caraway seeds
1/2 teaspoon dill seed
2 cups water
1/4 teaspoon sea salt

Drain soaked grains. Place all ingredients in a pressure cooker and secure lid. Over medium heat, bring up to pressure. Reduce heat to medium low and place a flame deflector under the cooker. Cook for 45-50 minutes. Remove from the heat.

Tomato Sauce

2 teaspoons grapeseed oil
1/4 cup onion, finely chopped
28-ounce can peeled and seeded Italian tomatoes
1 bay leaf
1/2 teaspoon dried thyme or marjoram
sea salt and freshly ground black pepper, to taste

Preheat oven to 350 F.

While the mixed grains are cooking, prepare the tomato sauce. In a large saucepan, heat oil and sauté onion until translucent. Add tomatoes, bay leaf and thyme. Break up tomatoes with the back of a wooden spoon. Bring to a boil and then reduce heat to a gentle simmer. Cook for 30 minutes. Season to taste and set aside.

12 large cabbage leaves, coarse veins removed
1 cup seitan, chopped
1/2 cup mixed fresh herbs (chives, parsley, dill), finely chopped
chopped fresh parsley, for garnish

Blanch cabbage leaves in boiling water until tender. Drain leaves and stack them.

To prepare the filling, place the cooked mixed grains in a large bowl. Add seitan and chopped herbs. Mix to incorporate. Season to taste.

Place 1/4 cup of rice-seitan mixture in the middle of a cabbage leaf. Fold into a cabbage roll and place roll in a baking dish. Repeat process until all cabbage leaves are filled. Cabbage rolls should be arranged in a single layer without any overlap.

Pour tomato sauce over cabbage rolls and bake for 30-40 minutes. Garnish with chopped parsley.

[serves 6]

Nutrition Per Serving: Calories 215, Total Fat 3g, Saturated Fat trace, Cholesterol 0mg, Sodium 293mg, Potassium 646mg, Total Carbohydrate 39g, Dietary Fiber 8g, Protein 11g, Calcium 131mg, Iron 3mg, Zinc 1mg, Vitamin C 40mg, Vitamin A 3096 IU, Vitamin B6 .3mg, Thiamin B1 .2mg, Riboflavin B2 .1mg, Folacin 54mcg, Niacin 3mg

Baked Millet Samosas

The Diet Doctor's Wife: In Singapore, samosas are often served with afternoon tea. They are a truly wonderful treat, yet in my experience, an unfortunate cause of tummy trouble. The traditional deep-fried dough with its rich potato filling is a lethal combination for me. I have created a much lower fat version that is equally delicious. My samosas are baked, not fried, and stuffed with a spiced millet mixture.

1 cup whole wheat flour
1 cup chickpea flour or white unbleached flour
3 1/2 tablespoons grapeseed oil
1/4 teaspoon sea salt
1/2 cup water
1/2 head cauliflower, cut in florets, steamed or boiled
1 medium turnip, cut in 1/2-inch cubes, steamed or boiled
*1 cup cooked millet
1 onion, minced
1 cup shelled peas
1 tablespoon fresh ginger root, grated
1 small fresh hot green chili pepper, finely chopped
3 tablespoons fresh coriander leaves, finely chopped
1 teaspoon sea salt
1/2 teaspoon ground coriander
1/2 teaspoon Couscous Seasoning (page 334) or garam masala
1/2 teaspoon ground cumin
pinch of ground cayenne pepper

2 tablespoons freshly squeezed lemon juice
grapeseed oil, for brushing dough
chutney (optional)

Preheat oven to 350 F.

To make dough, put flours, 3 tablespoons oil and sea salt in a food processor. Pulse until mixture is crumbly. Add water gradually until dough forms. Add a bit more water if the dough doesn't come together. Form dough into a ball and then cover in plastic wrap. Refrigerate.

To make stuffing, mash together cooked cauliflower, turnip and millet. Set aside. In a wok, heat the rest of the oil and sauté onions until golden brown. Add peas, ginger, chili pepper, fresh coriander and 1/4 cup water. Cover, lower heat and simmer until peas are cooked (about 5 minutes). Add water, if necessary. Add millet mixture, salt, spices and lemon juice. Stir to integrate and continue cooking over gentle heat for 3 minutes.

Remove dough from the refrigerator. Divide into 12 equal pieces and form into balls. Keep balls covered with a damp towel or plastic wrap. Lightly flour work surface. Roll out one of the dough balls into a 6-inch round. Place 2-3 tablespoons of stuffing in the center of the round. Join the edges of the dough to form a half circle. Flute the edges.

Brush samosas lightly with oil. Place samosas on a baking sheet lined with parchment paper. Bake for 30 minutes.

Samosas are generally served with chutney.

[serves 12]

Nutrition Per Serving: Calories 142, Total Fat 5g, Saturated Fat 1g, Cholesterol 0mg, Sodium 224mg, Potassium 204mg, Total Carbohydrate 20g, Dietary Fiber 4g, Protein 5g, Calcium 19mg, Iron 1mg, Zinc 1mg, Vitamin C 17mg, Vitamin A 132 IU, Vitamin B6 .1mg, Thiamin B1 .1mg, Riboflavin B2 .1mg, Folacin 53mcg, Niacin 1mg

*Note: To cook millet, bring 3 cups of water to a boil. Add a pinch of salt and 1 cup of millet. Simmer , covered, for 30 minutes. Yields 3-3 1/2 cups cooked millet.

Polenta with Herbs

The Diet Doctor's Wife: I hardly ever make polenta since Bill is allergic to corn. But when the mood strikes, I cook up a pot just for myself. The miso adds a lactose-free, cheesy flavor that should not be missed.

4 1/2 cups water
1/2 teaspoon sea salt
1 cup Italian cornmeal
1 tablespoon yellow miso
2 tablespoons fresh herbs (rosemary, parsley, thyme, etc.), chopped

Combine water and salt in a saucepan. Bring to a boil and then reduce heat to simmer. Slowly add cornmeal, continually stirring with a wooden spoon until completely blended. Reduce heat to low and cook for 30 minutes, stirring occasionally. The polenta is cooked when it falls away from the sides of the pan. Blend miso with 1/3 cup of polenta. Add miso mixture to the pot. Add chopped herbs and stir to incorporate. Check for seasoning. The polenta can now be served hot as porridge.

If polenta cakes are desired, do the following: Pour polenta porridge on a flat surface and spread out to form a cake about 3/4-inch thick. Let stand for 1 hour. Then cut polenta into strips or triangles and bake on a lightly greased baking sheet for 10 minutes per side at 375 F. Alternatively, lightly brush the polenta pieces with extra virgin olive oil and grill 3 minutes each side, until crisp and brown.

[serves 4]

Nutrition Per Serving: Calories 141, Total Fat 1g, Saturated Fat trace, Cholesterol 0mg, Sodium 399mg, Potassium 79mg, Total Carbohydrate 29g, Dietary Fiber 3g, Protein 4g, Calcium 29mg, Iron 2mg, Vitamin C 1mg, Vitamin A 198 IU, Vitamin B6 .1mg, Thiamin B1 .3mg, Riboflavin .2mg, Folacin 18mcg, Niacin 2mg

Bill's Oatmeal with Raisins

The Diet Doctor's Wife: Bill makes oatmeal on the weekends. The addition of raisins at the end of cooking is his simple secret.

1 cup rolled oats
4 cups water
pinch of sea salt
1/4 cup raisins

Bring water to a boil. Add oats and a pinch of salt and stir until oats start to thicken. Turn heat down and simmer for 1/2 hour, stirring occasionally. Stir in raisins and remove from the heat.

[serves 4]

Nutrition Per Serving: Calories 105, Total Fat 1g, Saturated Fat trace, Cholesterol 0mg, Sodium 9mg, Potassium 139mg, Total Carbohydrate 21g, Dietary Fiber 3g, Protein 4g, Calcium 20mg, Iron 1mg, Zinc 1mg, Vitamin A 21 IU, Thiamin B1 .2mg, Folacin 7mcg

Crockpot Oatmeal

The Diet Doctor: This is the perfect way to wake up to a healthy breakfast, particularly if you are not a morning person. Rice porridge can be made exactly the same way.

1 cup steel cut oats
4 cups water
pinch of sea salt

Place all ingredients in a crockpot and cook overnight.

[serves 4]

Nutrition Per Serving: Calories 150, Total Fat 2g, Saturated Fat trace, Cholesterol 0mg, Sodium 127mg, Total Carbohydrate 26g, Dietary Fiber 4g, Protein 4g, Calcium 20mg, Iron 1mg

Mochi Waffles

The Diet Doctor's Wife: Mochi waffles are quick and easy to make, and completely fat free. There is no batter to prepare, and no mess to clean up. All you have to do is cut the mochi, and place it in a waffle iron.

12-ounce package brown rice mochi

Cut mochi into 4 equal pieces (3 1/2" x 2 1/2" rectangles). Then half the thickness of each piece by making a cross-section cut.

Place a piece of mochi in each section of a dry waffle iron (preferable nonstick). Cook until puffed up and slightly crispy, about 4 minutes. Repeat until all mochi are cooked.

Place each mochi waffle on a plate. Eat just plain or top with Apple Sauce I (page 300), Apple Sauce II (page 301), Apple Pudding (page 302), Winter Fruit Compote (page 310), fresh fruit or maple syrup.

[serves 8]

Nutrition Per Serving: Calories 110, Total Fat 1g, Saturated Fat 0g, Cholesterol 0mg, Sodium 0mg, Total Carbohydrate 24g, Dietary Fiber 2g, Protein 2g, Iron 1mg

Pasta

PASTA

Bill and I love to eat pasta and noodles. We prefer to make our own when we have the time, but also enjoy store-bought varieties. In general, we recommend any European or Asian style pasta that does not contain eggs.

European style pasta comes in many shapes and sizes, and is most commonly made from durum wheat or semolina flour and water. Varieties flavored with spinach, tomato, garlic and herbs are available in gourmet shops and specialty food stores. Pasta made from whole grain flours (whole wheat, rye, kamut, spelt) can be found in most health food stores.

Asian style noodles also come in a variety of shapes, sizes and flavors. Our favorite is the flat Japanese soba noodle, which is available in most health food and Asian markets. Soba noodles are made from buckwheat flour, salt and water. Sometimes other ingredients are added to the buckwheat flour such as powdered green tea, mugwort and wild mountain potato flour. Other tasty Japanese noodles are somen and udon. Somen are very thin, delicate noodles made from whole wheat or high gluten white flour, salt and water. They are served cold or warmed in broth. Udon are thicker noodles made from various combinations of whole wheat flour, white flour, salt and water. Udon are wonderful in broths, soups and casseroles. Asian vermicelli are very thin noodles usually made from rice or mung bean flour, salt and water. They are also referred to as saifun, bean threads or glass noodles. Rice sticks or baifun are made from rice flour, wild potato starch, salt and water. Both Asian vermicelli and rice sticks are available in most grocery stores in the Asian food section. Ramen is a deep-fried dried noodle that comes in the instant miso or Asian soup packets found in most health food stores (the ramen found in most grocery stores is often deep-fried in animal fat). Banh Trang is a type of Vietnamese pasta made from wheat flour and water. Banh Trang is used to make fresh spring rolls and is available in most Asian markets.

Couscous is a type of pasta used in Mediterranean and North African cooking. It is very small-grained and made from semolina flour. Whole wheat varieties are available in most health food stores.

HOW TO COOK PASTA

To cook European style dried pasta, add water to a large pot until it is two-thirds full. Add 1 tablespoon of sea salt per pound of pasta to be cooked. (For sodium reduced diets, use less salt. Refer to page 52.) Bring to a rolling boil and add pasta. For small pasta, such as fusilli or macaroni, stir to prevent sticking. For longer spaghetti or linguini, use a wooden spoon to gently spread out and push down the noodles until they are totally immersed in the cooking water. To test for doneness, pasta should be slightly firm and the same color all the way through. Use the directions on the package as a guide to determine cooking time. Drain the pasta as soon as it has finished cooking.

Homemade pasta needs very little cooking time, anywhere from 30 seconds to 3 minutes. Cooking time depends on the thickness of the noodle.

To cook Japanese soba, udon or somen noodles, follow the directions on the package. Do not add salt to the cooking water. To cook baifun or ramen, follow the instructions on the package.

Asian vermicelli are not cooked, but rather soaked in boiling water for approximately 20 minutes and then drained. Banh Trang are paper-like rounds used as the outer wrapping for fresh spring rolls. Banh Trang do not need to be cooked. They simply need to be dipped in water for 30-60 seconds until they are completely reconstituted. Couscous needs to be soaked in water and then steamed.

Homemade Pasta

The Diet Doctor: Gabrielle and I really get into making our own pasta. It is a true team effort that takes up an entire evening. I am responsible for the first step, which is making the dough. After it has had a chance to sit for at least a half hour, Gabrielle enters the scene. She takes a piece of the dough and cranks it through one side of our pasta machine as I catch it on the other side. This process continues for a while until the dough is ready to be cut into noodles. With the flip of a switch, the flat strips of dough turn into linguini, fettuccini or spaghetti. At this point, the freshly cut noodles must be transferred to a drying rack. The trick is not to let the noodles overlap. It's a messy process, but great fun. And the flavor is sensational. Once you've tried homemade pasta, you'll never be satisfied with the packaged varieties.

3 cups semolina or any other flour
1 cup sparkling mineral water

Combine ingredients until a dough is formed. Knead 10 minutes, sprinkling with flour when needed. Allow the dough to rest in a covered bowl for about one half hour or refrigerate overnight.

Cut the dough in half. Flatten one half into a rectangle and keep the other half covered with a damp towel.

Follow the directions in your pasta machine manual. If you are using an Atlas machine, do the following: Take the flattened dough and pass it through your pasta machine on the thickest setting, 1. Dust the dough with flour and fold it into thirds. Pass the folded dough through the machine at the same setting, dusting with flour afterwards. Repeat this process twice more until the dough has the texture of an ear lobe. Dust the dough with flour but this time, do not fold it.

Change the setting to the next level, 2, and pass dough through the machine. Dust dough with flour. Adjust the setting to 3 and pass dough through the machine. Dust with flour. Continue this process until you have passed the dough through setting 5 or 6, depending on desired thickness.

Then choose the type of pasta shape you want and adjust to the appropriate setting. Pass the dough through the machine and allow the pasta to dry on a drying rack or lay pasta flat on a clean dishtowel.

Repeat entire procedure with the second half of the dough.

For best flavor, make the noodles and cook them within an hour. If you prefer to store the noodles, form them into nests and allow them to dry completely. Then place the nests in an airtight container.

[1 pound pasta, 6 servings]

Nutrition Per Serving: Calories 301, Total Fat 1g, Saturated Fat trace, Cholesterol 0mg, Sodium 1mg, Potassium 155mg, Total Carbohydrate 61g, Dietary Fiber 3g, Protein 11g, Calcium 15mg, Iron 4mg, Zinc 1mg, Vitamin B6 .1mg, Thiamin B1 .7mg, Riboflavin B2 .5mg, Folacin 129mcg, Niacin 5mg

Linguini with Tuna

The Diet Doctor: I call this a pantry dish since it's made with ingredients that you always have around the house. The fridge can be empty and the grocery store closed, and you can still pull it off. Plus, the preparation is a snap, which is why this is one of my specialties.

2 tablespoons extra virgin olive oil
2 cloves garlic
1/4 teaspoon red pepper flakes
1/4 cup fresh parsley leaves, chopped
sea salt and freshly ground black pepper, to taste
7 ounces canned water-packed tuna, drained and flaked
12 ounces linguini

Warm oil on medium low in a medium saucepan. Add garlic, red pepper flakes and parsley. Sauté for 1 minute. Add tuna and continue to cook for 10 minutes. Taste for seasoning. Add salt if necessary and plenty of freshly ground black pepper.

Meanwhile cook the pasta until al dente. Drain pasta, reserving a bit of the cooking liquid. Immediately add the pasta to the tuna mixture. Stir to coat the pasta and cook for a minute or two. If the pasta is too dry, add a splash of the pasta cooking liquid and continue to cook for another minute or two.

[serves 4]

Nutrition Per Serving: Calories 436, Total Fat 9g, Saturated Fat 1g, Cholesterol 15mg, Sodium 176mg, Potassium 282mg, Total Carbohydrate 64g, Dietary Fiber 2g, Protein 24g, Calcium 29mg, Iron 4mg, Zinc 1mg, Vitamin C 6mg, Vitamin A 229 IU, Vitamin B6 .3mg, Vitamin B12 1.5mcg, Thiamin B1 .9mg, Riboflavin B2 .4mg, Folacin 23mcg, Niacin 13mg

Fresh Spring Rolls

The Diet Doctor's Wife: I have never been a lover of the deep fried spring rolls or egg rolls served in Asian restaurants. But fresh spring rolls are a totally different story. The first time I tasted one was at a delightful Thai restaurant in Toronto. I was wowed by the aromatic hit of mint and coriander and the explosive fresh flavors. Unfortunately my memories of this exciting first are mixed. My dinner companion was a man I had dated two or three times. I clearly was not interested and was having a hard time letting him know. But in spite of the uneasiness I felt, I can't help but be grateful to him for expanding my culinary horizons.

Dipping Sauce

2 teaspoons grapeseed oil or light vegetable oil
4 cloves garlic, minced
1/3 cup hoisin sauce
1 tablespoon Thai fish sauce (optional)
1 tablespoon maple syrup or 2 tablespoons rice syrup
1/4 teaspoon hot pepper paste or a pinch of ground cayenne pepper
1/2 cup Basic Vegetable Stock (page 94)
1/4 cup unsalted, dry-roasted peanuts, chopped

To make the dipping sauce, heat oil in a small saucepan. Add garlic and cook for about 30 seconds. Add hoisin, Thai fish sauce, maple syrup and chili paste, and stir together.

Whisk in stock and cook for about 30 seconds. Add peanuts and allow to cool.

Filling

1/4 pound dried bean thread noodles
2 teaspoons Thai fish sauce
1/4 teaspoon maple syrup
pinch of freshly ground white pepper
12 cooked medium-size shrimp
1/2 cup carrot, finely julienned
1/2 cup jicama, finely julienned
1/2 cup cucumber, finely julienned
1/2 teaspoon maple syrup
12 dried Banh Trang
12 bibb lettuce leaves, coarse rib removed
12 mint leaves
12 coriander leaves

Place dried noodles in a large bowl. Pour boiling water over the noodles and soak for 20 minutes. Drain. Add noodles to a pot of boiling water and cook for 1 minute until noodles are clear. Pour into a colander and rinse under cold running water. Drain well and coarsely chop. Set aside.

In a small bowl, toss shrimp with Thai fish sauce, white pepper and 1/4 teaspoon maple syrup. Set aside to marinate for at least 1/2 hour.

Combine carrot, jicama, and cucumber in another small bowl. Toss with 1/2 teaspoon maple syrup.

To make the spring rolls, place 1 banh trang in a shallow dish of water. Allow to soak for 30 seconds until softened. Gently pat dry with a clean dish towel. Lay on a flat surface and place 1 lettuce leaf on the lower third of the round. Put a bit of the vegetable mixture in the center of the lettuce leaf. Top with 2 tablespoons of the chopped noodles and a mint leaf.

Fold the lower edge of the banh trang over the filling, half covering it to begin the log. Fold in the sides to close both ends. Place 1 piece of shrimp and 1 coriander leaf across the top of the log and continue rolling to close. Moisten the ends with water to seal the seam. Cover with a damp kitchen towel until you are ready to serve.

Serve with the dipping sauce.

[serves 12]

Nutrition Per Serving: Calories 118, Total Fat 3g, Saturated Fat trace, Cholesterol 19mg, Sodium 375mg, Potassium 206mg, Total Carbohydrate 18g, Dietary Fiber 2g, Protein 5g, Calcium 46mg, Iron 2mg, Vitamin C 12mg, Vitamin A 1758 IU, Vitamin B6 .1mg, Vitamin B12 .1mcg, Thiamin B1 .1mg, Folacin 21mcg, Niacin 1mg

Coucous in a Pinch

The Diet Doctor's Wife: You can cook couscous in the microwave. Of course, if you have the time, couscous tastes best prepared in a couscoussier.

1 cup whole wheat couscous
1/4 teaspoon sea salt
1 tablespoon extra virgin olive oil
1 1/2 cups water

Combine couscous and salt in a shallow bowl. Add olive oil and mix through. Fluff couscous with a fork. Add water and let sit for 15 minutes, fluffing with a fork every 5 minutes or so. Cover dish in plastic wrap and microwave on high for 2 minutes. Serve immediately.

[serves 6]

Nutrition Per Serving: Calories 120, Total Fat 3g, Saturated Fat trace, Cholesterol 0mg, Sodium 98mg, Total Carbohydrate 30g, Dietary Fiber 42g, Protein 4g, Calcium 2mg, Iron 1mg

Steamed Couscous the Traditional Way

1 cup whole wheat couscous
1/4 teaspoon sea salt
1 cup water
1 teaspoon extra virgin olive oil

Pour couscous in a large shallow dish. Add salt and water. Leave to soak for 1 hour, stirring occasionally.

One hour and 15 minutes before serving, put couscous in the upper part of the couscoussier. Fit over simmering stew, tagine (see page 169) or water, covered, and steam for 15 minutes. Make sure the seal between the upper and lower parts of the couscoussier is tight. If not, create a seal by fitting a damp rag that has been soaked in a mixture of flour and water between the upper and lower sections of the couscoussier.

Tip couscous into a large shallow dish and fluff grains with a fork and allow to rest. When cool enough to handle, add 1/4 cup water and mix the couscous with your hands. Leave to rest 15 minutes.

Put couscous back in the steamer insert of the couscoussier, cover and steam for another 15 minutes.

Once again, tip couscous into a large shallow dish and fluff grains with a fork and allow to rest. When cool enough to handle, add 1/4 cup water and mix the couscous with your hands. Leave to rest 15 minutes.

Return couscous to the couscoussier, cover and steam for 10 minutes. Tip couscous into a large shallow dish and fluff grains with a fork and allow to rest. When cool enough to handle, add 1/4 cup water and mix the couscous with your hands. Leave to rest 15 minutes. Drizzle a teaspoon of olive oil over the couscous. Fluff with a fork to coat.

[serves 6]

Nutrition Per Serving: Calories 107, Total Fat 1g, Saturated Fat trace, Cholesterol 0mg, Sodium 87mg, Total Carbohydrate 30g, Dietary Fiber 42g, Protein 4g, Calcium 1mg, Iron 1mg

Moroccan Root Vegetable Tagine

Tagine

2 teaspoons extra virgin olive oil, Clarified Butter (page 346) or combination
1 1/2 teaspoons Couscous Seasoning (page 334)
1 large onion, chopped
6 large carrots, cut in large chunks
3 parsnips, cut in large chunks
1/2 pound rutabaga, cut in large chunks
4-inch chunk daikon, cut in quarters
1 head cauliflower, cut in florets
1 1/2 cups cooked chickpeas
1/3 cup raisins
1/2 cup mixed fresh parsley and coriander leaves, chopped
2 cups Basic Vegetable Stock (page 94), water, or chickpea cooking liquid
1 teaspoon sea salt
*Steamed Couscous the Traditional Way (page 168) or Couscous in a Pinch (page 167)

Heat oil in the bottom of a large couscoussier or saucepan. Add couscous seasoning and onion. Sauté to coat and cook until onion softens. Add carrots, parsnips, rutabaga, daikon, cauliflower, chickpeas, raisins, parsley, coriander and stock. Bring to a boil. Reduce heat and gently simmer for 30 minutes to 1 1/4 hours. Add salt and simmer 3-5 more minutes. Serve with couscous and hot sauce on the side.

Hot Sauce

1 teaspoon Harissa (page 335)
1/2-1 cup broth from tagine

1 tablespoon freshly squeezed lemon juice
2 tablespoons fresh parsley, chopped
2 tablespoons fresh coriander, chopped

To make sauce, combine ingredients in a small saucepan. Make sure harissa is well mixed through. Bring to a boil and then remove from the heat. Serve in condiment-size bowls.

[serves 6]

*Nutrition Per Serving: Calories 263, Total Fat 3g, Saturated Fat trace, Cholesterol 0mg, Sodium 387mg, Potassium 1171mg, Total Carbohydrate 55g, Dietary Fiber 12g, Protein 7g, Calcium 129mg, Iron 3mg, Zinc 2mg, Vitamin C 63mg, Vitamin A 20830 IU, Vitamin B6 .4mg, Thiamin B1 .3mg, Riboflavin B2 .2mg, Folacin 198mcg, Niacin 2mg

*Note: The nutritional information does not account for the couscous. Refer to the couscous recipes on pages 167 and 168, and make the necessary adjustments.

Penne Puttanesca

The Diet Doctor's Wife: Penne Puttanesca has been in my dinner party repertoire since the mid-eighties. Bill just loves it and usually requests that I make it for his birthday or any other special occasion he can think of.

The Diet Doctor: If I eat tomatoes on a regular basis, I seem to develop symptoms of arthritis. However, a rare indulgence doesn't seem to cause me any trouble. And this dish is tops on my list of rare indulgences.

2 teaspoons extra virgin olive oil
1/3 cup onion, finely chopped
2 cloves garlic, finely chopped
1 tablespoon capers, rinsed and drained
1/3 cup green olives, pitted and halved
1/3 cup black olives, pitted and halved
2 cups Basic Tomato Sauce (page 330) or 28-ounce can
  Italian tomatoes, drained and chopped
1/4-1/2 teaspoon dried red pepper flakes
1 pound penne

Heat olive oil in a medium saucepan. Add onion and garlic, and sauté for 1-2 minutes. Add capers, olives, tomato sauce and red pepper flakes. Bring the mixture to a boil. Reduce heat and simmer, stirring occasionally, for 15 minutes.

Meanwhile cook pasta in salted boiling water as per instructions on package. Drain pasta. Pour pasta directly into saucepan. Toss to coat pasta with sauce.

[serves 6]

Nutrition Per Serving: Calories 349, Total Fat 5g, Saturated Fat 1g, Cholesterol 0mg, Sodium 341mg, Potassium 333mg, Total Carbohydrate 64g, Dietary Fiber 5g, Protein 11g, Calcium 59mg, Iron 1mg, Vitamin C 21mg, Vitamin A 852 IU, Vitamin B6 .1mg, Thiamin B1 .1mg, Folacin 15mcg, Niacin 1mg

Penne All'Arabiata

The Diet Doctor's Wife: I was turned on to this dish in Toronto. My friend Enid and I would often have dinner at the Monte Carlo on Eglinton West, and order their fiery Penne All'Arabiata with a simple Italian dinner salad and lots of red wine. Since leaving the city, I had to come up with a home version of this treasured pasta treat or else suffer from intense withdrawal. For a perfect result, warm the red pepper flakes for no longer than 30 seconds, otherwise you'll get an unpleasant burnt flavor.

The Diet Doctor: This dish is a real winner, especially for garlic lovers. And there is just enough hot pepper to create a little fire without making you sweat.

2 teaspoons extra virgin olive oil
6 cloves garlic, finely minced
1/2 teaspoon red pepper flakes, or more to taste
2 cups Basic Tomato Sauce (page 330)
1/4 teaspoon sea salt
1 pound penne
chopped fresh parsley, for garnish

In a saucepan, heat oil on medium low. Sauté garlic until golden, about 5 minutes. Add red pepper flakes and warm about 30 seconds. Add tomato sauce and bring to a boil. Reduce heat to a gentle simmer and cook for 15 minutes. Add salt. Taste for seasoning.

Meanwhile cook pasta in salted boiling water as per package instructions. Drain pasta. Pour pasta directly into saucepan. Toss to coat pasta with sauce. Garnish with chopped parsley.

[serves 6]

Nutrition Per Serving: Calories 331, Total Fat 4g, Saturated Fat trace, Cholesterol 0mg, Sodium 275mg, Potassium 326mg, Total Carbohydrate 63g, Dietary Fiber 4g, Protein 11g, Calcium 48mg, Iron 1mg, Vitamin C 20mg, Vitamin A 796 IU, Vitamin B6 .2mg, Thiamin B1 .1mg, Riboflavin B2 .1mg, Folacin 13mcg, Niacin 1mg

Spaghetti with Tomato and Mushroom Sauce

2 teaspoons extra virgin olive oil
2 cloves garlic, finely chopped
10 ounces cremini mushrooms, cut in 1/4-inch thick slices
2 cups Basic Tomato Sauce (page 330)
3 fresh basil leaves, finely chopped
sea salt and freshly ground black pepper, to taste
1 pound spaghetti or linguini
chopped fresh basil or parsley, for garnish

Warm olive oil in a large sauté pan over medium heat. Add garlic and cook for 2 minutes until softened. Add mushrooms and cook until softened, about 5 minutes. If the pan gets too dry while the mushrooms are softening, reduce heat slightly or add a couple of tablespoons of water.

Add tomato sauce and chopped basil. Bring to a boil and then reduce heat, and simmer about 15 minutes. Season to taste with salt and pepper.

Meanwhile, cook spaghetti al dente and drain. Pour spaghetti directly into the sauté pan. Toss together with sauce until pasta is coated. Garnish with fresh chopped parsley or basil.

[serves 6]

Nutrition Per Serving: Calories 350, Total Fat 5g, Saturated Fat trace, Cholesterol 0mg, Sodium 203mg, Potassium 611mg, Total Carbohydrate 66g, Dietary Fiber 4g, Protein 12g,

Calcium 61mg, Iron 4mg, Zinc 1mg, Vitamin C 21mg, Vitamin A 797 IU, Vitamin B6 .2mg, Thiamin B1 .9mg, Riboflavin B2 .6mg, Folacin 36mcg, Niacin 8mg

Angel Hair Pasta with Tomato Basil Sauce

2 teaspoons extra virgin olive oil
2 cloves garlic, minced
2 cups Basic Tomato Sauce (page 330)
10 basil leaves, cut in thin strips
sea salt and freshly ground black pepper, to taste
1 pound angel hair pasta

Warm oil in a saucepan. Add garlic and sauté for 1-2 minutes. Add tomato sauce and bring to a boil. Reduce heat to simmer for 15 minutes. Add basil leaves. Season to taste.

Fill a pasta pot two-thirds full of cold water. Add 1 tablespoon of sea salt (for sodium reduced diets, use less). Bring to a boil. Cook pasta according to the instructions on the package. Drain, reserving some of the cooking liquid.

Pour fresh cooked pasta directly into the tomato sauce. Toss to coat. Add a few tablespoons of pasta cooking liquid and continue cooking for about 1 minute until liquid has almost completely evaporated. Serve immediately.

[serves 6]

Nutrition Per Serving: Calories 339, Total Fat 5g, Saturated Fat trace, Cholesterol 0mg, *Sodium 202mg, Potassium 444mg, Total Carbohydrate 64g, Dietary Fiber 3g, Protein 11g, Calcium 59mg, Iron 4mg, Zinc 1mg, Vitamin C 20mg, Vitamin A 820 IU, Vitamin B6 .2mg, Thiamin B1 .8mg, Riboflavin B2 .4mg, Folacin 27mcg, Niacin 6mg

*Note: The sodium value in the nutritional analysis does not include the salt used in the pasta cooking water. The reason is that it is hard to determine how much of that salt is absorbed by the pasta.

Other pasta recipes: Japanese Tofu Nabe (page121), Japanese Fish Nabe (page 122), Chilled Somen with Sweet and Spicy Tofu and Baby Bok Choy (page 216), Seitan Chow Mein (page 225), Wakame and Glass Noodle Salad (page 277)

Bread

Walnut, Pear and Raisin Bread

The Diet Doctor's Wife: This is a simple and delicious tea bread based on a recipe by Maida Heatter. Great with marmalade or left just plain, it is best eaten the day it is made.

1/2 cup raisins
1 cup unbleached white flour
2 cups whole wheat flour
1 teaspoon sea salt
3/4 teaspoon baking soda
2 1/2 teaspoons aluminum-free baking powder
1 1/2 cups soy milk, rice milk or water
1/2 cup maple syrup
1/2 cup walnut meats, coarsely chopped
1 pear, cored and sliced in chunks

Adjust rack to the lower third of the oven and preheat to 275 F. Grease a 9" x 5" x 3" loaf pan.

Pour boiling water over raisins and let sit 5 minutes. Drain and allow to cool.

Into the large bowl of an electric mixer, sift together the two flours, salt, baking soda and baking powder. Add soy milk and maple syrup and beat on low speed until you get a smooth batter. With a wooden spoon, stir in raisins, nuts and chunks of pear.

Pour batter into a prepared pan and smooth top. Bake for 1 hour and 20 minutes, or until tester comes out clean.

[serves 12]

Nutrition Per Serving: Calories 206, Total Fat 4g, Saturated Fat trace, Cholesterol 0mg, Sodium 365mg, Potassium 251mg, Total Carbohydrate 39g, Dietary Fiber 4g, Protein 6g, Calcium 88mg, Iron 2mg, Zinc 1mg, Vitamin C 1mg, Vitamin A 28 IU, Vitamin B6 .1mg, Thiamin B1 .3mg, Riboflavin B2 .1mg, Folacin 13mcg, Niacin 2mg

Whole Wheat and Rosemary Beer Bread

The Diet Doctor's Wife: Beer bread is so easy to make. There is no need to wait for the dough to rise. Just combine the ingredients and pop it in the oven. One hour later you have fresh homemade bread.

1 1/2 cups self-rising flour
1 1/2 cups whole wheat pastry flour
1 1/2 teaspoons aluminum-free baking powder
1/2 teaspoon sea salt
1 tablespoon fresh rosemary, chopped
12 ounces beer, preferably nonalcoholic
1/4 cup honey or maple syrup

Preheat oven to 350 F.

In a large bowl, combine flours, baking powder, sea salt and rosemary. Stir in beer and honey until a batter is formed.

Pour into a lightly greased 8" x 4" x 3" loaf pan.

Bake loaf for 60-75 minutes until firm when pressed gently in the center.

[serves 16]

Nutrition Per Serving: Calories 105, Total Fat trace, Saturated Fat trace, Cholesterol 0mg, Sodium 255mg, Potassium 70mg, Total Carbohydrate 22g, Dietary Fiber 2g, Protein 3g, Calcium 73mg, Iron 1mg, Vitamin A 6 IU, Thiamin B1 .1mg, Riboflavin B2 .1mg, Folacin 9mcg, Niacin 2mg

Caraway Beer Bread

2 cups self-rising flour
1 cup dark rye flour, sifted
1 teaspoon aluminum-free baking powder
1/2 teaspoon sea salt
1 tablespoon caraway seeds

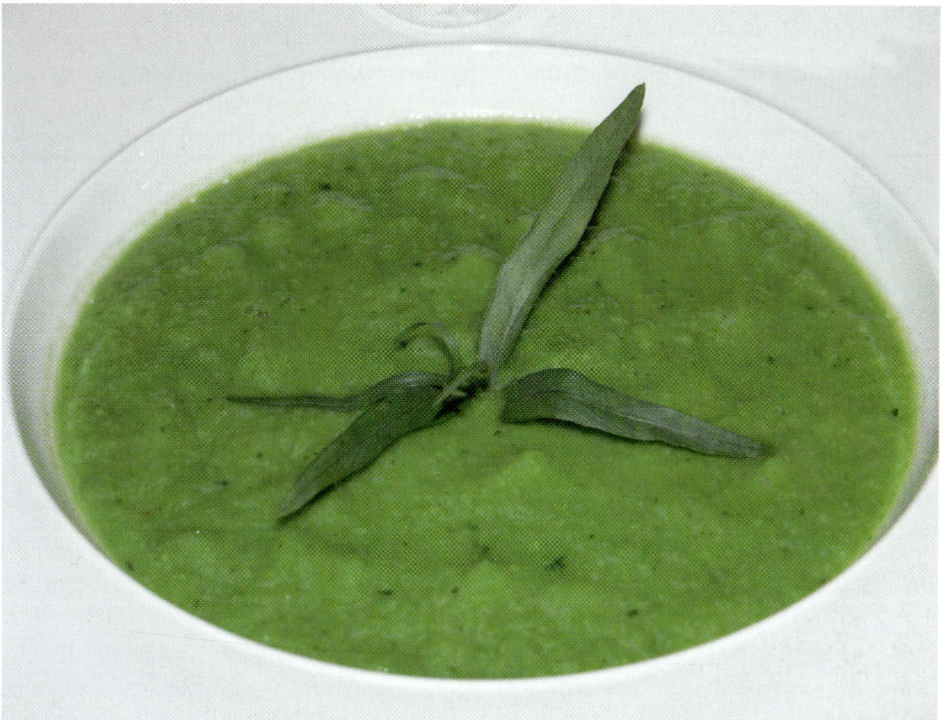

Fresh Pea Soup with Tarragon (page 104)

Cool Weather Miso Soup (page 118)

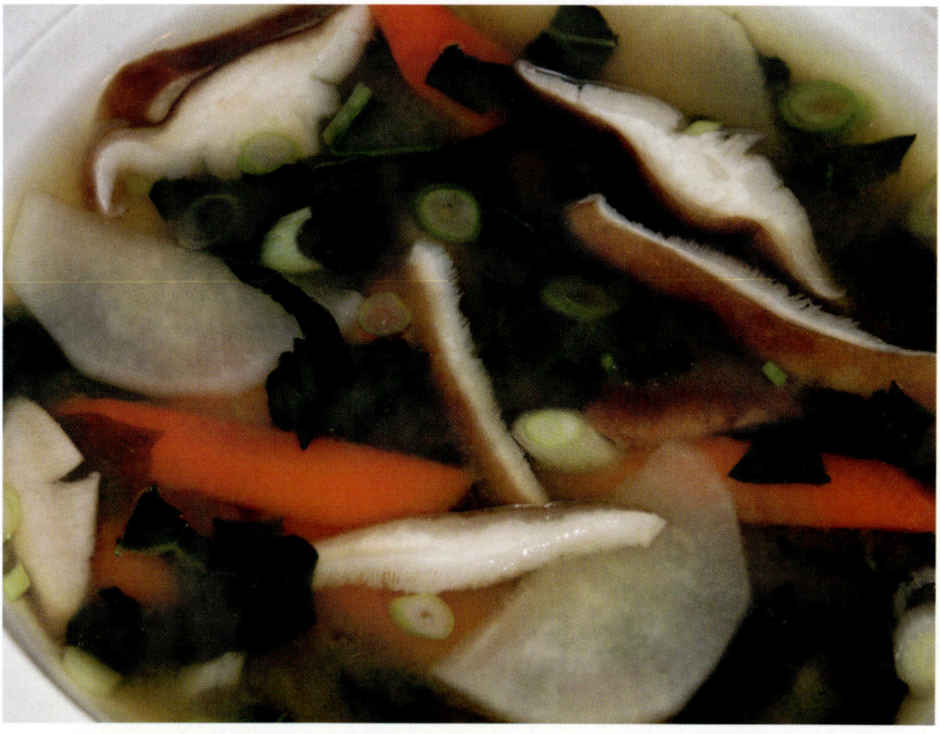

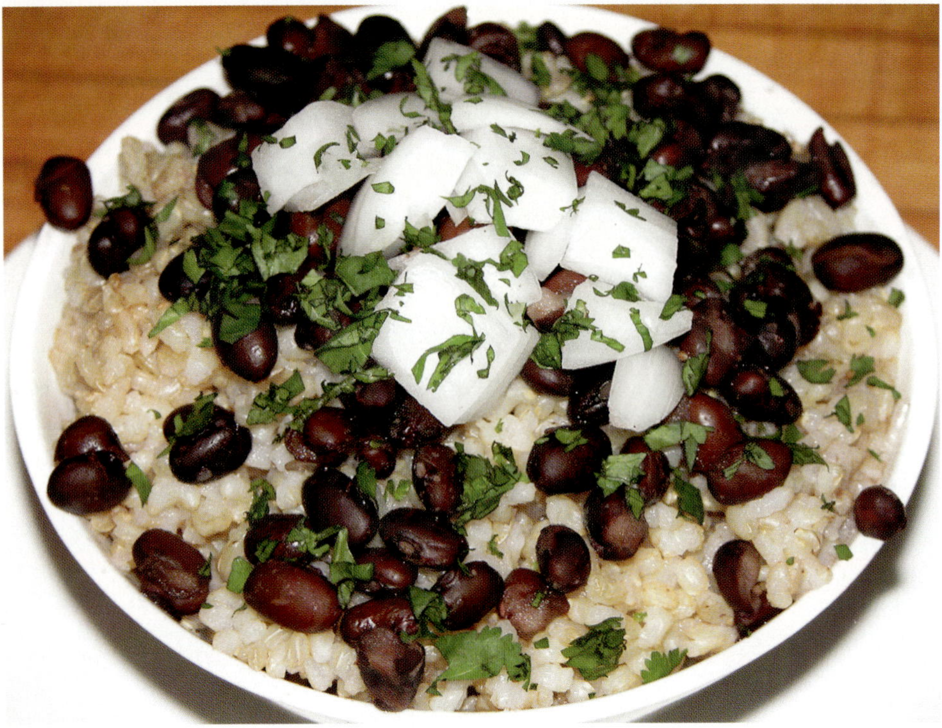

Cuban Black Beans II (page 193) with Pressure Cooked Brown Rice (page 132)

Morrocan Root Vegetable Tagine (page 169) with Couscous in a Pinch (page 167)

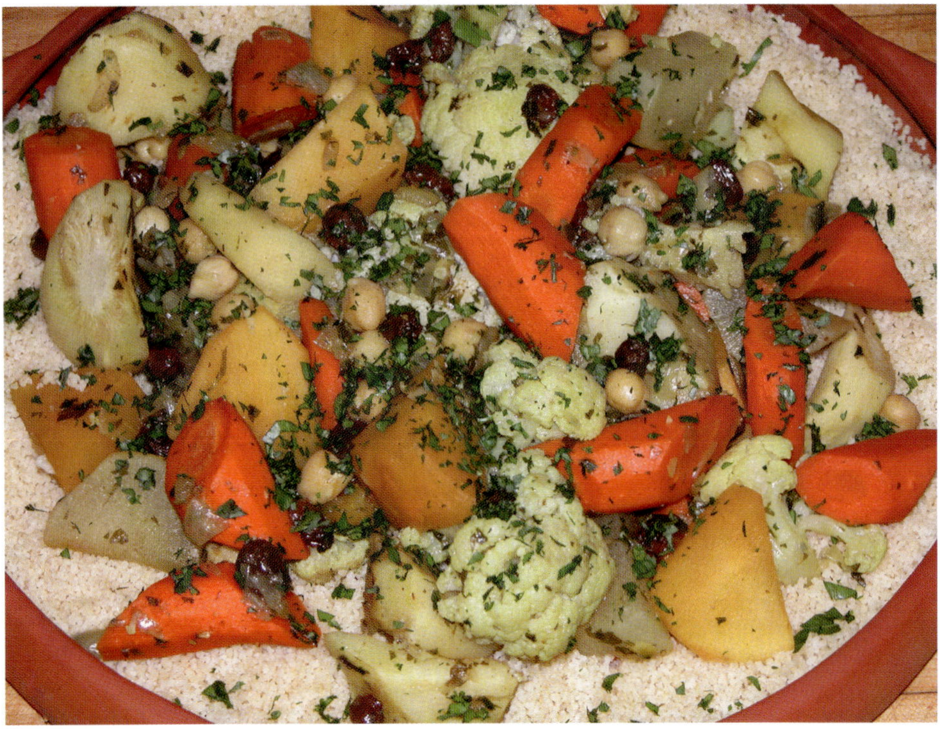

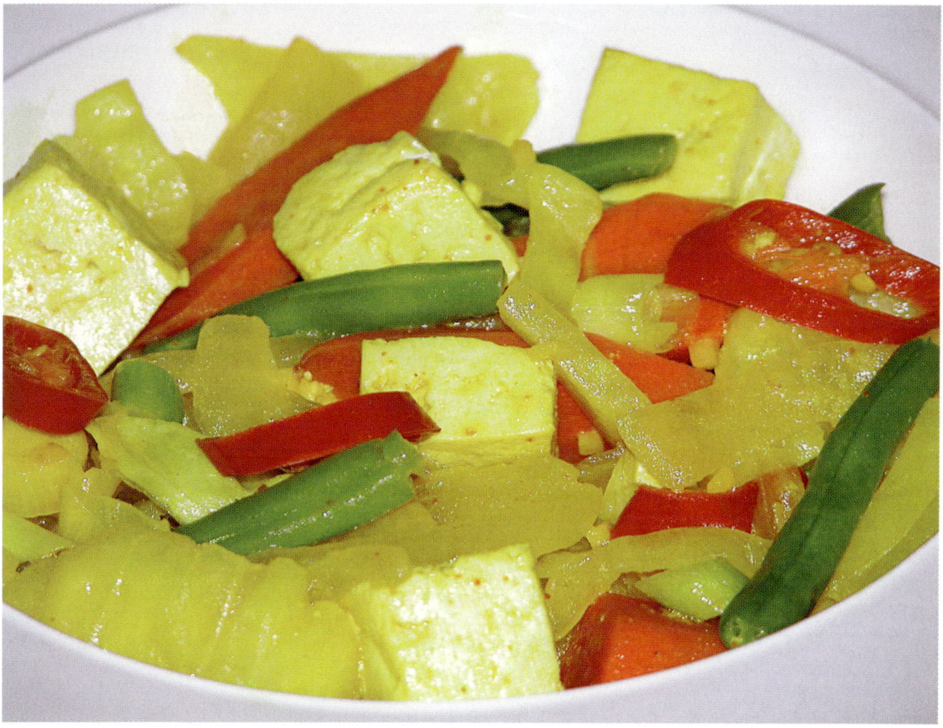

Indonesian Simmered Tofu with Lemongrass and Coconut Milk (page 219)

Bill's Throw-it-in-a-Pan Salmon (page 245)

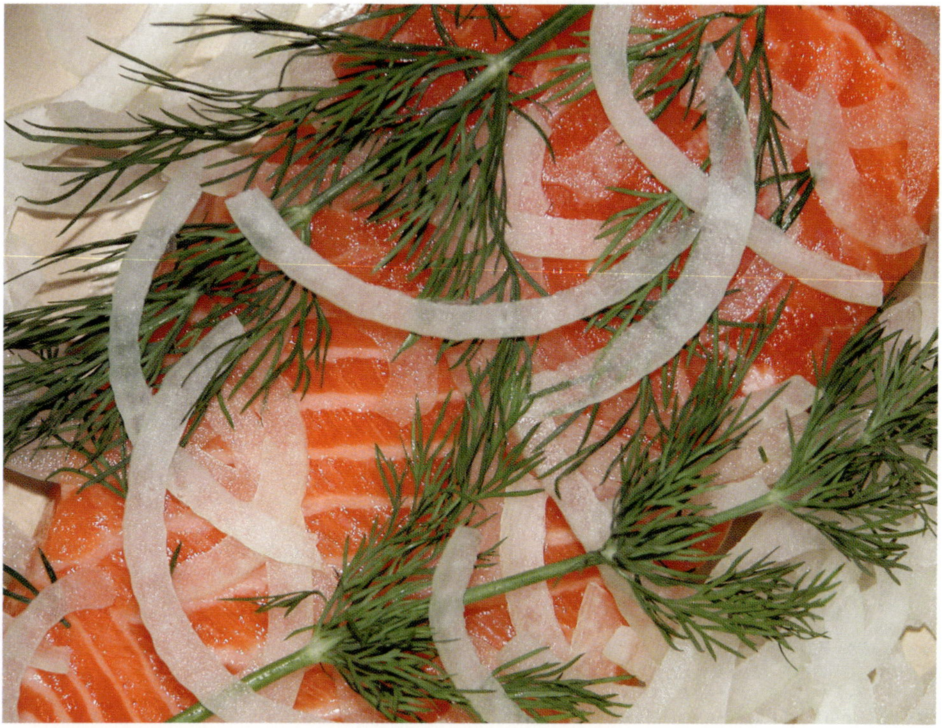

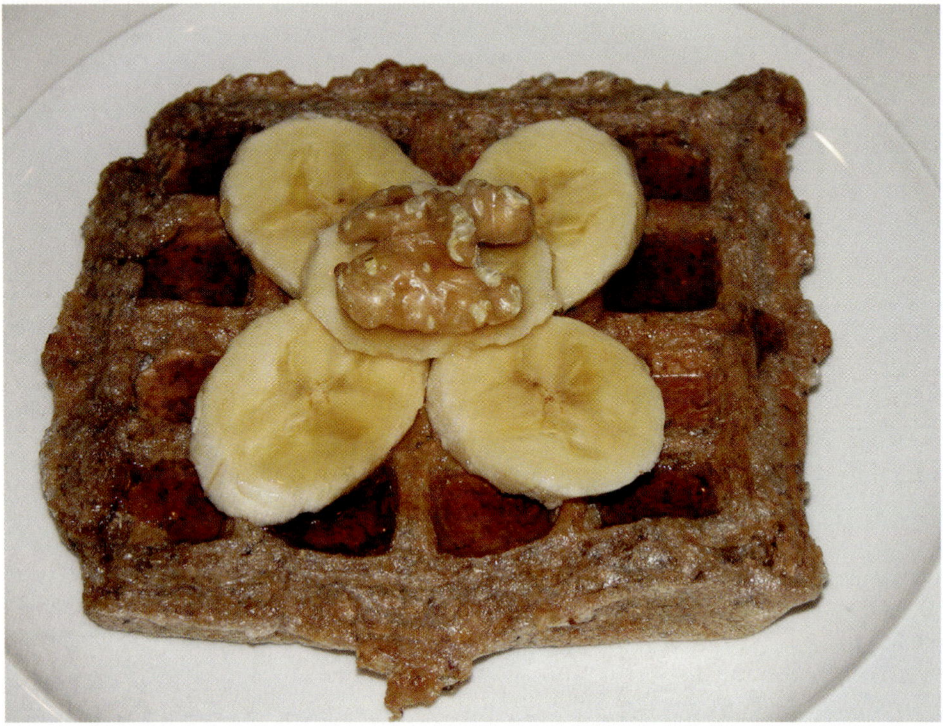

Mochi Waffles (page 159)

Gado Gado (page 87)

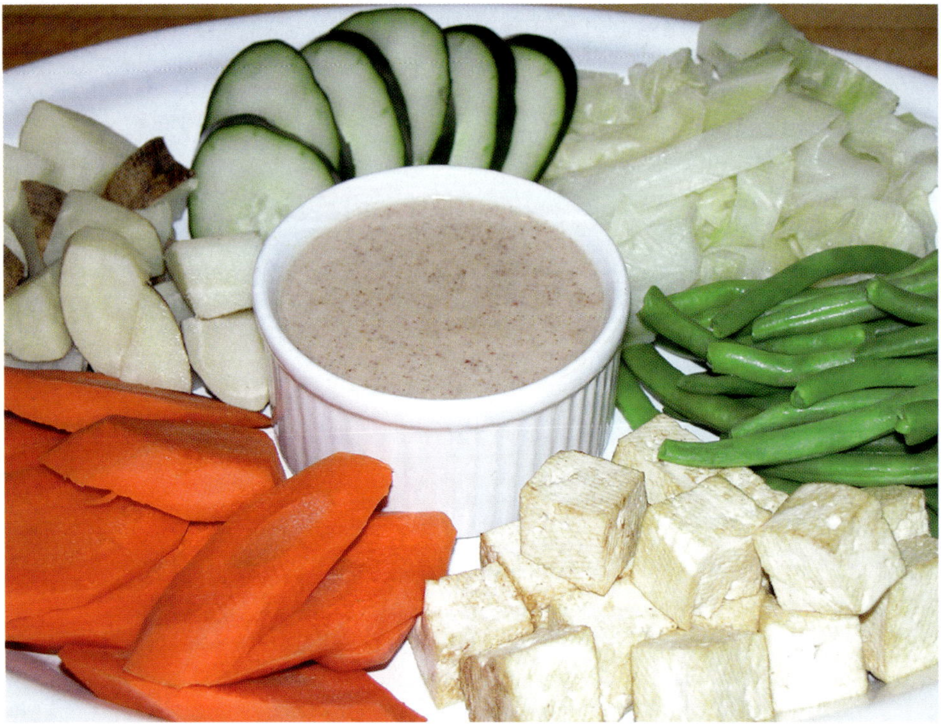

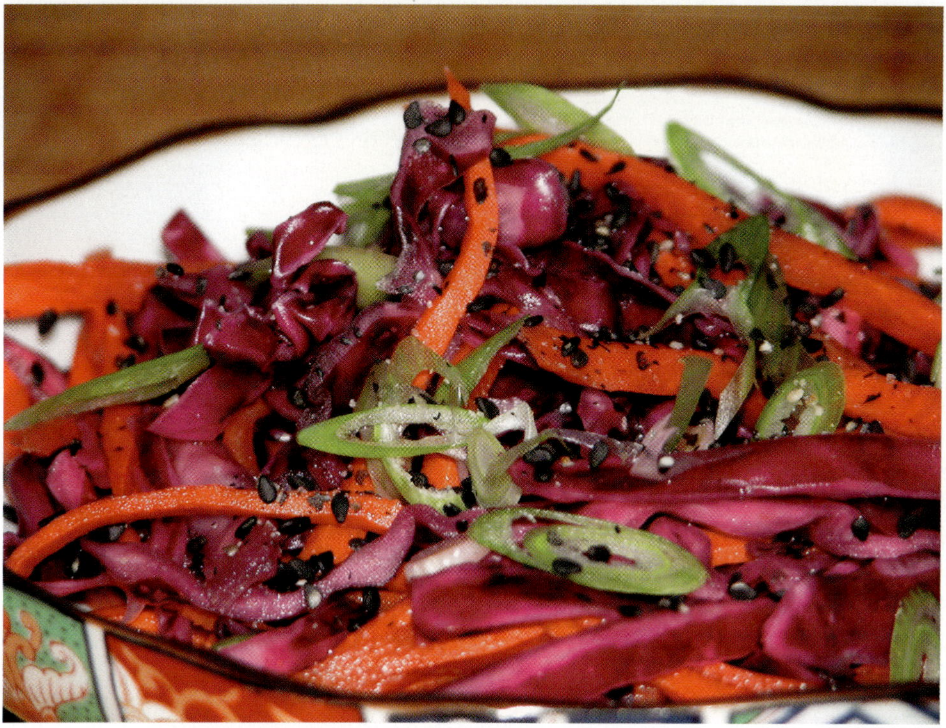

Pressed Salad (page 285) with Sesame Salt (page 327)

Chocolate Chip Cookies (page 315)

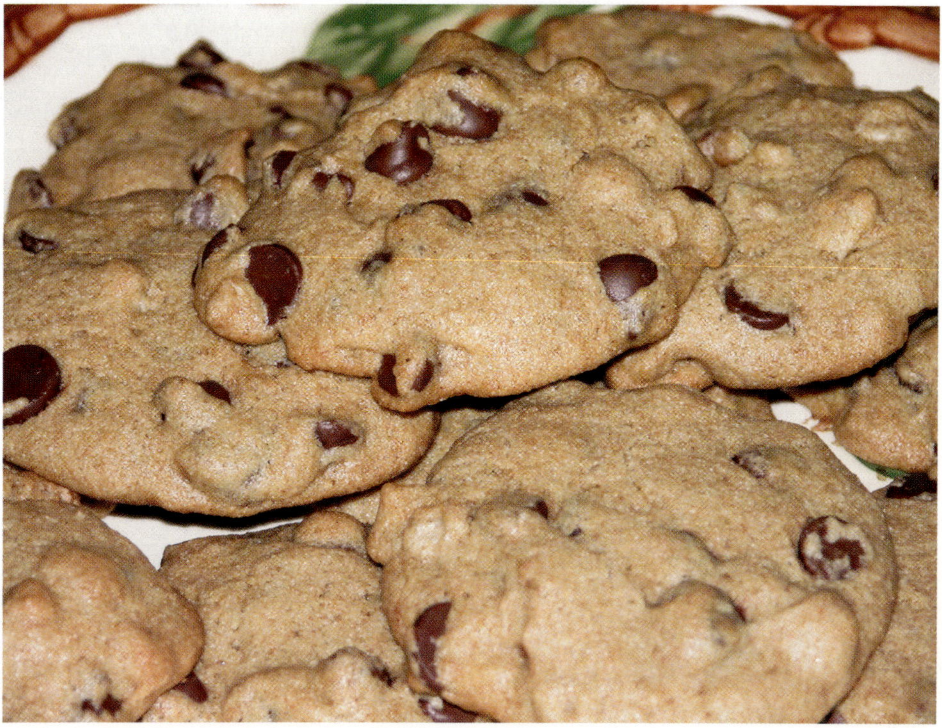

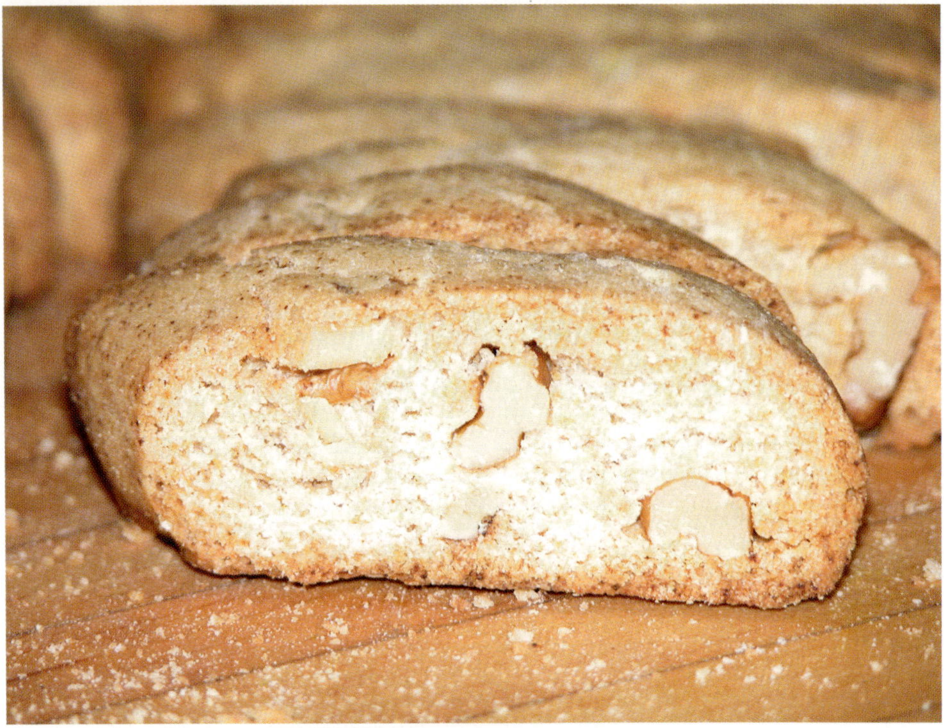

Mandelbroit with Walnuts (page 313)

Apple, Onion and Rosemary Scones (page 180)

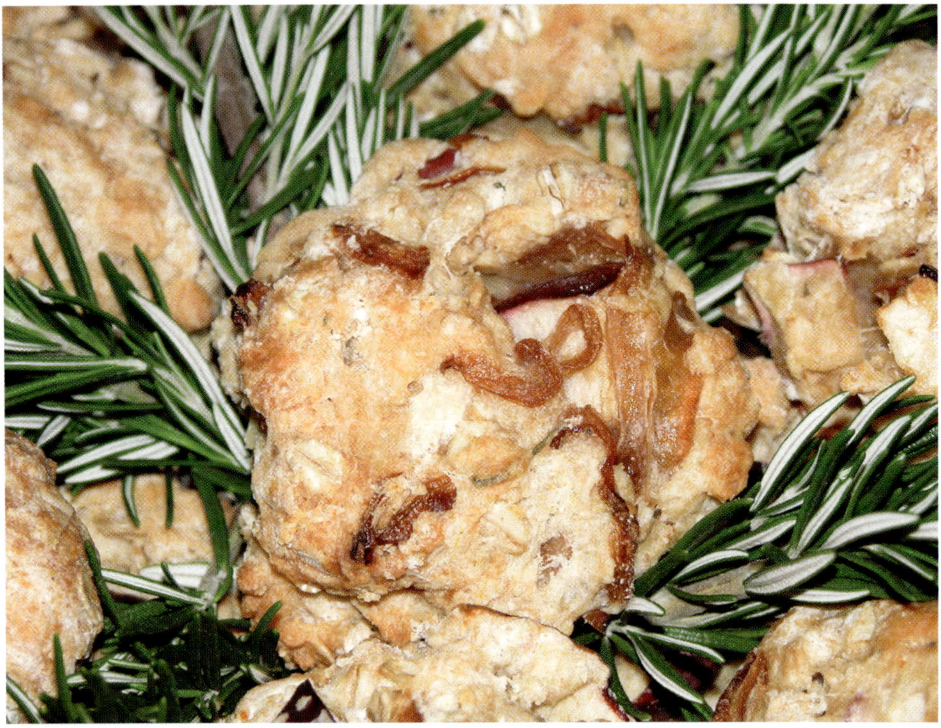

12 ounces beer, preferably nonalcoholic
1/4 cup maple syrup

Preheat oven to 350 F.

In a large bowl, combine flours, baking powder, salt and caraway seeds. Stir in beer and maple syrup until a batter is formed.

Pour into a lightly greased 8" x 4" x 3" loaf pan.

Bake loaf for 60-75 minutes until firm when pressed gently in the center.

[serves 16]

Nutrition Per Serving: Calories 100, Total Fat trace, Saturated Fat trace, Cholesterol 0mg, Sodium 289mg, Potassium 58mg, Total Carbohydrate 21g, Dietary Fiber 1g, Protein 2g, Calcium 78mg, Iron 1mg, Vitamin A 1 IU, Thiamin B1 .1mg, Riboflavin B2 .1mg, Folacin 9mcg, Niacin 1mg

Beer Stollen

The Diet Doctor's Wife: Bill loves the rich, buttery taste of Christmas Stollen. I came up with a more healthful version that is super easy to make, absolutely delicious and nowhere near as fattening as the traditional fare. Lovely with marmalade, Beer Stollen is best eaten the day it is baked.

3 cups self-rising flour
1 1/2 cups mixed candied fruit or dried fruit
1/2 cup slivered almonds
12 ounces light beer, preferably nonalcoholic
1/4 cup honey or maple syrup
1 teaspoon vanilla extract
1/4 teaspoon almond extract

Preheat oven to 350 F.

In a large bowl, combine flour, fruit and nuts. In a separate bowl, combine wet ingredients and whisk together. Empty wet mixture into flour mixture. Stir until well incorporated.

Pour batter into a lightly greased 8" x 4" x 3" loaf pan. Bake for 60-75 minutes until firm when pressed gently in the center.

[serves 12]

Nutrition Per Serving: Calories 217, Total Fat 4g, Saturated Fat trace, Cholesterol 0mg, Sodium 414mg, Potassium 135mg, Total Carbohydrate 41g, Dietary Fiber 2g, Protein 4g, Calcium 127mg, Iron 2mg, Thiamin B1 .2mg, Riboflavin B2 .2mg, Folacin 17mcg, Niacin 2mg

Whole Wheat Bread

1 1/2 cups lukewarm water
2, .25-ounce dry yeast packets
2 tablespoons barley malt syrup
2 tablespoons grapeseed oil
3 cups whole wheat bread flour
1 cup unbleached white bread flour
1 1/4 teaspoons sea salt

Pour 1/2 cup water into the large bowl of an electric mixer that is fitted with a dough hook. Add yeast and barley malt syrup. Blend and allow to sit for 5 minutes until yeast gets creamy.

Add the rest of the water, oil, flours and salt. Mix at a low speed so that flour doesn't fly all over your kitchen. Continue to mix until dough comes together. Process 2-3 minutes more.

If you don't have a mixer with a dough hook attachment, mix ingredients by hand until dough comes together. Then knead dough on a lightly floured surface for 5-10 minutes, adding flour if necessary.

Shape dough into a ball and place in a large, lightly oiled bowl. Flip ball so that entire surface is coated in oil. Cover with a damp dish towel. Let dough rise at room temperature for 20 minutes, until dough becomes light and spongy.

On a lightly floured surface, knead dough for 10 minutes. Place dough in a greased 8 1/2" x 4 1/2" x 3" loaf pan. Using a sharp knife, make 3 diagonal cuts in the top of the dough so that the tip of the knife touches the bottom of the loaf pan. Brush dough surface lightly with oil. Cover loaf with a damp dish towel and let rise for 20 minutes.

Preheat oven to 375 F. Bake loaf for 35-45 minutes until golden brown. To test if the bread is finished baking, tip it out of the pan and tap the bottom. It should sound hollow.

[serves 12]

Nutrition Per Serving: Calories 125, Total Fat 2g, Saturated Fat trace, Cholesterol 0mg, Sodium 149mg, Potassium 118mg, Total Carbohydrate 23g, Dietary Fiber 3g, Protein 4g, Calcium 10mg, Iron 1mg, Zinc 1mg, Thiamin B1 .2mg, Riboflavin B2 .1mg, Folacin 29mcg, Niacin 2mg

Chinese Flat Bread

1 1/2 cups unbleached all-purpose white flour
1 1/2 cups whole wheat pastry flour
2 teaspoons aluminum-free baking powder
1 teaspoon sea salt
1/2 cup boiling water
1/2 cup cold water
4 teaspoons grapeseed oil
1 teaspoon Sesame Salt (page 327)
1 cup scallions, finely chopped
vegetable oil spray

Place first 4 ingredients in a food processor fitted with a dough blade. Pulse a few seconds. While the motor is running, pour boiling water in a thin stream through the feed tube. Then add the cold water in a thin stream. Process until the mixture forms a ball, adding 1-2 tablespoons of cold water, if necessary. Turn the dough out onto a lightly floured surface. Knead 3 minutes and then cover with a clean dish towel. Let sit for 15 minutes.

Divide dough into 8 equal pieces. Take one piece and cover the others with a clean dish towel. On a lightly floured surface, roll out dough into an 8-inch circle. Spread 1/2 teaspoon of oil on the top surface of the circle. Then sprinkle on 1/8 teaspoon of Sesame Salt, followed by 2 tablespoons of the chopped scallions. Taking one edge of the circle, form a tight roll. Stretch out the roll a bit to lengthen. Taking one end of the stretched out roll, shape into a tight coil. Flatten the coil with the palm of your hand. Roll out the flattened coil to a 6-inch circle with the thickness of 1/4-inch.

Heat a heavy skillet over medium heat. Lower heat to medium low and coat the surface of the skillet with vegetable oil spray. Place the bread in the skillet. Cook for 3 minutes until bottom is lightly browned, then turn over and cook 3 minutes longer until the other side is lightly browned. Transfer to a cooling rack and cover with a clean dish towel.

Continue in the same way with the 7 other pieces of dough. Serve warm.

[serves 8]

Nutrition Per Serving: Calories 182, Total Fat 2g, Saturated Fat trace, Cholesterol 0mg, Sodium 365mg, Potassium 150mg, Total Carbohydrate 35g, Dietary Fiber 4g, Protein 6g, Calcium 89mg, Iron 2mg, Zinc 1mg, Vitamin C 2mg, Vitamin A 46 IU, Thiamin B1 .3mg, Riboflavin B2 .2mg, Folacin 50mcg, Niacin 3mg

Apple, Onion and Rosemary Scones

The Diet Doctor's Wife: These sweet and savory scones make wonderful dinner rolls or elegant snacks.

7 tablespoons extra virgin olive oil
1 medium onion, peeled and cut in 1/8-inch half-moons
2 tablespoons balsamic vinegar
2 apples, cored and cubed
sea salt and freshly ground black pepper, to taste
1 cup whole wheat pastry flour
3 cups unbleached white flour
1 cup rolled oats
1/2 teaspoon sea salt
1 1/2 tablespoons aluminum-free baking powder
1 tablespoon fresh rosemary leaves, chopped
1 1/2 cups apple juice

Preheat oven to 350 degrees F. Lightly grease a cookie sheet or set a piece of parchment paper on a dry cookie sheet.

In a nonstick pan, heat 1 tablespoon of oil on medium low. Sauté onions until caramelized, about 30 minutes. Add 1 tablespoon of balsamic vinegar and the apples. Stir to incorporate. Allow balsamic vinegar to cook away. Season with salt and pepper. Stir to incorporate. Remove from the heat.

In a large bowl, combine dry ingredients. Add rosemary. Stir to incorporate. Add onions and apples to the dry ingredients. Stir to incorporate.

In a separate bowl, whisk together the remaining oil and balsamic vinegar. Add the apple juice and whisk to incorporate. Empty wet ingredients into dry mixture. With a wooden spoon, mix to form a soft dough. If the dough is too dry, add a tablespoon or two of water.

Divide the dough into 20 pieces. Shape each piece into a scone and place on the cookie sheet.

Bake 30 to 45 minutes, until the edges of the scones become golden brown.

[serves 20]

Nutrition Per Serving: Calories 166, Total Fat 5g, Saturated Fat 1g, Cholesterol 0mg, Sodium 158mg, Potassium 108mg, Total Carbohydrate 26g, Dietary Fiber 2g, Protein 4g, Calcium 72mg, Iron 2mg, Vitamin C 1mg, Vitamin A 14 IU, Thiamin B1 .2mg, Riboflavin B2 .1mg, Folacin 9mcg, Niacin 2mg

Mushroom and Onion Scones

The Diet Doctor's Wife: I like to serve these savory scones on New Years Eve. They go great with champagne.

7 tablespoons plus 2 teaspoons extra virgin olive oil
1 medium onion, peeled and cut in 1/8-inch half-moons
3 tablespoons dry sherry
sea salt and freshly ground black pepper
8 ounces cremini or white button mushrooms, sliced
1 teaspoon tamari
2 tablespoons fresh thyme leaves
1 cup whole wheat pastry flour
3 cups unbleached white flour
1 cup rolled oats
1/2 teaspoon sea salt
1 1/2 tablespoons aluminum-free baking powder
1 1/2 cups apple juice

Preheat oven to 350 degrees F. Lightly oil a cookie sheet or set a piece of parchment paper on a dry cookie sheet.

In a saucepan, heat 1 tablespoon of extra virgin olive oil on medium low. Sauté onions until caramelized, about 30 minutes. Add 2 tablespoons sherry and cook until liquid is evaporated. Season with a pinch of sea salt. Set aside.

In a nonstick pan, heat 2 teaspoons extra virgin olive oil over medium heat. Add mushrooms, a pinch of salt and a few grinds of pepper. Sauté until browned. When the juices are almost completely evaporated add tamari. Cook until liquid is evaporated. Add 1 tablespoon sherry and cook until liquid is evaporated. Transfer mushrooms to a bowl and add thyme. Stir to combine and set aside.

In a large bowl, combine flours, oats, sea salt and baking powder. Add mushrooms and onions. Stir to incorporate.

In a separate bowl, whisk together the apple juice and remaining oil. Empty into the flour mixture. With a wooden spoon, mix to form a soft dough. If the dough is too dry, add a small amount of water.

Divide the dough into sixteen pieces. Shape each piece into a scone and place on the cookie sheet.

Bake 30 to 45 minutes, until the edges of the scones become golden brown.

[serves 16]

Nutrition Per Serving: Calories 209, Total Fat 7g, Saturated Fat 1g, Cholesterol 0mg, Sodium 234mg, Potassium 167mg, Total Carbohydrate 31g, Dietary Fiber 3g, Protein 5g, Calcium 90mg, Iron 2mg, Zinc 1mg, Vitamin 2mg, Vitamin A 20 IU, Thiamin B1 .3mg, Riboflavin B2 .2mg, Folacin 14mcg, Niacin 3mg

Olive Scones

1 cup chickpea flour
3 cups unbleached white flour
1/2 teaspoon sea salt
1 1/2 tablespoons aluminum-free baking powder
1 tablespoon fresh thyme leaves, chopped
grated zest of 1 orange
1/2 cup cracked olives, pitted and halved
1/4 cup extra virgin olive oil
1 1/2 cups water, rice milk or soy milk

Preheat oven to 350 F. Lightly oil a cookie sheet or set a piece of parchment paper on a dry cookie sheet.

In a large bowl, combine dry ingredients. Stir in thyme, zest and olives.

In a separate bowl, whisk together wet ingredients. Empty wet ingredients into dry mixture. With a wooden spoon, mix to form a soft dough. If dough is too dry, add a small amount of water.

Divide the dough into twelve pieces. Shape each piece into a scone and place on the cookie sheet.

Bake 30 to 45 minutes, until the edges of the scones become golden brown.

[serves 12]

Nutrition Per Serving: Calories 191, Total Fat 6g, Saturated Fat 1g, Cholesterol 0mg, Sodium 317mg, Potassium 103mg, Total Carbohydrate 29g, Dietary Fiber 2g, Protein 5g, Calcium 123mg, Iron 3mg, Vitamin C 1mg, Vitamin A 42 IU, Vitamin B6 .1mg, Thiamin B1 .3mg, Riboflavin B2 .2mg, Folacin 43mcg, Niacin 2mg

Coconut Curry Scones

1 cup whole wheat pastry flour
3 cups unbleached white flour
1/2 teaspoon sea salt
1 1/2 tablespoons aluminum-free baking powder
3/4 cup unsweetened shredded coconut
2 1/2 teaspoons curry powder
1/3 cup dried currants
1/4 cup grapeseed oil
1 1/2 cups soy or rice milk
1/4 cup maple syrup

Preheat oven to 350 F. Lightly grease a cookie sheet or line a dry cookie sheet with parchment paper.

In a medium-size bowl, combine dry ingredients. Mix well. Add currants and stir to combine.

In a separate bowl, whisk together wet ingredients.

Pour wet ingredients into dry mixture. Lightly mix with a wooden spoon until dough comes together. Be careful not to over-mix.

Divide dough into 12 pieces. Shape each piece into a scone and place on the cookie sheet.

Bake for 35 minutes, until edges of scones are golden brown.

[serves 12]

Nutrition Per Serving: Calories 246, Total Fat 7g, Saturated Fat 2g, Cholesterol 0mg, Sodium 268mg, Potassium 191mg, Total Carbohydrate 40g, Dietary Fiber 4g, Protein 6g, Calcium 124mg, Iron 3mg, Zinc 1mg, Vitamin A 17 IU, Thiamin B1 .4mg, Riboflavin B2 .2mg, Folacin 14mcg, Niacin 3mg

Beans

WASHING BEANS

Beans must be sorted for stones and twigs, and washed thoroughly before cooking. An easy way to sort beans is to place them in a large jellyroll pan and spread them around so that each bean is in full view. To wash beans, just place them in a large pot and cover with water. Swish the beans around. This will likely make the water turn cloudy. Drain the beans and repeat the washing procedure as many times as necessary until the water runs clear. Drain the beans. Note that the same techniques are used for washing and sorting lentils.

SOAKING BEANS

After beans are washed, they must be soaked. Do not cook beans without soaking them first. Proper soaking makes beans much easier to digest. Eating beans that have not been adequately soaked can cause terrible gastric problems. Soaking liquid should be discarded and not used for cooking (adzuki soaking liquid is the only exception). Lentils do not need to be soaked.

I prefer the following two methods of soaking:

1) Regular Presoak Method

Place beans in a large bowl. Add enough cold water to cover the beans by at least 2 inches. Let sit for 6-8 hours. Drain and discard soaking liquid. Start cooking.

Soaking Times

Adzuki	**6-8 hours**
Black Turtle	**6-8 hours**
Chickpeas	**6-8 hours**
Great Northern	**6-8 hours**
Lentils	**no soaking required**
Navy	**6-8 hours**
Pinto	**6-8 hours**

2) The Quick Soak Method

To quick soak, just place washed beans in a pot. Add enough cold water to cover the beans by at least 2 inches. Bring to a boil over medium heat. Cook at a rolling boil for 1 minute. Turn off heat and allow beans to sit in the hot water for 1 hour. Drain and discard soaking liquid. Start cooking.

COOKING METHODS

Beans may be boiled or pressure-cooked. I prefer to use a pressure-cooker as it takes much less time and I don't have to keep tabs on the water level throughout the cooking process. Cooking times vary according to the size of the bean.

Cooking Time in Minutes *

	Pressure Cooking	Boiling
Adzuki	30 minutes	30 - 60 minutes
Black Turtle	30 minutes	1 - 1 1/2 hours
Chickpeas	45 minutes	2 - 2 1/2 hours
Great Northern	30 minutes	1 - 1 1/2 hours
Lentils	--------------	1/2 hour
Navy	30 minutes	1 - 1 1/2 hours
Pinto	45 minutes	2 - 2 1/2 hours

* For firmer texture (preferable for bean salads), shorten cooking time. For softer texture, lengthen cooking time.

ADDING SALT

Beans should be salted at the end of the cooking process. Salting at the beginning creates toughness and a shriveled skin.

STORING BEANS

Dried beans should be stored in airtight containers and kept in a dark, cool place. To ensure freshness, shop at a market that sells a lot of dried beans. Markets that cater to vegetarians are always a good bet. Also be realistic about the quantity. Don't buy more dried beans than you'll cook within a six-month period.

Humus

The Diet Doctor's Wife: Homemade humus is simple to make and wonderful to have on hand. Spread it on rice cakes or use it as a vegetable dip. It is a no-fuss hors d'oeuvre served with marinated olives and pita wedges.

1 1/2 cups cooked chickpeas
1 tablespoon tahini
juice of 1 lemon
1-2 cloves garlic, finely minced
1/8-1/4 teaspoon sea salt
paprika or ground cayenne pepper (optional)

Combine first 5 ingredients in a food processor and puree. Place in a serving bowl. Sprinkle with paprika or cayenne, if desired.

[serves 6]

Nutrition Per Serving: Calories 84, Total Fat 2g, Saturated Fat trace, Cholesterol 0mg, Sodium 45mg, Potassium 139mg, Total Carbohydrate 12g, Dietary Fiber 2g, Protein 4g, Calcium 33mg, Iron 1mg, Zinc 1mg, Vitamin C 3mg, Vitamin A 29 IU, Vitamin B6 .1mg, Thiamin B1 .1mg, Folacin 74mcg

Middle Eastern Lentils and Rice

The Diet Doctor's Wife: This recipe is a much lower fat version of the Lebanese dish, Mujadra. I use a pressure cooker to create richness without the use of much oil.

1 tablespoon extra virgin olive oil
2 large onions, coarsely chopped
sea salt and freshly ground black pepper, to taste
2 cups long grain brown rice
1 cup brown or green lentils
4 1/2 cups water
1/2 teaspoon sea salt
1 teaspoon cumin
juice of 1 lemon

In a medium saucepan, heat 1 tablespoon of oil. Add onions and sauté slowly over low heat until they soften and turn a rich golden brown. This will take about 30 minutes.

Remove half the onions and place them in a pressure cooker. Place the second half in a bowl. Season the onions in the bowl with sea salt and freshly ground pepper. Set aside.

Add rice, lentils and water to the onions in the pressure cooker. Bring to a slow boil over low heat. Add 1/2 teaspoon sea salt and cumin. Secure lid and turn flame on high. Bring up to pressure and then reduce heat to medium low. Place a flame deflector under the cooker. Cook 45 to 50 minutes. Remove from heat and allow pressure to come down. Remove lid and let rice mixture rest for 5 minutes. Add lemon juice and mix. Taste for seasoning. Serve with remaining onions on top.

[serves 8]

Nutrition Per Serving: Calories 280, Total Fat 3g, Saturated Fat 1g, Cholesterol 0mg, Sodium 143mg, Potassium 375mg, Total Carbohydrate 52g, Dietary Fiber 9g, Protein 11g, Calcium 34mg, Iron 3mg, Zinc 2mg, Vitamin C 6mg, Vitamin A 14 IU, Vitamin B6 .4mg, Thiamin B1 .3mg, Riboflavin B2 .1mg, Folacin 119mcg, Niacin 3mg

Lentil Salad

The Diet Doctor's Wife: I usually have a container of Lentil Salad sitting in my fridge. It's terrific on it's own, with rice or spread on crackers. Add a few tablespoons to a green salad for an extra hit of protein.

1 cup green or brown lentils
1 medium onion, stuck with 1 whole clove
1 clove garlic
bouquet garni (6 sprigs parsley, 2 sprigs thyme, 5 chives and
 1 bay leaf, tied together with string)
1/2 teaspoon sea salt
1/4 cup Gingery Vinaigrette (page 343)

1/4 cup shallots, chopped
1/4 cup fresh parsley, chopped

Place lentils, onion, garlic and bouquet garni in a large pot. Add cold water to cover lentils by 1-2 inches. Bring to a boil and then lower heat to simmer for 40 minutes. Add a bit of water once or twice throughout cooking, if necessary. Add salt and simmer 1 more minute. Drain lentils. Remove onion, garlic and bouquet garni. Cool to room temperature. Transfer to a serving bowl.

Drizzle vinaigrette over lentils. Garnish with shallots and parsley.

[serves 6]

Nutrition Per Serving: Calories 171, Total Fat 6g, Saturated Fat 1g, Cholesterol 0mg, Sodium 163mg, Potassium 357mg, Total Carbohydrate 22g, Dietary Fiber 10g, Protein 9g, Calcium 27mg, Iron 3mg, Zinc 1mg, Vitamin C 8mg, Vitamin A 975 IU, Vitamin B6 .2mg, Thiamin B1 .2mg, Riboflavin B2 .1mg, Folacin 149mcg, Niacin 1mg

Cuban Black Beans I

The Diet Doctor's Wife: Believe it or not, Bill introduced me to this completely vegetarian dish. We were visiting his parents in St. Petersburg, Florida. Bill could barely wait to take me to his favorite local Cuban restaurant. He recommended that I try the black beans. What came to the table was a simple preparation of spiced beans served on a bed of white rice, topped with coarsely chopped onions. It was a humble yet remarkably delicious meal.

1 1/2 cups dried black beans, soaked 6-8 hours or quick-soaked
1 medium onion, chopped
2 cloves garlic, chopped
1/2 - 1 teaspoon ground cumin
1/8 teaspoon ground cayenne pepper
1/2 teaspoon sea salt
1/8 teaspoon freshly ground black pepper
1 cup onion, chopped

Drain soaked beans and put in a pressure cooker. Add water to cover beans by 1-2 inches. Secure lid. Bring beans up to pressure over medium heat. Reduce heat to low and cook for 30 minutes. Allow pressure to release and remove lid.

Add onions, garlic, cumin, cayenne, salt and pepper to the beans. Stir to combine. Secure lid and bring up to pressure over medium heat. Reduce heat to low and cook for 30 minutes.

Remove from heat and let pressure release naturally. Let bean mixture sit for at least 15 minutes before serving.

Serve beans on top of cooked rice and top with chopped onion. Garnish with Mexican Salsa (page 330) or Zen Salsa (page 329), if desired.

[serves 6]

Nutrition Per Serving: Calories 185, Total Fat 1g, Saturated Fat trace, Cholesterol 0mg, Sodium 182mg, Potassium 798mg, Total Carbohydrate 35g, Dietary Fiber 8g, Protein 11g, Calcium 73mg, Iron 3mg, Zinc 2mg, Vitamin C 3mg, Vitamin A 26 IU, Vitamin B6 .2mg, Thiamin B1 .5mg, Riboflavin B2 .1mg, Folacin 224mcg, Niacin 1mg

Cuban Black Beans II

2 cups dried black beans, soaked 6-8 hours or quick-soaked
1 sprig fresh thyme or oregano
1 bay leaf
2 teaspoons extra virgin olive oil
6 scallions, finely chopped
4 cloves garlic, finely chopped
1 1/2 teaspoons ground cumin
3/4 teaspoon sea salt
1/8 teaspoon freshly ground black pepper

Drain soaked beans and put in a pressure cooker. Add water to cover beans by 1-2 inches. Add thyme and bay leaf.

Secure lid and bring beans up to pressure over medium heat. Reduce heat to low and cook for 45 minutes. Allow pressure to release and remove lid. Remove thyme sprig and bay leaf.

In a sauté pan, heat oil on medium low. Sauté scallions, garlic and cumin 8-10 minutes. Add scallion mixture to the beans. Season with salt and pepper. Bring up to pressure again over medium heat. Reduce heat to low and cook for 15 minutes.

Remove from heat and let pressure release naturally. Let bean mixture sit for at least 15 minutes before serving.

Serve on top of cooked rice.

[serves 8]

Nutrition Per Serving: Calories 184, Total Fat 2g, Saturated Fat trace, Cholesterol 0mg, Sodium 205mg, Potassium 768mg, Total Carbohydrate 32g, Dietary Fiber 8g, Protein 11g, Calcium 86mg, Iron 4mg, Zinc 2mg, Vitamin C 3mg, Vitamin A 78 IU, Vitamin B6 .2mg, Thiamin B1 .4mg, Riboflavin B2 .1mg, Folacin 224mcg, Niacin 1mg

Black Bean Puree

The Diet Doctor's Wife: A great way to turn leftovers into a tasty appetizer. Serve as a sandwich spread or dip.

2 cups Cuban Black Beans I or II
1/2 cup onion, finely minced
pinch of sea salt

Puree black beans. Add onion and salt. Stir to combine.

[16 servings]

Nutrition Per Serving with Cuban Black Beans I: Calories 33, Total Fat trace, Saturated Fat trace, Cholesterol 0mg, Sodium 37mg, Potassium 93mg, Total Carbohydrate 6g, Dietary Fiber 2g, Protein 2g, Calcium 8mg, Vitamin C 1mg, Vitamin A 5 IU, Thiamin B1 .1mg, Folacin 34mcg

Nutrition Per Serving with Cuban Black Beans II: Calories 35, Total Fat trace, Saturated Fat trace, Cholesterol 0mg, Sodium 60mg, Potassium 97mg, Total Carbohydrate 6g, Dietary Fiber 2mg, Protein 2g, Calcium 16mg, Iron 1mg, Vitamin C 1mg, Vitamin A 24 IU, Thiamin B1 .1mg, Folacin 36mcg

Mexican Beans

The Diet Doctor's Wife: I make Mexican Beans a lot. The long pressure-cooking creates the richness of refried beans, minus the fat. I serve Mexican Beans with rice or use them to make burritos or nachos.

2 cups dried pinto beans, soaked 6-8 hours or quick-soaked
1 small onion, cut in wedges
1 large clove garlic
2 tablespoons chili powder
1/2 teaspoon ground cumin
1 teaspoon sea salt

Drain beans and discard soaking water. Put beans in a pressure cooker. Add enough water to cover beans by 2 inches. Add onion and garlic clove. Secure lid and bring up to pressure. Lower temperature to moderate heat and cook for 45 minutes. Remove from heat and allow pressure to release naturally. Remove 1/4 cup of bean cooking liquid from the pressure cooker and mix together with chili powder and cumin. Add spice mixture to the beans and stir to incorporate. Pressure-cook for another 30 minutes. Add salt and stir to incorporate. Break up bean mixture with a potato masher. Check for seasoning.

[serves 8]

Nutrition Per Serving: Calories 176, Total Fat 1g, Saturated Fat trace, Cholesterol 0mg, Sodium 259mg, Potassium 702mg, Total Carbohydrate 33g, Dietary Fiber 13g, Protein 11g, Calcium 70mg, Iron 3mg, Zinc 1mg, Vitamin C 6mg, Vitamin A 659 IU, Vitamin B6 .3mg, Thiamin B1 .3mg, Riboflavin B2 .1mg, Folacin 249mcg, Niacin 1mg

Burritos

8 whole wheat tortillas

1 recipe Mexican Beans (page 195), warmed or at room temperature
2 cups lettuce, shredded
2 cups tomatoes, chopped
2 cups onion, chopped
1/2 cup black olives, chopped
Mexican Salsa (page 330) or Zen Salsa (page 329) (optional)
Guacamole (page 333) (optional)
tofu sour cream (optional)
corn chips (optional)

Heat a dry skillet on medium low. Place a tortilla in the skillet and heat until soft and pliable. Remove the tortilla from the skillet. Place 1/2 cup of Mexican Beans a little below the center of the tortilla. Add a little shredded lettuce, some tomato, onion and black olives. Fold sides of tortilla over filling toward the center. Fold bottom over filling and roll up, enclosing filling completely. Repeat with the remaining tortillas.

Serve with Mexican Salsa or Zen Salsa, Guacamole, tofu sour cream and corn chips, if desired.

[serves 8]

Nutrition Per Serving: Calories 345, Total Fat 5g, Saturated Fat trace, Cholesterol 0mg, Sodium 752mg, Potassium 903mg, Total Carbohydrates 64g, Dietary Fiber 18g, Protein 16g, Calcium 97mg, Iron 12mg, Zinc 1mg, Vitamin C 20mg, Vitamin A 1247 IU, Vitamin B6 .4mg, Thiamin B1 .3mg, Riboflavin B2 .2mg, Folacin 270mcg, Niacin 1mg

Nachos

The Diet Doctor: Although this nacho recipe is radically lower in fat and calories than the standard, it is still incredibly fattening. Gabrielle has calculated the nutritional information for the most Spartan version of this dish. Note the serving size, only 3 chips per person. Add tofu cheese, shredded mochi, guacamole or tofu sour cream, and the calories and fat content skyrocket. Pretty scary. Even so, if nachos are your thing, this is the healthiest way to eat them.

24 baked unsalted tortilla chips
1 1/2 cups Mexican Beans (page 195)
1 cup onion, chopped
1 recipe Mexican Salsa (page 330) or double recipe of Zen Salsa (page 329)
1/2 cup tofu cheese or mochi, shredded (optional)
1/4 cup Guacamole (page 333) (optional)
1/4 cup tofu sour cream (optional)

Preheat oven to 350 degrees F. Place tortilla chips on the bottom of a baking pan. Spoon beans over the chips. Top with onions, and if desired, add shredded tofu cheese or mochi. Bake until warmed through (if using cheese or mochi, bake until cheese or mochi melts). Top with salsa, and if desired, add a few tablespoons of guacamole and tofu sour cream. Accompaniments can also be served on the side.

[serves 8]

Nutrition Per Serving: Calories 397, Total Fat 3g, Saturated Fat trace, Cholesterol 0mg, Sodium 225mg, Potassium 462mg, Total Carbohydrate 79g, Dietary Fiber 10g, Protein 13g, Calcium 210mg, Iron 2mg, Zinc 2mg, Vitamin C 11mg, Vitamin A 534 IU, Vitamin B6 .4mg, Thiamin B1 .2mg, Riboflavin B2 .2mg, Folacin 73mcg, Niacin 2mg

White Beans Provencal

The Diet Doctor's Wife: I often have White Beans Provencal for lunch with a tossed salad.

2 cups navy beans, soaked 6-8 hours or quick-soaked
1/2 head garlic, unpeeled
3 sprigs fresh rosemary
2 teaspoons freshly squeezed lemon juice or red wine vinegar
2 tablespoons extra virgin olive oil
1 clove garlic, minced
1/2 teaspoon sea salt
freshly ground pepper, to taste

Place beans, 1/2 head of garlic and rosemary in a pressure cooker. Cover with water. Secure lid and bring up to pressure over medium heat. Reduce heat to medium low and cook for 30 minutes. Allow pressure to be released naturally. Let beans sit in the pot covered for 15 minutes. Remove garlic and sprigs of rosemary. Drain the beans and set aside.

Whisk together lemon juice, olive oil, chopped garlic, salt and pepper. Add dressing to the beans. Toss gently to combine.

[serves 8]

Nutrition Per Serving: Calories 209, Total Fat 4g, Saturated Fat 1g, Cholesterol 0mg, Sodium 126mg, Potassium 609mg, Total Carbohydrate 33g, Dietary Fiber 13g, Protein 12g, Calcium 98mg, Iron 4mg, Zinc 1mg, Vitamin C 3mg, Vitamin A 41 IU, Vitamin B6 .2mg, Thiamin B1 .3mg, Riboflavin .1mg, Folacin 192mcg, Niacin 1mg

Variation: For less intense flavor, leave out the rosemary and add 2-3 tablespoons of chopped parsley to the dressing.

White Bean Puree

The Diet Doctor's Wife: The first time I had this bean puree was at a Jimmy Schmidt restaurant in Ann Arbor. It came with the breadbasket in place of the butter. I loved it so much that I had to create a home version.

1 cup navy beans, soaked 6-8 hours or quick-soaked
1/2 head garlic, unpeeled
3 sprigs fresh rosemary
1 tablespoon extra virgin olive oil
1 clove garlic, finely chopped
1/4 teaspoon sea salt
freshly ground black pepper, to taste

Place beans, 1/2 head of garlic and rosemary in a pressure cooker. Cover with water. Secure lid and bring up to pressure over medium heat. Reduce heat to medium low and cook for 30 minutes. Allow pressure to be released naturally. Let beans sit in the pot, covered, for 15 minutes.

Remove the garlic and sprigs of rosemary. Drain, reserving some of the cooking water. Place drained beans, olive oil, chopped garlic, salt and pepper in a food processor and puree. For a more liquid consistency, add some of the cooking water.

[serves 16]

Nutrition Per Serving: Calories 53, Total Fat 1g, Saturated Fat trace, Cholesterol 0mg, Sodium 32mg, Potassium 155mg, Total Carbohydrate 8g, Dietary Fiber 3g, Protein 3g, Calcium 29mg, Iron 1mg, Vitamin C 1mg, Vitamin A 20 IU, Vitamin B6 .1mg, Thiamin B1 .1mg, Folacin 48mcg

Variation: Combine 2 cups cooked navy beans with 1-2 cloves minced garlic, 1 teaspoon minced rosemary leaves, 1 tablespoon extra virgin olive oil, sea salt and pepper. Puree.

Vegetarian Cassoulet

The Diet Doctor's Wife: This dish is so rich and full of flavor, and so much lower in fat than the traditional non-vegetarian version (containing duck fat, sausage, lamb and other carnivorous goodies). If you don't have Onion Confit on hand, sauté a couple of large onions over low heat for about 30 minutes until they caramelize. Don't forget to season with salt and pepper.

2 cups navy beans, soaked 6-8 hours or quick-soaked
bouquet garni (6 sprigs parsley, 5 sage leaves and 2 sprigs thyme, tied together with string)
1/2 head garlic, unpeeled
1/2 teaspoon sea salt
2 cups Onion Confit (page 332)
1 tablespoon tomato paste
1 tomato, peeled, seeded, and diced
1/4 teaspoon sea salt
1/8 teaspoon freshly ground white pepper
2 tablespoons fresh thyme, finely chopped
2 tablespoons fresh parsley, finely chopped
1/2 cup fresh whole wheat bread crumbs
2 cloves garlic, finely chopped
1 tablespoon extra virgin olive oil or melted Clarified Butter (page 346)

Preheat oven to 400 F.

Place beans, bouquet garni and 1/2 head of garlic in a pressure cooker. Add enough water to cover beans by 2 inches. Secure lid and bring up to pressure over medium heat. Reduce heat to medium low and cook for 30 minutes. Allow pressure to release naturally. Remove garlic and bouquet garni. Add 1/2 teaspoon sea salt. Stir and let beans sit for 5 minutes. Drain, reserving the liquid.

Heat a large, flameproof casserole on medium. Add confit, tomato paste, tomato, 1/4 teaspoon sea salt, pepper and 1/2 the chopped herbs. Cook 1 minute, stirring until the mixture is well incorporated. Add the drained beans and 1/2 cup of reserved bean cooking liquid. Stir gently to combine. Cook 1 more minute. Remove from the heat. Taste for seasoning.

In a small bowl, combine breadcrumbs, the rest of the chopped herbs, garlic and oil. Sprinkle the top of the beans with the breadcrumb mixture.

Bake in the oven, uncovered, for 15-20 minutes, until golden brown and crusty.

[serves 8]

Nutrition Per Serving: Calories 291, Total Fat 5g, Saturated Fat 1g, Cholesterol 0mg, Sodium 270mg, Potassium 937mg, Total Carbohydrate 47g, Dietary Fiber 16g, Protein 15g, Calcium 150mg, Iron 6mg, Zinc 2mg, Vitamin C 28mg, Vitamin A 1045 IU, Vitamin B6 .5mg, Thiamin B1 .4mg, Riboflavin B2 .2mg, Folacin 246mcg, Niacin 2mg

Chulent with Kishka

The Diet Doctor's Wife: When I was child, I was often invited to my friend Ruthy Rosenzweig's house for Sabbath lunch. It was always a great time as Ruthy is one of the funniest people I know, and her mother one of the best cooks. Everything Ruthy's mother made was stupendous. I could go on for hours about her pastries, her chicken dishes and even her coleslaw. But her chulent was extra special. Chulent is a bean, barley and beef stew cooked overnight at a very low temperature. Usually it is prepared with kishka, a yummy and extremely fatty dumpling. Believe me when I say that it tastes much better than it sounds. The memory of Mrs. Rosenzweig's chulent has inspired me to create this recipe. Mine still sticks to your ribs without all the fat and meaty bits.

Kishka

2 cups whole-grain flour (combination of barley, buckwheat and whole wheat flours)
3/4 cup onion, chopped
4 tablespoons extra virgin olive oil
1/4 teaspoon sea salt
generous pinch of freshly ground black pepper
1 teaspoon aluminum-free baking powder
1/4 cup (or more) water, to bind

Combine ingredients. Add enough water to bind the dough. Shape into a large dumpling and set aside. (For a richer dumpling, add 1 free-range egg. You will need less water.)

Chulent

2 cups white beans, soaked for 6-8 hours or quick soaked
1 1/2 cups barley, soaked for 4-8 hours
2 cups Onion Confit (page 332) or 2 large onions, sliced
4 medium turnips, peeled and halved, or 1 rutabaga, peeled and cut in large chunks
4 medium carrots, peeled and halved
1 tablespoon tomato paste, diluted in 1/4 cup water
6 cloves garlic, peeled and smashed with the side of a knife
1 tablespoon sweet paprika
1 teaspoon sea salt
1 tablespoon low sodium tamari
1/2 teaspoon freshly ground black pepper

Drain beans and barley, and set aside.

Place onion confit in a large flameproof casserole. Add beans, barley, turnips, carrots, tomato paste, garlic and seasonings. Add water to cover. Bring to a boil and simmer for 20 minutes. Place kishka in the casserole. Tightly cover and transfer to the oven. Bake at 200 F overnight (for at least 12 hours). Serve hot.

[serves 12]

Nutrition Per Serving for Kishka: Calories 117, Total Fat 5g, Saturated Fat 1g, Cholesterol 0mg, Sodium 82mg, Potassium 107mg, Total Carbohydrate 17g, Dietary Fiber 2g, Protein 3g, Calcium 32mg, Iron 1mg, Zinc 1mg, Vitamin C 1mg, Vitamin B6 .1mg, Thiamin B1 .1mg, Folacin 8mcg, Niacin 1mg

Nutrition Per Serving for Chulent: Calories 266, Total Fat 2g, Saturated Fat trace, Cholesterol 0mg, Sodium 264mg, Potassium 800mg, Total Carbohydrate 49g, Dietary Fiber 15g, Protein 13g, Calcium 100mg, Iron 4mg, Zinc 2mg, Vitamin C 13mg, Vitamin A 7150 IU, Vitamin B6 .5mg, Thiamin B1 .4mg, Riboflavin B2 .2mg, Folacin 156mcg, Niacin 2mg

Gentle White Bean Stew

The Diet Doctor's Wife: This dish is simple and tasty. You can serve it on its own or as a side dish. Garnished with slivers of fresh black truffles, this humble stew turns into a gourmet delight (see variation note at the end of the recipe).

1 1/2 cups dried navy beans, soaked 6-8 hours or quick-soaked
2 teaspoons grapeseed oil
3 large cloves garlic, chopped
1/2 medium onion, chopped
1/2 medium carrot, diced
1/2 rib celery, diced
1 teaspoon tomato paste
bouquet garni (6 sprigs parsley, 2 sprigs thyme and 1 bay leaf, tied together with string)
sea salt and freshly ground white pepper, to taste
1 tablespoon fresh parsley, chopped

Drain beans and set aside.

Heat oil in a pressure cooker on medium. Add garlic, onion, carrot, celery, tomato paste and bouquet garni. Cook until vegetables are softened, about 5 minutes. Stir in beans and cover with water by 1-2 inches. Secure lid and bring up to pressure. Lower heat and cook for 30 minutes. Allow to sit for 20 minutes, covered. Remove bouquet garni. Season with salt and pepper. Spoon beans onto 4 serving plates. Sprinkle with chopped parsley.

[serves 4]

Nutrition Per Serving: Calories 310, Total Fat 4g, Saturated Fat 1g, Cholesterol 0mg, Sodium 48mg, Potassium 1156mg, Total Carbohydrate 53g, Dietary Fiber 21g, Protein 19g, Calcium 196mg, Iron 8mg, Zinc 2mg, Vitamin C 47mg, Vitamin A 4226 IU, Vitamin B6 .4mg, Thiamin B1 .5mg, Riboflavin B2 .2mg, Folacin 344mcg, Niacin 2mg

Variation: For an elegant twist, you can garnish this dish with slivers of fresh black truffles when they are in season, or you can drizzle the top of the beans with truffle oil.

Mom's Tuna and White Bean Salad

The Diet Doctor's Wife: My mother serves this as an hors d'oeuvre whenever she has guests over. Spread on Belgium endive, lavash crackers or small rye rounds, it is a simple elegant treat.

6-ounce can white tuna, water packed, drained and flaked
2 cups cooked white beans
1/3 cup pitted black olives, coarsely chopped
1/2 red onion, sliced in thin half-moons
1/3-1/2 cup marinated artichoke hearts, rinsed and drained, cut in quarters
1/4 cup Basic Vinaigrette (page 342)

Combine ingredients.

[serves 10]

Nutrition Per Serving: Calories 122, Total Fat 5g, Saturated Fat 1g, Cholesterol 6mg, Sodium 74mg, Potassium 259mg, Total Carbohydrate 11g, Dietary Fiber 3g, Protein 8g, Calcium 39mg, Iron 2mg, Zinc 1mg, Vitamin C 1mg, Vitamin A 390 IU, Vitamin B6 .1mg, Vitamin B12 1.6mcg, Thiamin B1 .1mg, Riboflavin B2 .1mg, Folacin 31mcg, Niacin 2mg

Chickpea Salad

The Diet Doctor's Wife: When my friend Enid and I were single, we would often prepare meals together. Usually very simple fare with nice, bold flavors. This chickpea salad was one of our favorites.

2 cups cooked chickpeas
1 tablespoon fresh rosemary, chopped
1 tablespoon extra virgin olive oil
1 tablespoon freshly squeezed lemon juice
sea salt and freshly ground black pepper, to taste

Combine ingredients.

[serves 4]

Nutrition Per Serving: Calories 168, Total Fat 6g, Saturated Fat 1g, Cholesterol 0mg, Sodium 6mg, Potassium 251mg, Total Carbohydrate 23g, Dietary Fiber 3g, Protein 7g, Calcium 51mg, Iron 3mg, Zinc 1mg, Vitamin C 3mg, Vitamin A 49 IU, Vitamin B6 .1mg, Thiamin B1 .1mg, Riboflavin B2 .1mg, Folacin 142 mcg

Adzuki Beans

The Diet Doctor's Wife: Although adzuki beans are highly recommended on the macrobiotic diet for their high protein and low fat properties, they are not at the top of my list of favorites. However, the Sunflower Cafe in Ann Arbor has helped to change my tune. Their adzuki beans are sweetened with root vegetables and onions. I have tried to replicate the recipe and am very pleased with the results. Note that the beans are boiled not pressure-cooked since adzuki beans turn out a bit sweeter when you boil them. Of course, if you want to speed up cooking time, pressure-cook the beans for 30 minutes.

2 teaspoons grapeseed oil
1/2 cup onions or shallots, chopped
1 cup carrots, cubed
2 cups adzuki beans, soaked 6-8 hours in 6 cups of water
1/4 teaspoon sea salt, or more to taste

In a large heavy pot, heat oil over medium heat, and add onions and carrots. Sauté 1-3 minutes until vegetables start to release their juices. Add adzuki beans and soaking liquid. (Soaking liquid for adzuki beans can be used for cooking. This is not the case for other beans.) Bring to a boil. Cover and reduce heat to simmer. Cook for 1 hour until beans are tender. Check water level from time to time. Add sea salt to taste and simmer another 5 minutes. Allow to sit for 10 minutes before serving.

[serves 8]

Nutrition Per Serving: Calories 183, Total Fat 1g, Saturated Fat trace, Cholesterol 0mg, Sodium 67mg, Potassium 685mg, Total Carbohydrate 33g, Dietary Fiber 7g, Protein 10g, Calcium 39mg, Iron 3mg, Zinc 3mg, Vitamin C 2mg, Vitamin A 4529 IU, Vitamin B6 .2mg, Thiamin B1 .2mg, Riboflavin B2 .1mg, Folacin 310mcg, Niacin 1mg

Beans, Swiss Chard and Rice

1 cup white beans or chickpeas, soaked 6-8 hours or quick-soaked
2 teaspoons extra virgin olive oil
1 medium onion, finely chopped
2 cloves garlic, finely chopped
1/4 teaspoon red pepper flakes
3 cups Basic Vegetable Stock (page 94)
1 cup long grain brown rice
3 fresh sage leaves
1 bay leaf
1 bunch Swiss chard leaves (stems removed), chopped
sea salt and freshly ground black pepper, to taste

Drain beans and set aside.

In a pressure cooker, heat oil on medium low. Sauté onion, garlic and red pepper flakes until vegetables soften. Stir in stock, beans, rice, sage and bay leaf. Secure lid on cooker and bring mixture up to pressure over medium heat. Reduce heat to medium low and cook for 45 minutes. Run cold water over cooker to release pressure. Remove lid and add chard. Simmer for another 10 minutes. Add water or broth if necessary and cook until warmed through. Remove bay leaf and sage. Season to taste.

[serves 6]

Nutrition Per Serving: Calories 259, Total Fat 3g, Saturated Fat trace, Cholesterol 0mg, Sodium 35mg, Potassium 750mg, Total Carbohydrate 49g, Dietary Fiber 7g, Protein 11g, Calcium 98mg, Iron 4mg, Zinc 2mg, Vitamin C 4mg, Vitamin A 269 IU, Vitamin B6 .3mg, Thiamin B1 .3mg, Riboflavin B2 .1mg, Folacin 141mcg, Niacin 2mg

Connie's South Indian Lentil Burgers

The Diet Doctor's Wife: When I was living in Singapore, my friend and colleague, Connie Singham, would often invite me over for dinner. She was incredibly hospitable and such wonderful company. I particularly liked assisting her in the kitchen where she taught me a great deal about Southeast Asian cooking. Connie could whip up the most delightful meals without ever consulting a cookbook. Her lentil burgers are a fine example. I have tried to work out her recipe from memory.

vegetable oil spray
1 small onion, finely chopped
1/2 teaspoon fresh chili pepper, finely chopped
pinch of fenugreek
sea salt, to taste
6 curry leaves
2 cups cooked lentils

Coat a nonstick sauté pan with a thin film of vegetable oil spray and heat on medium. Add onion, chili pepper, fenugreek, salt and curry leaves. Sauté 1 minute and reduce heat to medium low. Cook until onion browns slightly.

Add onion mixture to the lentils. Mash together and taste for seasoning.

Form patties and either bake for 20-30 minutes at 350 degrees F, or pan fry (using oil spray) 4-5 minutes per side.

[serves 4]

Nutrition Per Serving: Calories 126, Total Fat trace, Saturated Fat trace, Cholesterol 0mg, Sodium 3mg, Potassium 410mg, Total Carbohydrate 22g, Dietary Fiber 8g, Protein 9g Calcium 24mg, Iron 3mg, Zinc 1mg, Vitamin C 4mg, Vitamin A 11 IU, Vitamin B6 .2mg, Thiamin B1 .2mg, Riboflavin B2 .1mg, Folacin 184mcg, Niacin 1mg

Prepared Vegetable Proteins

Prepared Vegetable Proteins

There are many types of prepared vegetable proteins. They are listed below:

TOFU

Tofu is a protein rich vegetarian food that is made from soaked, ground and cooked soybeans. Tofu can be boiled, steamed, baked, broiled, fried and even pickled. It comes in a variety of textures: soft, firm, extra firm, silken and dried. Tofu is available in any health food market as well as most grocery stores.

TEMPEH

Tempeh is a fermented soybean product that is high in protein. Tempeh can be prepared in a number of ways. It can be boiled, steamed, pressure-cooked, fried, baked and broiled. Tempeh is available in most health food markets.

SEITAN

Seitan or wheat meat is made from high gluten flour. Seitan is a wonderful vegetarian source of protein that is also rich in calcium and niacin. Like tofu and tempeh, seitan can be prepared in many different ways. Seitan is available in most health food markets.

OTHERS

There are many other prepared vegetable proteins that are available in the frozen food section of most health food markets as well as some grocery stores. Examples are vegetarian burgers, GimmeLean™ and tofu hotdogs.

Tofu Cheese

The Diet Doctor: The miso coating gives simple tofu a delicious cheese-like quality. Note that the serving size is small as the flavor is pretty intense.

8-ounce block tofu
1 tablespoon miso (preferably barley)
2 tablespoons hot water

Whisk together miso and hot water.

Cover block of tofu with miso puree. Place in a covered container and leave to ferment at room temperature for 24 hours.

Cut in thin slices just as you would with cheese. Scrape off miso for a less intense flavor.

[serves 8]

Nutrition Per Serving: Calories 26, Total Fat 1g, Saturated Fat trace, Cholesterol 0mg, Sodium 80mg, Potassium 38mg, Total Carbohydrate 1g, Protein 3g, Calcium 31mg, Iron 2mg, Vitamin A 26 IU, Folacin 5mcg

Eggless Salad

The Diet Doctor: I love egg salad. My mother made it all the time for us when we were kids. She slathered it on slices of whole wheat bread and added chopped raw onion. I add chopped raw onion to Gabrielle's eggless version, and I am a kid again.

1 pound firm tofu, extra water pressed out
2 teaspoons grapeseed oil
2 tablespoons shallot, minced
3 tablespoons celery, minced
1 tablespoon Dijon mustard

1 tablespoon pickle relish
1 tablespoon fresh dill, chopped
pinch of ground cayenne pepper
pinch of turmeric
sea salt, to taste

Combine all ingredients in a food processor and puree until smooth. Season to taste.

[serves 8]

Nutrition Per Serving: Calories 60, Total Fat 4g, Saturated Fat trace, Cholesterol 0mg, Sodium 46mg, Potassium 120mg, Total Carbohydrate 3g, Protein 5g, Calcium 96mg, Iron 1mg, Vitamin C 1mg, Vitamin A 334 IU, Thiamin B1 .1mg, Riboflavin B2 .6mg, Folacin 21mcg

Tofu Spread

The Diet Doctor: This is a great snack. I spread it on celery. Gabrielle puts it on rice crackers.

1 pound firm tofu, extra water pressed out
3 tablespoons shallots, minced
1 tablespoon tamari
1 tablespoon ume vinegar
1 tablespoon tahini
1-2 tablespoons fresh dill, chopped

Combine ingredients in a food processor. Puree until smooth. Taste for seasoning.

[serves 8]

Nutrition Per Serving: Calories 59, Total Fat 4g, Saturated Fat 1g, Cholesterol 0mg, Sodium 264mg, Potassium 125mg, Total Carbohydrate 3g, Protein 5g, Calcium 102mg, Iron 1mg, Zinc 1mg, Vitamin A 479 IU, Thiamin B1 .1mg, Riboflavin B2 .6mg, Folacin 22mcg

Herbed Tofu Lyonnais

The Diet Doctor's Wife: This is a vegan adaptation of a marvelous recipe by Patricia Wells. I have substituted tofu for cheese, and added a few other ingredients to give normally bland tofu a bit more zip. The end result is a hit. So much so, that my mom who is less than a fan of tofu, asked me for the recipe. Serve as a spread or dip.

12 ounces firm tofu, crumbled
1/4 cup shallots, minced
2 teaspoons garlic, minced
3 tablespoons fresh chives, chopped
3 tablespoons fresh tarragon leaves, chopped
3 tablespoons fresh parsley leaves, chopped
1/2 teaspoon fresh thyme leaves, chopped
1 tablespoon tahini
1 tablespoon tamari
sea salt and freshly ground black pepper, to taste
1 tablespoon dry white wine
1 teaspoon sherry vinegar or ume vinegar
1 teaspoon extra virgin olive oil

Place tofu, shallots, garlic, herbs, tahini and tamari in a food processor. Pulse briefly just to blend. Season to taste. Pulse a few more seconds.

Transfer tofu mixture to cheesecloth-lined mesh strainer and place strainer over a bowl. Cover and refrigerate overnight.

Remove tofu mixture from the refrigerator. Discard liquid in the bowl. Place tofu mixture in a food processor. Add the remaining ingredients. Pulse to blend. Taste for seasoning.

[serves 6]

Nutrition Per Serving: Calories 77, Total Fat 5g, Saturated Fat 1g, Cholesterol 0mg, Sodium 177mg, Potassium 167mg, Total Carbohydrate 4g, Dietary Fiber 1g, Protein 6g, Calcium 114mg, Iron 1mg, Zinc 1mg, Vitamin C 4mg, Vitamin A 1013 IU, Vitamin B6 .1mg, Thiamin B1 .1mg, Riboflavin B2 .6mg, Folacin 28mcg

Japanese Simmered Tofu

The Diet Doctor's Wife: Don't be fooled by the simplicity of this dish. The array of condiments adds just the right zing to make things interesting.

The Diet Doctor: This is my favorite thing to order in a Japanese restaurant. But I prefer Gabrielle's version. It's also good cold.

2-inch piece kombu
24 ounces firm tofu, cut into 1-inch cubes

Dipping Sauce

1 cup Japanese Stock (page 95)
1/4 cup low sodium tamari or low sodium soy sauce
2 tablespoons sake
2 tablespoons mirin

Condiments

1/4 ounce loose bonito flakes
2 scallions, finely chopped, water squeezed out
1 sheet sushi nori, crumbled
2 tablespoons fresh ginger root, grated

Pour 6 cups of water into a pot. Add kombu and bring to a boil. Add tofu and lower heat to simmer until tofu starts to float.

While the tofu is simmering, prepare the dipping sauce. Combine stock, tamari, sake and mirin. Bring to a boil and reduce heat to low.

When tofu is ready, serve it immediately with individual bowls of dipping sauce. Season dipping sauce with condiments, according to taste.

[serves 8]

Nutrition Per Serving: Calories 86, Total Fat 4g, Saturated Fat 1g, Cholesterol 1mg, Sodium 312mg, Potassium 190mg, Total Carbohydrate 4g, Dietary Fiber 1g, Protein 8g, Calcium 146mg, Iron 2mg, Zinc 1mg, Vitamin C 1mg, Vitamin A 88 IU, Vitamin B6 .1mg, Thiamin B1 .1mg, Riboflavin B2 .9mg, Folacin 36mcg

Scrambled Tofu with Spinach

The Diet Doctor: Sometimes I miss bacon and eggs. To satisfy my cravings, Gabrielle whips up Scrambled Tofu and Spinach. She substitutes chipotle pepper for the red pepper flakes to create the smoky, meaty flavor I love so much. To reduce the fat (even further), she uses low fat tofu.

2 teaspoons extra virgin olive oil
2 cloves garlic, minced
1/8 teaspoon red pepper flakes
1 bunch spinach or other greens, chopped
1 pound tofu, crumbled
2 teaspoons tamari
1 teaspoon freshly squeezed lemon juice
sea salt and freshly ground black pepper, to taste

Heat olive oil in a nonstick pan on medium. Add garlic and red pepper flakes, and sauté for 30 seconds. Add spinach and allow to wilt. Crumble tofu over the spinach. Cover pan and reduce heat to medium low. Cook for 4 minutes. Add tamari and lemon juice, and cover once again. Continue to cook for 1-2 minutes. Remove cover and mix well to incorporate. Season to taste.

[serves 4]

Nutrition Per Serving: Calories 112, Total Fat 8g, Saturated Fat 1g, Cholesterol 0mg, Sodium 182mg, Potassium 193mg, Total Carbohydrate 3g, Dietary Fiber 2g, Protein 10g, Calcium 130mg, Iron 6mg, Zinc 1mg, Vitamin C 3mg, Vitamin A 604 IU, Vitamin B6 .1mg, Thiamin B1 .1mg, Riboflavin B2 .1mg, Folacin 32mcg

Tofu Frittata

The Diet Doctor: Eighty-five percent of the calories of a traditional frittata come from saturated fat (eggs, butter and cheese). That is not the

case for this tofu frittata. It tastes great, possibly even better than an egg frittata, and has less than a tenth of the calories and fat. Plus it doesn't give me indigestion.

10 dried shitake mushrooms
5 fresh shitake mushrooms
1 stalk broccoli
vegetable oil spray
2 large cloves garlic, minced
2 shallots, minced
1 carrot, diced
1/2 cup daikon, diced
3 drops tamari
1 pound firm tofu, crumbled
1 tablespoon kuzu
1/8-1/4 teaspoon freshly ground white pepper
sea salt, to taste
1/4 teaspoon toasted sesame oil

Soak the dried mushrooms in 2-3 cups of hot water. Remove mushrooms after 1/2 hour, squeezing out excess liquid. Reserve soaking liquid.

Cut off and discard stems of both reconstituted and fresh mushrooms. Slice caps thinly. Set aside.

Strain mushroom soaking liquid to get rid of any dirt particles. Set aside.

Cut flower head off broccoli stalk. Cut flower head into small bite-size florets, and set aside. Cut a 3 to 4 inch section of the stalk and peel away fibrous outer layer. Slice the inner tender portion into 1/8-inch rounds, and set aside.

Spray a thin coat of oil in a wok over medium heat. Add half the garlic and shallots. Sauté for 30 seconds. Add broccoli (florets and stalk slices), carrot and daikon. Sauté for 1 minute. Add the mushroom liquid and a pinch of sea salt. Boil for 1-2 minutes. Remove vegetables from the wok with a slotted spoon and set aside. Pour out cooking liquid and set aside as well.

Rinse off wok and dry it. Spray a thin coat of oil in the wok. Over medium heat, warm remaining garlic and shallots, and sauté for 30 seconds. Add the mushroom slices. Sauté for 30 seconds until mushrooms begin to sweat. Add a few drops of tamari and sauté a few seconds. Add a couple of tablespoons of mushroom liquid and cook until liquid evaporates. Add tofu and a few drops of tamari. Sauté to warm tofu. Add 1/3 cup more of mushroom liquid. Cover and continue cooking for 1 minute.

Meanwhile, combine kuzu with 3 tablespoons mushroom liquid (or water) and whisk together. Pour kuzu liquid into tofu-mushroom mixture. Add the broccoli-carrot-daikon mixture. Season with sea salt, white pepper and toasted sesame oil. Stir to incorporate. Cover and cook for 1 minute. Taste for seasoning.

[serves 4]

Nutrition Per Serving: Calories 199, Total Fat 6g, Saturated Fat 1g, Cholesterol 0mg, Sodium 95mg, Potassium 944mg, Total Carbohydrate 27g, Dietary Fiber 8g, Protein 15g, Calcium 206mg, Iron 8mg, Zinc 3mg, Vitamin C 147mg, Vitamin A 10344 IU, Vitamin B6 .5mg, Thiamin B1 .2mg, Riboflavin B2 .4mg, Folacin 154mcg, Niacin 3mg

Chilled Somen with Sweet and Spicy Tofu and Baby Bok Choy

The Diet Doctor's Wife: I love Japanese-style chilled noodle dishes, especially in the summer. This one makes a terrific lunch that is both satisfying and light.

The Diet Doctor: This dish is relatively high in sodium. Make sure to keep your salt intake low for the rest of the day, and drink a lot of water.

1/4 cup low sodium tamari
1/4 cup mirin

1/2 teaspoon toasted sesame oil
1 tablespoon fresh ginger root, grated
1/4 teaspoon fresh hot chili pepper, minced
1 clove garlic, minced
12 ounces firm tofu, cut in 1/4-inch strips
8 ounces dried somen
4 baby bok choy or 4 cups mixed chopped greens
vegetable oil spray
1 tablespoon kuzu
chopped scallion and coriander leaves, for garnish

In a medium bowl, whisk together tamari, mirin and toasted sesame oil. Roll grated ginger pulp into a ball and squeeze juice into the bowl. Discard pulp. Stir in chili and garlic. Add tofu strips. Marinate 1 hour. Drain and reserve liquid.

While tofu is marinating, cook somen in a large pot of boiling water, according to the directions on the packet. Stir in greens at the last minute of cooking. Drain somen and greens, and transfer to a bowl of ice water. When cold, drain again.

Heat vegetable oil spray in a nonstick pan or wok and sauté tofu strips 2-3 minutes per side. Set aside.

Heat reserved marinade in a small saucepan until it comes to a gentle simmer. Stir kuzu in 3 tablespoons of water until smooth. Add kuzu mixture to the simmering marinade. Stir until thickened. Remove from heat.

Combine, tofu, noodles, greens and warmed marinade. Garnish with chopped scallions and coriander.

[serves 4]

Nutrition Per Serving: Calories 330, Total Fat 6g, Saturated Fat 1g, Cholesterol 0mg, *Sodium 735mg, Potassium 491mg, Total Carbohydrate 49g, Dietary Fiber 4g, Protein 17g, Calcium 237mg, Iron 4mg, Zinc 2mg, Vitamin C 32mg, Vitamin A 2108 IU, Vitamin B6 .2mg, Thiamin B1 .3mg, Riboflavin B2 1mg, Folacin 77mcg, Niacin 3mg

*Note: This is a high sodium dish. Be sure to watch your sodium intake for the rest of the day, and drink lots of water.

Tofu and Vegetable Cobbler

16 dried shitake mushrooms, soaked in 2 cups hot water for 1/2 hour
1 cup Basic Vegetable Stock (page 94)
2 tablespoons tamari
1 tablespoon extra virgin olive oil
2 tablespoons dry sherry
sea salt and freshly ground black pepper, to taste
1 cup onion, coarsely chopped
8 cloves garlic
2 large carrots, cut in 1-inch chunks
2 cups cabbage, chopped
3 sprigs thyme
2 bay leaves
1 pound firm tofu, cut in 1-inch cubes
1 tablespoon whole wheat flour
1/4 cup fresh parsley, finely chopped

Preheat oven to 400 F. Remove mushrooms from soaking water and squeeze out excess liquid. Reserve the liquid. Remove mushroom stems and discard. Cut caps in half and set aside.

Strain mushroom soaking liquid to remove any dirt particles. Add enough vegetable stock to the strained mushroom soaking liquid to create a volume of 2 1/2 cups. Set aside.

In a small bowl, combine tamari, oil, sherry, salt and pepper. Set aside.

Put mushrooms, onions, garlic, carrots, cabbage, thyme and bay leaves in a medium-size roasting pan. Add tamari mixture and toss to incorporate. Roast for 20 minutes, stirring occasionally. Add tofu cubes. Stir in flour. Add stock and parsley. Continue roasting for 10 minutes. Remove bay leaves and thyme. Remove pan and lower heat to 375 F. Place a rack on the top shelf of the oven. Prepare the cobbler topping.

Cobbler Topping

1 cup unbleached white flour
1/2 cup whole wheat pastry flour
1 1/2 teaspoons aluminum-free baking powder
1/2 cup fresh parsley, finely chopped
1/4 teaspoon sea salt
pinch of freshly ground black pepper
3/4 cup water
1/2 cup applesauce or apple juice
2 tablespoons extra virgin olive oil
1 teaspoon balsamic vinegar

To make cobbler topping, combine dry ingredients. In a separate bowl, combine wet ingredients. Add wet ingredients to dry ingredients. Stir to combine.

Spoon batter over the tofu and vegetable mixture. It is okay if there are spaces. They will fill in as the cobbler cooks. Bake on the top shelf for 35 minutes. Test for doneness with a toothpick.

[serves 6]

Nutrition Per Serving: Calories 318, *Total Fat 11g, Saturated Fat 1g, Cholesterol 0mg, Sodium 451mg, Potassium 616mg, Total Carbohydrate 46g, Dietary Fiber 6g, Protein 12g, Calcium 243mg, Iron 4mg, Zinc 2mg, Vitamin C 24mg, Vitamin A 7205 IU, Vitamin B6 .3mg, Thiamin B1 .4mg, Riboflavin B2 1.1mg, Folacin 80mcg, Niacin 4mg

*Note: To reduce fat, use low fat tofu.

Indonesian Simmered Tofu with Lemongrass and Coconut Milk

The Diet Doctor's Wife: Although reduced fat coconut milk is used in this recipe, the fat content may still be higher than you want. If you are really concerned, cut the coconut milk with water or stock. You will still get the desired effect with less guilt.

2 teaspoons grapeseed oil or other light vegetable oil
1 fresh red chili pepper, sliced in thin rounds
2 teaspoons fresh ginger root, minced
1 large onion, sliced in 1/8-inch thick half-moons
2 stalks lemongrass, lower 3 inches, each chopped in 3 pieces
1/2 teaspoon turmeric
1 cup reduced fat coconut milk
1/2 cup water
1/2 teaspoon sea salt
1/2 pound tofu, cut in 1 1/2-inch cubes
1 large carrot, thinly sliced
2 cups white cabbage, coarsely chopped
1-2 cups green beans, trimmed and cut in half
3 scallions, cut in 1-inch pieces

Heat oil in a saucepan over medium heat. Add chili pepper, ginger, onions, lemongrass and turmeric. Sauté for 1 minute. Add coconut milk, water and salt. Bring to a boil. Lower heat to simmer and add tofu, carrots, cabbage and beans. Cover saucepan and cook until vegetables are tender. Add scallions and cook for 1 more minute. Taste for seasoning. Remove lemongrass pieces.

[serves 4]

Nutrition Per Serving: Calories 143, Total Fat 8g, Saturated Fat 1g, Cholesterol 0mg, Sodium 257mg, Potassium 425mg, Total Carbohydrate 14g, Dietary Fiber 4g, Protein 7g, Calcium 140mg, Iron 2mg, Zinc 1mg, Vitamin C 49mg, Vitamin A 5428 IU, Vitamin B6 .2mg, Thiamin B1 .1mg, Riboflavin B2 .6mg, Folacin 62mcg, Niacin 1mg

Szechwan Seitan

The Diet Doctor: I used to order Szechwan chicken every time I went to a Chinese restaurant. But I don't anymore. There is clearly no need. Gabrielle's vegetarian version is so good, I don't even miss the chicken.

Marinade

2 tablespoons low sodium tamari or low sodium soy sauce
2 tablespoons mirin or dry sherry
1 tablespoon brown rice syrup or maple syrup
1 teaspoon arrowroot powder
1 pound seitan, sliced or 1 pound tofu, cubed

Whisk together the first 4 ingredients. Add seitan and marinate for 1-24 hours in the refrigerator. Drain.

Sauce

1 tablespoon low sodium tamari or low sodium soy sauce
1 teaspoon brown rice vinegar
2/3 cup Basic Vegetable Stock (page 94) or water
2 tablespoons freshly squeezed orange juice
1 tablespoon brown rice syrup or maple syrup
1/2 teaspoon arrowroot powder

Whisk ingredients together and set aside.

Stir-fry

vegetable oil spray
1 tablespoon fresh ginger root, minced
1 1/2 tablespoons garlic, minced
2 tablespoons scallions, minced
1/2-1 teaspoon fresh hot chili pepper, minced or 1/4-1/2 teaspoon hot chili paste
zest of 1 orange
1 onion, sliced in half-moons
1 cup mushrooms, sliced
1 carrot, sliced on the diagonal and halved
2 cups broccoli florets or snow peas
1/2 red bell pepper, cut in strips (optional)

freshly ground white pepper, to taste
*1/4 cup unsalted dry-roasted peanuts or cashews (optional)

Warm oil in a wok over medium heat. If you use a nonstick wok, you will need less oil. Sauté seitan to lightly brown. Remove and set aside. Add ginger, garlic, scallions, chili pepper and zest to the wok, and warm for 30 seconds. Add onions and mushrooms, and sauté 3 minutes until onions are translucent. If the pan gets too dry, add a splash of water. Add carrots, broccoli, red bell pepper (if using) and browned seitan. Sauté about 1 minute. Add sauce and a generous amount of freshly ground white pepper. Stir to combine and cover. Cook 3-5 minutes. Serve on its own, or over rice or noodles. Garnish with unsalted dry-roasted peanuts, if desired.

[serves 4]

Nutrition Per Serving: Calories 196, Total Fat trace, Saturated Fat trace, Cholesterol 0mg, Sodium 474mg, Potassium 359mg, Total Carbohydrate 28g, Dietary Fiber 11g, Protein 19g, Calcium 92mg, Iron 3mg, Vitamin C 47mg, Vitamin A 6199 IU, Vitamin B6 .2mg, Riboflavin B2 .2mg, Folacin 47 mcg, Niacin 2mg

*Note: If you garnish this dish with nuts, the total fat goes up to 4-5g and the saturated fat goes up to 1g.

Bisteeya

The Diet Doctor's Wife: Bisteeya is a heavenly Moroccan pastry traditionally filled with pigeon meat and spiced with cinnamon-sugar. My interest in this sweet and savory pastry was inspired by a wonderful afternoon I spent in Paris a few years ago. While Bill was exploring a magic shop that he had read about, I seized the opportunity to rest my feet at a nearby café. Thankfully, I didn't have to look too hard. Right across the street was a charming Moroccan restaurant that was only serving drinks as it was late in the afternoon and still hours before dinner. I sat down and ordered a glass of Sauternes. As I was sipping my drink, the cook and one of the waiters came out of the kitchen carrying large mixing bowls and covered trays, which they spread across the table next to me. The cook sat down and proceeded to prepare the bisteeya for the evening meal. It was fascinating watching her handle the paper thin pastry leaves, assembling the bisteeya in such seamless motion. She made it look so easy that I vowed to try a vegetarian version at home.

The Diet Doctor: When I was a medical student living in San Francisco, a favorite treat was to go to one of the six Moroccan restaurants in the Bay area and order chicken bisteeya. The chicken was wrapped in steaming filo dough, dusted with powdered sugar and cinnamon. I ate it with my fingers, as is the custom, and loved every mouthful. Gabrielle has recreated a healthier, vegetarian version that is truly awesome.

vegetable oil spray
*2 tablespoons Clarified Butter (page 346) or ghee
1 small onion, finely chopped
1/2 pound seitan, chopped in small pieces
1 1/2 cups water or Basic Vegetable Stock (page 94)
2 cloves garlic, minced
1/3 cup fresh flat-leaf parsley leaves, finely chopped
pinch of saffron threads
1/8 teaspoon ground turmeric
1/4 teaspoon sea salt
1/8 teaspoon freshly ground black pepper
1 tablespoon fresh ginger root, grated
1 cinnamon stick
4 cups chopped Swiss chard leaves, stems removed
**1/2 cup whole almonds, lightly toasted
1/2 teaspoon ground cinnamon, plus extra for dusting
2 tablespoons confectioner's sugar, plus extra for dusting
1/4 cup dried currants
1 tablespoon freshly squeezed lemon juice
4 sheets whole wheat filo dough, thawed

Preheat oven to 375 F. Grease an 8-inch round baking pan with vegetable oil spray.

Coat the bottom of a large saucepan with vegetable oil spray. Add 1/4 teaspoon of Clarified Butter and set heat at medium low. Add the onions and cook until they begin to brown, 8 to 10 minutes. Add seitan, water, garlic, parsley, saffron, turmeric, salt, pepper, ginger and cinnamon stick. Cover and bring to a boil. Reduce the heat and simmer for 10 minutes. Add chard and simmer for another 5 minutes.

While the seitan mixture is cooking, place half the toasted almonds in a food processor and pulse until coarsely ground. Combine ground almonds with ground cinnamon and confectioner's sugar. Set aside. Coarsely chop the remaining almonds and set aside.

Uncover the seitan and chard mixture. Most of the liquid should be absorbed. Add the currants and lemon juice. Cook, stirring, another 2 to 3 minutes. Drain mixture and place in a bowl. Stir in chopped almonds and set aside.

Melt the rest of the Clarified Butter. Place 1 sheet of filo on a dry surface, and keep the remaining sheets covered with a clean, slightly damp towel. Brush the 1 sheet lightly with melted Clarified Butter and place in cake pan. Some of the dough will hang over the sides of the pan. Repeat the same process with the 3 other sheets, alternating the way the sheets are arranged so that there is equal overhang of dough all the way around the cake pan. Spread seitan mixture over the filo sheets. Sprinkle almond, sugar and cinnamon mixture on top. Fold the overhanging flaps of filo over the top of the filling to completely cover. Brush the top of the pastry with melted Clarified Butter.

Bake until the filo is golden, 30-35 minutes. Remove the bisteeya from the pan right away. Sprinkle the top with ground cinnamon and confectioner's sugar. Serve warm.

[serves 8]

Nutrition Per Serving: Calories 200, Total Fat 11g, Saturated Fat 3g, Cholesterol 9mg, Sodium 130mg, Potassium 308mg, Total Carbohydrate 19g, Dietary Fiber 6g, Protein 9g, Calcium 93mg, Iron 3mg, Zinc 1mg, Vitamin C 12mg, Vitamin A 876 IU, Vitamin B6 .1mg, Riboflavin B2 .1mg, Folacin 16mcg, Niacin 1mg

*Note 1: You may substitute the clarified butter with grapeseed oil or any other light vegetable oil.

**Note 2: To lightly toast almonds, place almonds on a cookie sheet and bake for 8 minutes at 350 degrees F.

Seitan Chow Mein

The Diet Doctor: Every Thursday evening, my father would come home from work with Chinese take-out from Chungs of downtown Detroit. We'd break out the chopsticks and feast on egg rolls, egg foo yung, and chicken chow mein. The chicken chow mein was my favorite. But these days I don't touch the stuff. Fortunately, Gabrielle's Seitan Chow Mein allows me to enjoy a stroll down Memory Lane without suffering the gastric consequences.

5 dried shitake mushrooms, soaked for 1/2 hour in hot water
1 onion, sliced in thin half-moons
1/2 pound seitan, cubed
1 cup celery, sliced diagonally
1 carrot, sliced diagonally and then halved lengthwise
1 cup Chinese cabbage, shredded
2 kale leaves, sliced in ribbons
2 tablespoons kuzu
1 tablespoon soy sauce
1 tablespoon fresh ginger root, grated
1 teaspoon fresh hot chili pepper, thinly sliced (optional)
sea salt to taste
1 pound noodles, cooked and drained
2 teaspoons peanut oil or grapeseed oil

Remove shitake mushrooms from soaking liquid, squeezing out excess liquid. Reserve soaking liquid and set aside. Remove mushroom stems and discard. Slice mushroom caps. Set aside.

Pour reserved soaking liquid through a mesh strainer lined with cheesecloth. Add water to the strained shitake broth to yield 4 cups. Bring the 4 cups of liquid to a boil. Add onion and sliced mushrooms. Reduce heat to low and simmer 7 minutes.

Add seitan and bring back to a boil. Reduce heat and simmer 5 minutes. Add celery, carrots, cabbage and kale. Dissolve kuzu in 1/3 cup of the simmering broth and then stir back into the vegetable mixture. Add soy sauce. Squeeze the grated ginger over the pot to extract juice. Discard ginger pulp. Simmer vegetable mixture until thickened, about 10 minutes.

Heat peanut oil in a frying pan. Sauté noodles until lightly coated with oil.

Place noodles in small serving bowls and cover with the seitan mixture.

[serves 4]

Nutrition Per Serving: Calories 313, Total Fat 3g, Saturated Fat 1g, Cholesterol 0 mg, Sodium 315mg, Potassium 468mg, Total Carbohydrate 56g, Dietary Fiber 9g, Protein 16g, Calcium 101mg, Iron 4mg, Zinc 1mg, Vitamin C 37mg, Vitamin A 10,641 IU, Vitamin B6 .3mg, Thiamin B1.1mg, Riboflavin B2 .4mg, Folacin 122mcg, Niacin 3mg

Cantaloupe Stuffed with Seitan Salad

The Diet Doctor: About fifteen years ago, I was invited to lunch at a trendy restaurant on Capital Hill with a seriously bizarre menu. I decided on the chicken salad, thinking it was the safest thing to order . But I was wrong. What came to the table was deep fried chicken served on top of iceberg lettuce. I took one heavenly bite, but couldn't bring myself to take another. I've never been able to do too much damage when it comes to deep fried food. The calorie counter in my head starts screaming and I just stop eating. Besides, who needs all that saturated fat. Thankfully, Gabrielle has come up with a very tasty and much healthier alternative.

whole wheat pastry flour, for dredging
sea salt and freshly ground white pepper, to taste
1/2 pound seitan, sliced in bite-size pieces
vegetable oil spray
1/4 cup sliced toasted almonds
1 rib celery, chopped
1/2 cup grapes, halved and seeded
2 cantaloupes, halved and seeded
1/4 cup Sweet Sesame Vinaigrette (page 345)

Season 1/2 cup of flour with a pinch of sea salt and ground white pepper. Dredge seitan in flour mixture.

Heat a nonstick pan and coat with vegetable oil spray. Sauté seitan pieces until they are browned, 2-3 minutes per side. Remove seitan pieces from the pan and pat with paper towels to remove excess oil.

Combine seitan pieces, almonds, celery and grapes in a bowl. Toss with vinaigrette. Divide seitan mixture in four and stuff cantaloupe halves.

[serves 4]

Nutrition Per Serving: Calories 315, Total Fat 12g, Saturated Fat 2g, Cholesterol 0mg, Sodium 61mg, Potassium 1033mg, Total Carbohydrate 41g, Dietary Fiber 8g, Protein 14g, Calcium 113mg, Iron 3mg, Zinc 1mg, Vitamin C 118mg, Vitamin A 8924 IU, Vitamin B6 .3mg, Thiamin B1 1.1mg, Riboflavin B2 .1mg, Folacin 63mcg, Niacin 2mg

Seitan Stew

The Diet Doctor: When I was a kid, my mother would make beef stew and serve it in ceramic pots. There were big chunks of beef, carrots and potatoes in a savory sauce. Gabrielle makes a vegetarian version that I like just as much. I don't even miss the ceramic pot.

2 teaspoons extra virgin olive oil
2 cups shallots or onion, chopped
1 large clove garlic, minced
10 dried shitake mushrooms, reconstituted in 3 cups hot water
1 tablespoon fresh thyme, finely chopped
1 tablespoon fresh rosemary, finely chopped
1 tablespoon fresh tarragon, finely chopped
1 teaspoon fresh sage, finely chopped
2 bay leaves
2 cups dry red wine
2 tablespoons sun-dried tomato paste
1 tablespoon Dijon mustard
1 turnip, peeled and cut in 1-inch cubes

2 parsnips, peeled and cut in 1/2-inch cubes
2 carrots, peeled and cut in 1/2-inch cubes
1 celery root, peeled and cut in 1/2–inch cubes
1 cup kabocha or buttercup squash, seeded and cut in 1-inch cubes
1 pound seitan, cut in 1-inch cubes
1/2 teaspoon freshly ground black pepper
1 tablespoon tamari
2 tablespoons kuzu, dissolved in 1/4 cup water
sea salt, to taste
chopped fresh parsley, for garnish

In a large saucepan, heat oil on medium low. Sauté shallots and garlic until lightly browned, about 5 minutes.

Remove mushroom stems and discard. Quarter mushroom caps and add them with the herbs to the shallots and garlic. Sauté for 2 minutes. Add remaining ingredients except the kuzu mixture and salt. Bring stew to a boil and lower heat to simmer for 30 minutes. Stir in kuzu mixture and continue cooking for 5 minutes. Season to taste. Garnish with parsley.

[serves 8]

Nutrition Per Serving: Calories 238, Total Fat 2g, Saturated Fat trace, Cholesterol 0mg, Sodium 228mg, Potassium 678mg, Total Carbohydrate 39g, Dietary Fiber 9g, Protein 11g, Calcium 91mg, Iron 2mg, Zinc 1mg, Vitamin C 21mg, Vitamin A 10691 IU, Vitamin B6 .3mg, Thiamin B1 .1mg, Riboflavin B2 .1mg, Folacin 73mcg, Niacin 2mg

Seitan Stew with Tahini Onion Sauce

The Diet Doctor: The tahini sauce adds richness to this simple seitan preparation.

light vegetable oil spray
1 pound seitan, cut in bite-size pieces
2 portabella mushroom caps, sliced 1/2-inch thick
1 onion, sliced in half-moons

1 medium carrot, cut in chunks
1 small parsnip, cut in chunks
1 medium turnip, cut in chunks or 1/2 small cauliflower, cut in florets
4 cups Basic Vegetable Stock (page 94)
couple handfuls coarsely chopped greens (collards, kale)
2 tablespoons kuzu
2 tablespoons low sodium tamari or low sodium soy sauce
sea salt and freshly ground pepper, to taste

Coat a large nonstick pot or wok with vegetable oil spray (or use a brush to lightly coat with oil). Sauté seitan over medium heat until lightly brown on both sides, 1-2 minutes per side. Remove from pan.

Respray pan if necessary and add mushroom slices. Sauté until juices are released and almost completely evaporated. Add a few drops of tamari and cook until liquid is almost completely evaporated.

Add seitan, onions, carrot, parsnip, turnip and stock to the mushrooms. Bring to a boil. Reduce heat and simmer 5 minutes. Add greens. Dissolve kuzu in 1/3 cup of the simmering broth and then pour back into the vegetable mixture. Stir to incorporate. Add tamari. Stir and simmer another 10 minutes. Season to taste.

Sauce

3 tablespoons tahini
1 tablespoon low sodium tamari
1 cup water
1 shallot, minced

While the stew is simmering, prepare the sauce. Combine ingredients in a small saucepan. Slowly bring to a boil, stirring occasionally. Reduce heat to low and stir mixture until a creamy pourable consistency is achieved (1-2 minutes). Do not overcook or sauce will separate.

Serve stew with tahini sauce drizzled on top. This stew goes well with rice or noodles.

[serves 4]

Nutrition Per Serving: Calories 320, Total Fat 7g, Saturated Fat 1g, Cholesterol 0mg, Sodium 528mg, Potassium 770mg, Total Carbohydrate 46g, Dietary Fiber 15g, Protein 22g, Calcium 170mg, Iron 4mg, Zinc 2mg, Vitamin C 29mg, Vitamin A 6071 IU, Vitamin B6 .3mg, Thiamin B1 .3mg, Riboflavin .5mg, Folacin 110mcg, Niacin 5mg

Seitan Paprikash

The Diet Doctor: My Hungarian grandmother loved to make chicken paprikash. She grew her own peppers, ground her own paprika, and loaded the dish with onions and chicken fat. Those were the days. You couldn't get up from the table after a plateful. Gabrielle's version is much lighter, more carefully prepared, and in my opinion, far better tasting. I'm half Hungarian, so I should know.

1 pound seitan, cut in thin slices
1/8 teaspoon sea salt
1/2 cup whole wheat pastry flour, for dredging
vegetable oil spray
1 medium onion, sliced in thin half-moons
2 cloves garlic, minced
1 1/2 tablespoons sweet Hungarian paprika
1 green pepper, cut in strips
1/3 cup tomato puree
1/2 cup Basic Vegetable Stock (page 94)
sea salt and freshly ground black pepper, to taste

Season seitan with salt and then dredge with flour. Coat a nonstick pan lightly with vegetable oil spray. Sauté seitan slices 2-3 minutes a side, just to brown a bit. Remove seitan from the pan.

In the same pan, heat oil spray over medium heat. Sauté onion and garlic until onions get translucent, about 3 minutes. Add paprika and stir until onions and garlic are evenly coated. Add seitan pieces and tomato puree. Stir to coat. Top with green pepper strips.

Add stock and bring to a boil. Cover and lower heat to a gentle simmer and cook for 10 minutes. Season to taste. Simmer 3-4 minutes longer.

[serves 4]

Nutrition Per Serving: Calories 195, Total Fat 1g, Saturated Fat trace, Cholesterol 0mg, Sodium 207mg, Potassium 312mg, Total Carbohydrate 29g, Dietary Fiber 12g, Protein 20g, Calcium 73mg, Iron 3mg, Zinc 1mg, Vitamin C 33mg, Vitamin A 2022 IU, Vitamin B6 .2 mg, Thiamin B1 .1mg, Riboflavin B2 .1 mg, Folacin 21mcg, Niacin 2mg

Note: This dish can also be made with tofu, tempeh, soymeat or fish.

Basic Tempeh

The Diet Doctor's Wife: I always have a container of Basic Tempeh in my fridge or freezer. The slow cooking and spicing make ordinary tempeh much more appetizing. Basic Tempeh is ready to use in any recipe. You can grill it, put it in a stir-fry or a stew. The possibilities are endless.

The Diet Doctor: Although the consistency of tempeh is like chopped meat, if left unadulterated, it has a slightly sour, earthy taste that I don't particularly care for. Gabrielle has found a way to prepare tempeh to eliminate that unpleasant taste so the great texture and heartiness shines through. Don't be alarmed by the amount of tamari used. Most of it is not absorbed in the cooking process.

2 pounds tempeh

Marinade

1 cup red wine
3 cups Basic Vegetable Stock (page 94) or water
1 cup apple juice
1/2 cup low sodium tamari
4 cloves garlic, minced

1 tablespoon Dijon mustard
pinch of nutmeg
pinch of red pepper flakes (optional)
5 fresh sage leaves
1 large sprig fresh thyme

Preheat oven to 350 F. Cut tempeh into 4-ounce servings and set aside.

Whisk together all the ingredients of the marinade except for the sage and thyme. Place tempeh in a large baking dish and cover with marinade. Add sage and thyme. Bake for 1 1/2 hours. Basic Tempeh can be refrigerated for up to 1 week or frozen for up to 3 months.

[serves 8]

Nutrition Per Serving: Calories 249, Total Fat 9g, Saturated Fat 1g, Cholesterol 0g, Sodium 241mg, Potassium 464mg, Carbohydrate 23g, Protein 22g, Calcium 123mg, Iron 3mg, Zinc 2mg, Vitamin A 803 IU, Vitamin B6 .4mg, Vitamin B2 1.1mcg, Thiamin B1 .2mg, Riboflavin B2 .1mg, Folacin 62mcg, Niacin 6mg

Korean Style Barbecued Tempeh

The Diet Doctor: I used to love barbecued chicken, and worried that my days of enjoying it were gone for good. This recipe has allayed my fears.

Marinade

2 tablespoons low sodium tamari
1 teaspoon toasted sesame oil
1 tablespoon crushed garlic
1 teaspoon fresh ginger root, minced
2 tablespoons maple syrup
2 tablespoons freshly squeezed orange juice
pinch of freshly ground black pepper

8 ounces tempeh, thinly sliced
vegetable oil spray

Whisk together first 7 ingredients and pour over tempeh slices. Marinate for at least 3 hours.

Drain and reserve marinade. Heat wok, coating with vegetable oil spray. Brown tempeh, 1-2 minutes per side. Resist the temptation to keep spraying with oil. If the wok gets too dry, add a bit of leftover marinade or water instead. Remember, less oil spray is required if using a nonstick wok.

Dipping Sauce

1 teaspoon garlic, crushed
1/2 teaspoon hot pepper paste
1 tablespoon mirin
1/2 teaspoon toasted sesame oil
2 tablespoons water
2 tablespoons low sodium tamari
1 teaspoon Sesame Salt (page 327)
1 tablespoon scallion, finely chopped

To prepare the dipping sauce, combine first seven ingredients in a small sauce pan and bring to a slow simmer. Remove from heat and add chopped scallion to garnish.

Serve tempeh with dipping sauce on the side.

This dish is lovely served with brown rice and Spicy Korean Cucumber Pickle (page 283).

[serves 3]

Nutrition Per Serving: Calories 238, Total Fat 8g, Saturated Fat 1g, Cholesterol 0g, *Sodium 824mg, Potassium 395mg, Total Carbohydrate 27g, Protein 16g, Calcium 101mg, Iron 2mg, Zinc 2mg, Vitamin C 7mg, Vitamin A 547 IU, Vitamin B6 .3mg, Vitamin B12 .8mcg, Thiamin B1 .1mg, Riboflavin B2 .1mg, Folacin 50mcg, Niacin 4mg

*Note: This dish has a relatively high sodium content. Be sure to watch sodium intake for the rest of the day and drink a lot of water.

Barbecued Tempeh

The Diet Doctor: Although lower in fat and calories than its chicken-and-ribs counterpart, I put Barbecued Tempeh in the junk food category. The reason is that the sauce is made from bottled preparations that are sweeter and saltier than what we recommend for the daily diet. But once in a while, Barbecued Tempeh is a healthy way to satisfy your cravings for a finger-licking-good treat.

2/3 cup hoisin sauce
3 tablespoons sake
3 tablespoons low sodium tamari
3 tablespoons ketchup
2 tablespoons maple syrup
1 tablespoon garlic, minced
1 pound tempeh, cut in 1/2-inch strips

To make the barbecue sauce, combine the first 6 ingredients. Place 1/2 cup of sauce in a large bowl. Save the rest for basting.

Add tempeh pieces to the sauce in the bowl and toss to coat. Cover and marinate in the refrigerator overnight.

Preheat oven to 400 F.

Pour tempeh mixture in a baking dish. Bake for 20 minutes, turning and basting occasionally.

[serves 4]

Nutrition Per Serving: Calories 382, Total Fat 10g, Saturated Fat 2g, Cholesterol 1g, *Sodium 1281mg, Potassium 577mg, Total Carbohydrate 50g, Dietary Fiber 1g, Protein 24g, Calcium 138mg, Iron 3mg, Zinc 2mg, Vitamin C 3mg, Vitamin A 897 IU, Vitamin B6 .4mg, Vitamin B12 1.1mcg, Thiamin B1 .2mg, Riboflavin B2 .2mg, Folacin 73mcg, Niacin 6mg

*Note: This is a very high sodium dish. Keep your sodium intake very low for the rest of the day and drink a lot of water.

Mediterranean Tempeh Stew

vegetable oil spray
1 red onion, minced
2 cloves garlic, minced
1/2 pound cremini mushrooms, thinly sliced
1 cup dry red wine
1 pound Basic Tempeh (page 231), crumbled
1 tablespoon fresh rosemary, minced
2 tablespoons fresh parsley, minced
1 cinnamon stick
pinch of freshly grated nutmeg
1/2 teaspoon ground cumin
1 bay leaf
sea salt and freshly ground black pepper, to taste
1 cup tomato puree

Coat the cooking surface of a large saucepan with vegetable oil spray. Heat saucepan on medium low and sauté onions for 2-3 minutes. Add garlic and mushrooms and sauté until mushrooms release their juices, another 3-4 minutes. Add wine. Bring to a boil and reduce heat to simmer for 10 minutes. Add tempeh, rosemary, parsley, cinnamon, nutmeg, cumin, bay leaf, salt, pepper and tomato puree. Bring to a boil, then lower heat to simmer. Cover and cook for 20 minutes. Remove cinnamon stick and bay leaf.

[serves 4]

Nutrition Per Serving: Calories 390, Total Fat 10g, Saturated Fat trace, Cholesterol 0mg, Sodium 299mg, Potassium 620mg, Total Carbohydrate 42g, Dietary Fiber 10g, Protein 27g, Calcium 75mg, Iron 3mg, Zinc 1mg, Vitamin C 14mg, Vitamin A 920 IU, Vitamin B6 .2mg, Thiamin B1 .1mg, Riboflavin B2 .3mg, Folacin 29mcg, Niacin 4mg

Variation: Pour stew into a baking dish and drizzle with Tahini Sauce (page 340). Add 1 tablespoon of dry roasted pine nuts if desired. Bake for 10 minutes at 400 F.

Chili Con Soy

The Diet Doctor: I used to live on Wendy's Chili. At least once a week, I'd pick up a large cup or two, and inhale it on the way home from the office. I loved the stuff so much that I asked Gabrielle to come up with a vegetarian version. She puts it in a thermos for me. I'm such a lucky guy.

2 teaspoons grapeseed oil
1 large onion, minced
2 cloves garlic, minced
1 pound GimmeLean™ or seitan or combination, cut in 1-inch cubes
3 cups water
14-ounce can whole peeled tomatoes
1/2 teaspoon celery seed
1/4 teaspoon ground cayenne pepper
1 teaspoon ground cumin
1 small bay leaf
2 tablespoons chili powder
1/8 teaspoon dried basil
sea salt, to taste
2 cups cooked red beans, drained

Heat oil in a stewpot. Add onion and garlic, and sauté until golden brown. Add GimmeLean™ or seitan and cook until lightly browned. Add water, tomatoes and seasonings. Bring to a boil. Reduce heat and gently simmer, uncovered, about 3 hours or until sauce is as thick as desired. Just before serving, add beans and cook until warmed through.

[serves 6]

Nutrition Per Serving: Calories 213, Total Fat 2g, Saturated Fat trace, Cholesterol 0mg, Sodium 446mg, Potassium 476mg, Total Carbohydrate 31g, Dietary Fiber 7g, Protein 18g, Calcium 109mg, Iron 5mg, Zinc 1mg, Vitamin C 16mg, Vitamin 1306 IU, Vitamin B6 .2mg, Thiamin B1 .1mg, Riboflavin B2 .1mg, Folacin 88mcg, Niacin 1mg

Goulash

The Diet Doctor: I remember my grandmother's goulash very well. It was loaded with big chunks of fatty beef, in a tomato sauce so thick and rich you could use it to pour concrete. I had to hibernate for a week after eating it. Gabrielle's version is much lighter of course. And it doesn't put me to sleep.

2 teaspoons grapeseed oil
1 large onion, coarsely chopped
1 tablespoon sweet paprika
1 pound GimmeLean$_{TM}$ or seitan, cut in 1-inch cubes
sea salt, to taste
1/4 cup tomato paste
1 cup water

In a heavy 2-quart saucepan, heat oil on medium. Add onions and sauté 5 minutes. Add paprika and GimmeLean$_{TM}$ or seitan, and sauté 1-2 minutes. Add remaining ingredients, and stir to combine. Bring to a boil. Reduce heat and simmer, covered, for 1/2 hour.

[serves 4]

Nutrition Per Serving: Calories 189, Total Fat 3g, Saturated Fat trace, Cholesterol 0mg, *Sodium 611mg, Potassium 237mg, Total Carbohydrate 23g, Dietary Fiber 4g, Protein 19g, Calcium 94mg, Iron 4mg, Vitamin C 14mg, Vitamin A 1446 IU, Vitamin B6 .1mg, Riboflavin B2 .1mg, Folacin 11mcg, Niacin 1mg

Note: This is a high sodium dish. Watch sodium intake for the rest of the day and remember to drink lots of water.

Fish

Miso Cured Black Cod

The Diet Doctor's Wife: When in Aspen, Bill and I do not miss an opportunity to go to Kenichi's and order their famous broiled black cod. The fish is marinated in miso, creating a richness that is indescribable. Below is my rendition.

The Diet Doctor: If you can't get fresh fish, don't even attempt this recipe. To play it extra safe, I ask the fishmonger to fillet a freshly caught whole fish right in front of me.

1 tablespoon red miso
3 tablespoons mirin
1 tablespoon maple syrup or 2 tablespoons brown rice syrup
6-ounce black cod fillet, very fresh and good quality

Combine first 3 ingredients. Pour over fish and marinate in the refrigerator overnight (at least 4 hours). Broil for 8-10 minutes.

[serves 2-4, as an appetizer]

Nutrition Per Serving: Calories 143, Total Fat 1g, Saturated Fat trace, Cholesterol 37mg, Sodium 361mg, Potassium 391mg, Total Carbohydrate 10g, Protein 16g, Calcium 31mg, Iron 1mg, Zinc 1mg, Vitamin C 1mg, Vitamin A 41 IU, Vitamin B6 .2mg, Vitamin B12 .8mcg, Thiamin B1 .1mg, Riboflavin B2 .1mg, Folacin 9mcg, Niacin 2mg

Broiled Striped Bass in Miso Marinade

1/3 cup sake
1/3 cup mirin
1/3 cup light miso
2 tablespoons low sodium tamari
1/4 teaspoon freshly ground black pepper
2 tablespoons maple syrup or 1/4 cup brown rice syrup
4, 6-ounce pieces striped bass

Whisk together the first six ingredients and pour over fish. Marinate 3-8 hours in the refrigerator. Broil the fish until done, 10-12 minutes per inch of thickness. Fish should flake easily when done. Do not allow to dry out.

[serves 4]

Nutrition Per Serving: Calories 296, Total Fat 5g, Saturated Fat 1g, Cholesterol 70mg, *Sodium 1253mg, Potassium 521mg, Total Carbohydrate 16g, Dietary Fiber 1g, Protein 35g, Calcium 46mg, Iron 1mg, Zinc 1mg, Vitamin A 333 IU, Vitamin B6 .7mg, Vitamin B12 .5mcg, Thiamin B1 .2mg, Riboflavin B2 .3mg, Folacin 17mcg, Niacin 3mcg

*Note: This dish is high in sodium. Make sure other food choices for the day are low in sodium. And remember to drink a lot of water.

Grilled Halibut Steak with Chermoula

Chermoula

4 cloves garlic, chopped
1 teaspoon sea salt
1/2 cup fresh cilantro leaves, chopped
1/2 cup fresh parsley leaves, chopped
1 teaspoon paprika
1 teaspoon ground cumin
1/8 teaspoon ground cayenne pepper
2 tablespoons extra virgin olive oil
2 lemons, juiced

6, 6-ounce halibut fillets
sea salt, to taste

To prepare the chermoula, place garlic and salt in a mortar and break up with a pestle. Add the herbs and spices, and pound until a paste is formed. Gradually add oil and lemon juice. Mix together until well integrated.

Season halibut fillets with sea salt. Rub halibut fillets with the Chermoula. Grill to desired doneness, about 10-12 minutes per inch of thickness.

If desired, make extra Chermoula to use as a condiment, or to flavor soups, grains, sandwiches or marinades.

[serves 6]

Nutrition Per Serving: Calories 238, *Total Fat 9g, Saturated Fat 1g, Cholesterol 54mg, Sodium 410mg, Potassium 840mg, Total Carbohydrate 3g, Protein 36g, Calcium 96mg, Iron 2mg, Zinc 1mg, Vitamin C 18mg, Vitamin A 852 IU, Vitamin B6 .6mg, Vitamin B12 2mcg, Thiamin B1 .1mg, Riboflavin B2 .1mg, Folacin 24mcg, Niacin 10mg

*Note: To cut down on fat, use less olive oil in the chermoula or use less chermoula.

Thai Roasted Halibut Fillets

6, 6-ounce halibut fillets
1/2 teaspoon sea salt
1/2 teaspoon freshly ground white pepper
2 tablespoons mirin
3 tablespoons Thai fish sauce
1/4 cup freshly squeezed lime juice
2 cloves garlic, crushed
6 scallions, halved
2 stalks lemongrass, lower 3 inches, each cut in 2-inch pieces and bruised with a meat-tenderizing mallet
1 jalapeno pepper, seeded and slivered
1/4 cup fresh ginger root, peeled and sliced in thin rounds
1/4 cup Thai or Italian basil leaves

Preheat oven to 400 degrees F.

Season fillets with salt and pepper, and place in a roasting pan. In a separate bowl, whisk together wine, fish sauce, lime juice and garlic. Evenly distribute the scallions, lemongrass, jalapeno pepper, ginger root and basil leaves over the fish fillets. Pour the liquid mixture over the fish. Roast fish for 15-18 minutes.

[serves 6]

Nutrition Per Serving: Calories 207, Total Fat 4g, Saturated Fat 1g, Cholesterol 54mg, Sodium 260mg, Potassium 848mg, Total Carbohydrate 4g, Dietary Fiber 1g, Protein 36g, Calcium 96mg, Iron 2mg, Zinc 1mg, Vitamin C 11mg, Vitamin A 355 IU, Vitamin B6 .6mg, Vitamin B12 2mcg, Thiamin B1 .1mg, Riboflavin B2 .1mg, Folacin 26mcg, Niacin 10mg

Roasted Salmon Japanese Style

The Diet Doctor: This preparation helped turn me on to salmon.

3 tablespoons low sodium tamari
1 tablespoon mirin
1 tablespoon sake
*2 pounds salmon or striped bass fillets

Preheat oven to 400 F.

Combine the first 3 ingredients and pour over the salmon to marinate for 1 hour.

Roast salmon for 15-18 minutes (10-12 minutes per inch of thickness).

[serves 6]

Nutrition Per Serving: Calories 187, Total Fat 5g, Saturated Fat 1g, Cholesterol 79mg, Sodium 401mg, Potassium 506mg, Total Carbohydrate 1g, Protein 31g, Calcium 21mg, Iron 1mg, Zinc 1mg, Vitamin A 179 IU, Vitamin B6 .3mg, Vitamin B12 4.5mcg, Thiamin B1 .3mg, Riboflavin B2 .2mg, Folacin 7mcg, Niacin 8mg

*Note: We recommend that you use wild-caught salmon instead of farm-raised salmon (see page 35).

Variation 1: To make a sauce, double or triple the marinade. Heat the extra marinade over medium heat and reduce to half the original volume. Drizzle over the cooked salmon.

Variation 2: You can also barbeque the fish and baste with extra marinade.

Zingy Poached Salmon for Two

The Diet Doctor's Wife: This recipe is quick and easy. It's an old dinner party standard.

vegetable oil spray
1 small onion, minced
2 cloves garlic, minced
1/2 teaspoon fresh hot chili pepper, minced
*2, 6-ounce salmon fillets or other firm-flesh fish fillets, skin removed
2 cups water
1 tomato, peeled, seeded and chopped
1 sprig thyme
juice of 1 lime
1 bay leaf
6 black peppercorns
sea salt, to taste
3 scallions, minced
1/4 cup fresh cilantro leaves, chopped

Coat pan lightly with vegetable oil spray. Sauté onion, garlic and chili for 1-2 minutes. Add fish, water, tomato, lime juice, thyme, bay leaf, peppercorns and salt. Bring to a boil and immediately reduce heat to simmer for 10 minutes. Remove fish and strain broth. Place fish in shallow serving bowls. Ladle some of the strained broth over the fish. Garnish with chopped scallions and cilantro.

[serves 2]

Nutrition Per Serving: Calories 269, Total Fat 6g, Saturated Fat 1g, Cholesterol 88mg, Sodium 130mg, Potassium 988mg, Total Carbohydrate 17g, Dietary Fiber 4g, Protein 37g, Calcium 116mg, Iron 5mg, Zinc 1mg, Vitamin C 87mg, Vitamin A 1062 IU, Vitamin B6 .6mg, Vitamin B12 5.1mcg, Thiamin B1 .4mg, Riboflavin B2 .3mg, Folacin 56mcg, Niacin 9mg

*Note: We recommend that you use wild-caught salmon instead of farm-raised salmon (see page 35).

No Fuss Poached Salmon for Two

*2, 6-ounce salmon fillets
1 tomato, halved
3 scallions, trimmed at both ends
3 sprigs fresh cilantro
1 fresh hot chili pepper, halved and seeded
sea salt and freshly ground black pepper, to taste
chopped fresh cilantro leaves, for garnish

Place ingredients in a saucepan. Add 2 cups water. Bring to a boil. Lower heat and simmer for 10 minutes. Remove fish and garnish with chopped cilantro leaves.

[serves 2]

Nutrition Per Serving: Calories 234, Total Fat 6g, Saturated Fat 1g, Cholesterol 88mg, Sodium 130mg, Potassium 946mg, Total Carbohydrate 8g, Dietary Fiber 2g, Protein 36g, Calcium 79mg, Iron 3mg, Zinc 1mg, Vitamin C 86mg, Vitamin A 1367 IU, Vitamin B6 .4mg, Vitamin B12 5.1mcg, Thiamin B1 .4mg, Riboflavin B2 .3mg, Folacin 36mcg, Niacin 9mg

*Note: We recommend that you use wild-caught salmon instead of farm-raised salmon (see page 35).

Roast Salmon in a Blanket of Lemon Balm

The Diet Doctor's Wife: This is a special recipe from my mother. The lemon balm, which she grows in her garden, imparts an exquisite, aromatic, citrus flavor that is indescribable. You must grow lemon balm in your garden so that you can include this dish in your repertoire.

*3-pound salmon roast
8-10 sprigs fresh lemon balm
juice of 1 lemon
1 cup Vermouth
1/2 cup water
sea salt and freshly ground black pepper, to taste

Preheat oven to 450 F.

Place half the lemon balm leaves on the bottom of a roasting pan. Place salmon, skin side down, on top of the leaves. Completely cover salmon with the rest of the lemon balm leaves. Add lemon juice, vermouth and water. Cover with aluminum foil. Poke a big air hole in the center of the foil. Roast for 15-18 minutes (approximately 10-12 minutes per inch of thickness).

Remove lemon balm from the top of the fish. Season with sea salt and freshly ground pepper.

[serves 8]

Nutrition Per Serving: Calories 243, Total Fat 6g, Saturated Fat 1g, Cholesterol 89mg, Sodium 123mg, Potassium 569mg, Total Carbohydrate 2g, Protein 34g, Calcium 26mg, Iron 1mg, Zinc 1mg, Vitamin C 4mg, Vitamin A 203 IU, Vitamin B6 .3mg, Vitamin B12 5.1mcg, Thiamin B1 .3mg, Riboflavin B2 .2mg, Folacin 8mcg, Niacin 9mg

*Note: We recommend that you use wild-caught salmon instead of farm-raised salmon (see page 35).

Bill's Throw-it-in-a-Pan Salmon

*2, 6-ounce salmon fillets
1/3 cup onion, thinly sliced
2 sprigs fresh dill
splash of Vermouth
sea salt and freshly ground black pepper, to taste

Preheat oven to 500 F.

Season salmon fillets with sea salt and freshly ground pepper. Place in an ovenproof skillet. Top salmon with onion slices and dill sprigs. Add a splash of vermouth and roast for 15-18 minutes. Remove from oven and discard dill sprigs.

[serves 2]

Nutrition Per Serving: Calories 257, Total Fat 6g, Saturated Fat 1g, Cholesterol 88mg, Sodium 129mg, Potassium 691mg, Total Carbohydrate 5g, Dietary Fiber 1g, Protein 35g, Calcium 83mg, Iron3mg, Zinc 1mg, Vitamin C 3mg, Vitamin A 382 IU, Vitamin B6 .4mg, Vitamin B12 5.1mcg, Thiamin B1 .4mg, Riboflavin B2 .2mg, Folacin 10mcg, Niacin 9mg

*Note: We recommend that you use wild-caught salmon instead of farm-raised salmon (see page 35).

Shrimp Cocktail

Cocktail Sauce

1/2 cup ketchup
2 tablespoons celery, chopped
1-2 tablespoons horseradish
juice of 1/2 lemon

iceberg lettuce leaves, chopped
20 medium to large cooked shrimp
lemon wedges and celery leaves, for garnish

Combine first 4 ingredients. In 4 small serving bowls, place a handful of chopped lettuce leaves. Top each mound of lettuce with 2 tablespoons of sauce. Surround the sauce in each bowl with 5 pieces of cooked shrimp. Garnish with lemon wedges and celery leaves.

[serves 4]

Nutrition Per Serving: Calories 84, Total Fat 1g, Saturated Fat trace, Cholesterol 95mg, Sodium 474mg, Potassium 283mg, Total Carbohydrate 10g, Dietary Fiber 1g, Protein 11g, Calcium 33mg, Iron 2mg, Zinc 1mg, Vitamin C 11mg, Vitamin A 452 IU, Vitamin B6 .1mg, Vitamin B12 .7mcg, Folacin 14mcg, Niacin 2mg

Shrimp in Garlic and Chive Vinaigrette

The Diet Doctor: Shrimp in Garlic and Chive Vinaigrette makes a nice little appetizer. As shrimp is high in cholesterol, you may want to keep your servings small. That way you can enjoy yourself without getting into trouble.

1 pound cooked shrimp
1/4 cup Garlic and Chive Vinaigrette (page 342)
1 head bibb lettuce, torn
chopped fresh chives, for garnish

In a large bowl, combine shrimp and vinaigrette. Allow to sit in the refrigerator for 1/2 hour.

On individual plates, place a small handful of torn lettuce leaves. Spoon an equal amount of marinated shrimp on top of each plate of lettuce. Garnish with chopped chives.

[serves 6]

Nutrition Per Serving: Calories 132, Total Fat 7g, Saturated Fat 1g, Cholesterol 148mg, Sodium 181mg, Potassium 213mg, Total Carbohydrate 1g, Protein 16g, Calcium 39mg, Iron 2mg, Zinc 1mg, Vitamin C 5mg, Vitamin 441 IU, Vitamin B6 .1mg, Vitamin B12 1.1mcg, Folacin 23mcg, Niacin 2mg

Sake Simmered Halibut

The Diet Doctor: Don't be alarmed by the amount of soy sauce used in this recipe. Most of it stays in the pot and is not absorbed by the fish. If you are still concerned about the sodium content, serve this dish as an appetizer and watch your sodium intake for the rest of the day. And remember to drink a lot of water.

1 1/2 cups sake
1 pound halibut steaks or salmon steaks, each cut in 1/2 lengthwise, spinal bone removed
3/4 cup mirin
3/4 cup low sodium soy sauce
1/3 cup fresh ginger root, peeled and thinly sliced
1 1/2 tablespoons maple syrup or 3 tablespoons brown rice syrup

Pour sake in a heavy saucepan and bring to a boil over medium heat. Add fish, skin side up. Bring back to a boil. Add mirin, soy sauce, ginger and maple syrup. Return to a boil. To ensure even cooking, weight the fish with an *otoshibuta. Lower heat just a bit and gently boil for 10 minutes.

Remove fish from the pan with a slotted spatula. Divide fish among 4 serving plates. Drizzle 1-2 tablespoons of sauce over each piece of fish. Garnish with ginger slices from the pan, if desired.

[serves 4]

Nutrition Per Serving: Calories 219, Total Fat 3g, Saturated Fat trace, Cholesterol 36mg, **Sodium 664mg, Potassium 602mg, Total Carbohydrate 10g, Protein 25g, Calcium 68mg, Iron 1mg, Zinc 1mg, Vitamin C 3mg, Vitamin A 176 IU, Vitamin B6 .4mg, Vitamin B12 1.3mcg, Thiamin B1 .1mg, Riboflavin B2 .1mg, Folacin 13mcg, Niacin 7mg

*Note 1: If you do not have an otoshibuta, you can weight the fish with a lid that fits inside your saucepan.

**Note 2: This is a high sodium dish. Remember to watch your salt intake for the rest of the day and drink lots of water.

Variation: For a more intense flavor, marinate fish before cooking in 3 tablespoons of soy sauce, 1 tablespoon of mirin and 1 tablespoon of sake. Note that this will increase the sodium content of the dish.

Boiled Fish

1 1/2 pounds halibut or cod fillet, skin removed
sea salt and freshly ground black pepper, to taste
1/4 cup Garlic and Chive Vinaigrette (342) or Lemon Vinaigrette (341)

Place fish in a skillet. Add water to cover and season with salt and pepper. Simmer on medium for 10-15 minutes until fish flakes. Drain fish. Dress with vinaigrette.

[serves 6]

Nutrition Per Serving: Calories 144, Total Fat 6g, Saturated Fat 1g, Cholesterol 49mg, Sodium 61mg, Potassium 472mg, Protein 20g, Calcium 19mg, Zinc 1mg, Vitamin C 2mg, Vitamin A 57 IU, Vitamin B6 .3mg, Vitamin B12 1mcg, Thiamin B1 .1mg, Riboflavin B2 .1mg, Folacin 8mcg, Niacin 2mg

Other fish recipes: Doc's Salad (page 82), Salad Nicoise (page 85), French Dejeuner Salad (page 88), Bonito Miso (page 120), Japanese Fish Nabe (page 122), Caldo Verde with Fresh Cod (page 124), Provencal Fish Stew (page 125), Fish Chowder (page 126), California Sushi Bowl (page 135), Outback Rice Dinner (page 140), Fish Porridge (page 148), Linguini with Tuna (page 164), Fresh Spring Rolls (page 165), Mom's Tuna and White Bean Salad (page 203)

Vegetables

Portabella Appetizer

The Diet Doctor's Wife: On a trip to NYC, I found myself ravenous for a vegetarian pick-me-up that wasn't loaded with cheese and fat. Luckily I came across a little gourmet market called Marche Madison and saw these lovely portabella mushroom appetizers. They really hit the spot, so much so that I had to go home and figure out the recipe.

4 teaspoons extra virgin olive oil
6 portabella mushrooms, stems removed
1 pound spinach leaves
2 cloves garlic, minced
1 cup Basic Tomato Sauce (page 330), Tomato Confit (page 331) or tomato puree
sea salt and freshly ground black pepper, to taste
fresh basil leaves, cut in strips, for garnish

Preheat oven to 400 F.

Brush mushroom caps with 2 teaspoons oil. Place in a small roasting pan, covered with foil. Bake for 20-30 minutes until mushrooms are cooked through. Season with salt and freshly ground pepper.

In a pot of salted boiling water, blanch spinach leaves for 1 minute. Drain, chop and set aside. Warm remaining oil and add garlic. Sauté 1 minute and add spinach. Sauté 2-3 minutes. Season with salt and freshly ground pepper.

To assemble, place caps so that gills are facing up. Divide spinach mixture in 6 and fill caps. Top each filled mushroom cap with 1 tablespoon of tomato sauce. Garnish with strips of fresh basil. Serve cold.

[serves 6]

Nutrition Per Serving: Calories 98, Total Fat 5g, Saturated Fat trace, Cholesterol 0mg, Sodium 163mg, Potassium 1044mg, Total Carbohydrate 12g, Dietary Fiber 4g, Protein 5g, Calcium 104mg, Iron 4mg, Zinc 1mg, Vitamin C 36mg, Vitamin A 5475 IU, Vitamin B6 .3mg, Thiamin B1 .2mg, Riboflavin B2 .7mg, Folacin 180mcg, Niacin 6mg

Braised Shitake Mushroom Caps

2 teaspoons toasted sesame oil
12 large fresh shitake mushrooms or reconstituted dried shitake mushrooms, caps only
1 tablespoon sake
1 tablespoon low sodium tamari

Heat oil in a skillet over medium heat. Add mushroom caps and sauté 3 minutes per side. Add sake and tamari, and sauté 10-15 seconds per side.

[serves 3-4]

Nutrition Per Serving: Calories 79, Total Fat 3g, Saturated Fat trace, Cholesterol 0mg, Sodium 202mg, Potassium 233mg, Total Carbohydrate 12g, Dietary Fiber 2g, Protein 2g, Calcium 3mg, Zinc 1mg, Vitamin B6 .1mg, Riboflavin B2 .2mg, Folacin 24mcg, Niacin 2mg

Simple Kale

The Diet Doctor's Wife: Adding a few drops of tamari to cooked greens is a simple trick that enhances flavor without adding calories or fat.

Place kale (or collards) in vigorously boiling, lightly salted water.

Boil greens for 2 minutes. Remove greens and drain in a colander. Immediately immerse in ice water.

After greens are chilled, drain again and gently squeeze out excess water. Cut in 1 1/2-inch squares. Just before serving, add 1/4 teaspoon of tamari for each 1/2 cup of cooked greens.

Nutrition Per Cup: Calories 38, Total Fat 1g, Saturated Fat trace, Cholesterol 0mg, Sodium 130mg, Potassium 302mg, Total Carbohydrate 8g, Dietary Fiber 3g, Protein 3g, Calcium 94mg, Iron 1mg, Vitamin C 53mg, Vitamin A 9620 IU, Vitamin B6 .2mg, Thiamin B1 .1mg, Riboflavin .1mg, Folacin 18mcg, Niacin 1mg

Stir-Fried Greens

1 teaspoon grapeseed oil
8 cups mixed greens (cabbage, kale, collards, mustard), chopped
2 teaspoons tamari

Heat oil in a nonstick pan. Sauté greens 1-2 minutes. Add tamari. Stir. Cover and simmer on low for 10-15 minutes. If the pan gets too dry, add a splash of water.

[serves 4]

Nutrition Per Serving: Calories 41, Total Fat 1g, Saturated Fat trace, Cholesterol 0mg, Sodium 196mg, Potassium 403mg, Total Carbohydrate 6g, Dietary Fiber 4g, Protein 3g, Calcium 116mg, Iron 2mg, Vitamin C 78mg, Vitamin A 5936 IU, Vitamin B6 .2mg, Thiamin B1 .1mg, Riboflavin B2 .1mg, Folacin 210mcg, Niacin 1mg

Napa Cabbage Sauté

The Diet Doctor's Wife: Bill liked this dish at the very start of our vegetarian journey.

1 teaspoon grapeseed oil
1/4 teaspoon fresh hot chili pepper, minced
2 teaspoons fresh ginger root, grated
1 pound Napa cabbage, shredded
1 medium carrot, julienned
1/2 cup fresh chives, cut in 2-inch pieces
sea salt, to taste
2 tablespoons mirin

Heat oil in a sauté pan over medium heat. Add chili and ginger, and warm for 30 seconds. Add the cabbage, carrots and chives. Season with sea salt and sauté for 3 minutes. Add mirin, cover and cook for 4 minutes. Uncover and cook until liquid evaporates.

[serves 6]

Nutrition Per Serving: Calories 30, Total Fat 1g, Saturated Fat trace, Cholesterol 0mg, Sodium 54mg, Potassium 246mg, Total Carbohydrate 3g, Dietary Fiber 1g, Protein 1g, Calcium 87mg, Iron 1mg, Vitamin C 38mg, Vitamin A 5821 IU, Vitamin B6 .2mg, Riboflavin B2 .1mg, Folacin 56mcg, Niacin 1mg

Soy Glazed Turnips and Greens

2 teaspoons grapeseed oil
2 pounds turnips, peeled and cut in 1 1/2-inch cubes
1 tablespoon low sodium tamari
1 tablespoon maple syrup
1 cup water
1/4 teaspoon toasted sesame oil
6 cups kale, turnip greens, collards or chard, chopped

Heat oil in a large saucepan on medium. Add turnips and sauté until lightly browned on all sides, about 5 minutes. Add tamari, maple syrup and water. Bring to a boil. Cover, reduce heat to low and simmer for 15 minutes. Add sesame oil and stir. Remove turnips from saucepan with a slotted spoon and set aside.

Bring leftover liquid to a boil. Add greens (and water, if necessary). Cover and cook for 3 minutes.

To serve, place greens on a serving plate. Place turnips on top.

[serves 4]

Nutrition Per Serving: Calories 138, Total Fat 3g, Saturated Fat trace, Cholesterol 0mg, Sodium 319mg, Potassium 819mg, Total Carbohydrate 25g, Dietary Fiber 5g, Protein 5g, Calcium 198mg, Iron 2mg, Zinc 1mg, Vitamin C 159mg, Vitamin A 8944 IU, Vitamin B6 .4mg, Thiamin B1 .2mg, Riboflavin .2mg, Folacin 57mcg, Niacin 2mg

Rutabaga Puree

The Diet Doctor's Wife: Cumin adds a splendid spark to the nutritious and hearty rutabaga. Have this dish on its own or get creative and mix it with mashed potatoes.

2 teaspoons grapeseed oil
1 1/2 pounds rutabaga, peeled and cubed
sea salt, to taste
1 teaspoon maple syrup
1 cup Basic Vegetable Stock (page 94)
1/2 teaspoon cumin seeds

In a large skillet, heat oil over medium heat. Add cubed rutabaga and a pinch of salt. Sauté for 5 minutes. Add maple syrup and vegetable stock. Cover skillet and reduce heat to simmer for 30 minutes. Uncover and turn up heat so that remaining liquid evaporates.

Transfer to a blender and add cumin. Pulse to puree and taste for seasoning.

[serves 4]

Nutrition Per Serving: Calories 92, Total Fat 3g, Saturated Fat trace, Cholesterol 0mg, Sodium 41mg, Potassium 582mg, Total Carbohydrate 16g, Dietary Fiber 4g, Protein 2g, Calcium 84mg, Iron 1mg, Zinc 1mg, Vitamin C 43mg, Vitamin A 991 IU, Vitamin B6 .2mg, Thiamin B1 .1mg, Riboflavin B2 .1mg, Folacin 36mcg, Niacin 1mg

Mashed Rutabaga and Greens

The Diet Doctor's Wife: This is a hearty, low fat dish that offers a huge source of Vitamin A. Mashed potatoes will seem boring by comparison.

2 pounds rutabaga
1 pound kale
2 teaspoons extra virgin olive oil

1 cup shallots or onions, minced
2 tablespoons garlic, minced
sea salt and freshly ground black pepper, to taste

Peel rutabaga and cut into 1-inch cubes. Place cubes in a medium saucepan with enough water to cover. Bring to a boil over medium heat. Reduce heat to a simmer and cook 25 minutes until tender. Drain and set aside.

Remove kale leaves from stems. Discard stems. Coarsely chop kale leaves.

Warm oil in a large sauté pan over medium heat. Add shallots and garlic. Sauté until shallots are translucent. Add kale and cook until wilted. Add salt and pepper. Puree kale mixture in a food processor. Add cooked rutabaga. Puree until smooth.

[serves 4]

Nutrition Per Serving: Calories 193, Total Fat 4g, Saturated Fat trace, Cholesterol 0mg, Sodium 100mg, Potassium 1423mg, Total Carbohydrate 38g, Dietary Fiber 8g, Protein 8g, Calcium 282mg, Iron 4mg, Zinc 1mg, Vitamin C 197mg, Vitamin A 16412 IU, Vitamin B6 .7mg, Thiamin B1 .3mg, Riboflavin B .2mg, Folacin 95mcg, Niacin 3mg

Braised Squash

The Diet Doctor's Wife: This is a sugar-free version of a classic Japanese dish. Bill loves it.

1 pound buttercup or other winter squash
sea salt
soy sauce

Cut open squash and remove seeds. Cut squash into large chunks. Leave skin on (unless the squash has a waxy coating). Place one layer of squash pieces, skin side down, in a medium heavy-bottomed pot. Sprinkle lightly with salt. Add water to cover squash by 1-2 inches. Bring to a boil over medium heat and cover with lid. Cook 10 minutes. Season with a dash of soy sauce. Cook away excess liquid.

[serves 4]

Nutrition Per Serving: Calories 43, Total Fat trace, Saturated Fat trace, Cholesterol 0mg, Sodium 4g, Potassium 336mg, Total Carbohydrate 11g, Dietary Fiber 2g, Protein 1g, Calcium 46mg, Iron 1mg, Vitamin C 20mg, Vitamin A 7437 IU, Vitamin B6 .1mg, Thiamin B1 .1 mg, Folacin 25mcg, Niacin 1mg

Roasted Root Vegetables with Mustard Oil

The Diet Doctor's Wife: When I serve Roasted Root Vegetables with Mustard Oil, Bill gives me the third degree. He swears that the dish is not truly vegetarian. He believes that I roast the vegetables with chicken and then hide the bird.

2 carrots
1 parsnip
1 large turnip
1 rutabaga
1 celery root
2 tablespoons Mustard Oil (page 343)
sea salt and freshly ground black pepper, to taste

Preheat oven to 475 F. Wash and peel vegetables. Cut carrots and parsnip in 1/4-inch slices. Cut turnip, rutabaga and celery root in quarters and then again in 1/4-inch slices.

Put vegetables in a bowl and toss with Mustard Oil.

Spread vegetables evenly in a roasting pan. Season with salt and pepper.

Roast vegetables for 10 minutes. Turn vegetables and continue roasting for another 10 minutes until crisped at the edges and tender in the center.

[serves 6]

Nutrition Per Serving: Calories 68, Total Fat 5g, Saturated Fat trace, Cholesterol 0mg, Sodium 44mg, Potassium 252mg, Total Carbohydrate 6g, Dietary Fiber 2g, Protein 1g, Calcium 32mg, Vitamin C 14mg, Vitamin A 6913 IU, Vitamin B6 .1mg, Thiamin B1 .1mg, Folacin 17mcg, Niacin 1mg

Pressure Cooked Root Vegetables

The Diet Doctor's Wife: This is a great winter dish, packed with nutrition and incredibly simple to prepare. The pressure-cooking creates a delightful complexity and heartiness. Add a potato if you like.

2 large carrots
1 large onion
1 large parsnip
1 large turnip
1 celery root
1 1/2 cups water
sea salt, to taste

Clean and peel vegetables. Cut vegetables in large, equal-size chunks. Place vegetables in a pressure cooker. Add water and salt. Cover and bring up to pressure. Reduce heat to low and cook for 10 minutes.

[serves 4-6]

Nutrition Per Serving: Calories 82, Total Fat trace, Saturated Fat trace, Cholesterol 0mg, Sodium 66mg, Potassium 517mg, Total Carbohydrate 19g, Dietary Fiber 5g, Protein 2g, Calcium 57mg, Iron 1mg, Zinc 1mg, Vitamin C 23mg, Vitamin A 10167 IU, Vitamin B6 .2mg, Thiamin B1 .1mg, Riboflavin B2 .1mg, Folacin 61mcg, Niacin 1mg

Cajun Collards

The Diet Doctor's Wife: Collards are under-appreciated greens. They are not only sweet and tender but also a good source of Vitamin A, Calcium and Folacin. Cook them just plain or Cajun style.

1 bunch collard greens
2 teaspoons grapeseed oil or Clarified Butter (page 346)
1 chipotle pepper
1/2 cup water
1 teaspoon brown rice vinegar
sea salt and freshly ground black pepper, to taste

Remove and discard stems from the collard greens. Chop leaves and place them in a medium saucepan with grapeseed oil, chipotle pepper and water. Cover saucepan and braise over low heat for 10-15 minutes. Remove from the heat. Season with vinegar, salt and pepper. Remove chipotle pepper.

[serves 4]

Nutrition Per Serving: Calories 27, Total Fat 2g, Saturated Fat trace, Cholesterol 0mg, Sodium 3mg, Potassium 53mg, Total Carbohydrate 2g, Calcium 15mg, Vitamin C 30mg, Vitamin A 431 IU, Folacin 18mcg

Braised Italian Kale

1 pound Italian kale
1 tablespoon extra virgin olive oil
2 cloves garlic, finely sliced
1/4 teaspoon red pepper flakes (optional)
sea salt and freshly ground black pepper, to taste

Remove stems from the kale leaves. Blanch in salted boiling water for 3 minutes. Drain and set aside.

Warm olive oil in a saucepan. Add garlic and red pepper flakes, and sauté over moderately low heat for 3-5 minutes, until garlic begins to color. Add kale and season with salt and pepper. Cover and cook for 5 minutes.

[serves 4]

Nutrition Per Serving: Calories 89, Total Fat 4g, Saturated Fat 1g, Cholesterol 0mg, Sodium 49mg, Potassium 514mg, Total Carbohydrate 12g, Dietary Fiber 2g, Protein 4g, Calcium 156mg, Iron 2mg, Zinc 1mg, Vitamin C 137mg, Vitamin A 10108 IU, Vitamin B6 .3mg, Thiamin B1 .1mg, Riboflavin B2 .1mg, Folacin 33mcg, Niacin 1mg

Steamed Vegetables with Dipping Sauce

The Diet Doctor's Wife: Dipping sauce adds a little zip to plain old steamed vegetables. And preparation is a snap. Just whisk the ingredients together and you're done.

steamed vegetables (cauliflower, broccoli, carrots, turnips, etc.)

Sesame Dipping Sauce (page 336), Ginger Soy Dipping Sauce (page 336), Soy Garlic Dipping Sauce (page 337), Soy Garlic Sherry Dipping Sauce (page 337), Basic Japanese Dipping Sauce (page 338) or Korean Dipping Sauce (page 338)

Nutrition Per Serving: The nutritional content for this dish depends on the vegetables you choose as well as the dipping sauce. Portion size is also a consideration. Sources with the nutritional values for given foods are available in bookstores, the library or on-line. Nutritional information for the dipping sauces listed above is indicated at the end of each recipe.

Italian Steamed Vegetables

fresh vegetables (cauliflower, broccoli, carrots, turnips, etc.), cut in equal-size pieces
garlic cloves, sliced paper thin (optional)
extra virgin olive oil
sea salt and freshly ground black pepper, to taste

Place vegetables in a bowl. Drizzle with good quality extra virgin olive oil. Sprinkle with salt and freshly ground pepper.

Place vegetables in a steamer and steam until tender.

Nutrition Per Serving: The nutritional content for this dish depends on the vegetables you choose as well as the amount of olive oil. Portion size is also a consideration. Sources with nutritional values for given foods are available in bookstores, the library or on-line. One tablespoon of extra virgin olive oil contains approximately 120 calories, 14g of total fat, 1.8g of saturated fat and no cholesterol.

Mexican Steamed Vegetables

fresh vegetables, cut in equal-size pieces
grapeseed oil
*dry-roasted cumin seeds
sea salt and freshly ground black pepper, to taste

Place vegetables in a bowl. Drizzle lightly with grapeseed oil.

Add a sprinkle of cumin seeds. Toss to incorporate. Season with sea salt and freshly ground pepper.

Place vegetables in a steamer and steam until tender.

Nutrition Per Serving: The nutritional content for this dish depends on the vegetables you choose as well as the amount of oil. Portion size is also a consideration. Sources with nutritional values for given foods are available in bookstores, the library or on-line. One tablespoon of grapeseed oil contains approximately 120 calories, 14g of total fat, 1.3g of saturated fat and no cholesterol.

*Note: To roast cumin seeds, heat a small skillet over medium heat. Add enough seeds to cover the bottom of the pan. Roast seeds 1-2 minutes until an aroma is released. Stir the seeds continuously with a wooden spoon to prevent them from burning. Allow seeds to cool off before using them.

Steamed Vegetables with Zatar

steamed vegetables
My Zatar (page 335)
extra virgin olive oil (optional)

Place zatar and olive oil in separate dipping bowls (one set per person or community style). Dip steamed vegetables in oil and then in the zatar. To reduce fat, you can skip the oil step entirely.

Nutrition Per Serving: The nutritional content for this dish depends on the type and quantity of vegetables as well as the amount of olive oil and zatar. Sources with nutritional values for given foods are available in bookstores, the library or on-line. One tablespoon of extra virgin olive oil contains approximately 120 calories, 14g of total fat, 1.8g of saturated fat and no cholesterol. The nutritional information for My Zatar is indicated at the end of the recipe on page 336.

Snow Peas and Carrots

1 pound snow peas
1 cup carrots, cut in julienne strips
1 tablespoon soy sauce or tamari
1 teaspoon maple syrup
1 teaspoon red wine vinegar
1 tablespoon grapeseed oil
1/4 teaspoon toasted sesame oil
2 teaspoons black or tan sesame seeds

In a pot of boiling water, blanch snow peas until they turn bright green, about 1 minute. Remove with a slotted spoon and refresh with cold water. Drain. Bring water to a boil once more. Add carrots and cook about 1 minute. Drain and refresh with cold water. Drain again.

To make dressing, whisk together soy sauce, maple syrup, vinegar and both oils.

Place snow peas and carrots in a bowl. Add dressing and toss gently to coat the vegetables. Sprinkle with sesame seeds.

[serves 4]

Nutrition Per Serving: Calories 111, Total Fat 5g, Saturated Fat 1g, Cholesterol 0mg, Sodium 269mg, Potassium 363mg, Total Carbohydrate 14g, Dietary Fiber 4g, Protein 4g, Calcium 63mg, Iron 3mg, Zinc 1mg, Vitamin C 71mg, Vitamin A 10292 IU, Vitamin B6 .2mg, Thiamin B1 .2mg, Riboflavin B2 .1mg, Folacin 54mcg, Niacin 1mg

Sweet Pea Puree

The Diet Doctor's Wife: This puree is truly delightful, especially if the peas are freshly plucked from the garden.

1 cup fresh green peas, shelled
1 teaspoon mild yellow miso
1 teaspoon extra virgin olive oil
1 teaspoon fresh tarragon, finely chopped
pinch of ground cayenne pepper
sea salt, to taste

Bring salted water to a boil. Add peas and simmer for 5-7 minutes. Drain peas and combine with the rest of the ingredients. Puree. Season to taste.

[serves 2]

Nutrition Per Serving: Calories 85, Total Fat 3mg, Saturated Fat trace, Cholesterol 0mg, Sodium 167mg, Potassium 184mg, Total Carbohydrate 11g, Dietary Fiber 4g, Protein 4g, Calcium 21mg, Iron 1mg, Zinc 1mg, Vitamin C 29mg, Vitamin A 469 IU, Vitamin B6 .1mg, Thiamin B1 .2mg, Riboflavin B2 .1mg, Folacin 48mcg, Niacin 2mg

Middle Eastern Eggplant Puree

1 pound eggplant
2 cloves garlic
sea salt, to taste
1 tablespoon tahini paste
juice of 1 lemon
1/4 teaspoon ground cumin or My Zatar (page 335)

Preheat oven to 400 F. Place whole eggplant(s) on a baking sheet. Pierce skin a few times with a knife. Bake for 40 minutes until eggplant gets all wrinkly. Turn occasionally to ensure even cooking. Remove from oven and allow to cool.

Cut open eggplant(s) and scoop out the flesh with a wooden spoon. Place flesh in a colander to release bitter juices.

Crush garlic. Place in a food processor. Add eggplant flesh, salt, tahini, lemon juice and cumin. Pulse a few times to combine. Taste for seasoning.

[2 cups]

Nutrition Per 2 Tablespoons: Calories 13, Total Fat 1g, Saturated Fat trace, Cholesterol 0mg, Sodium 2mg, Potassium 62mg, Total Carbohydrate 2g, Dietary Fiber 1g, Calcium 8mg, Vitamin C 2mg, Vitamin A 22 IU, Folacin 6mcg

Hotel Mushrooms

The Diet Doctor's Wife: In 1993, I met my cousin Michele in Amsterdam for a short little visit over the Christmas holidays. We had a marvelous time sightseeing, exploring and eating together. One of the "eating" highlights was the hotel breakfast buffet. The button mushrooms, in particular, grabbed my attention. They were prepared very simply, sautéed whole with a little butter and parsley. Each mouthful sent me humming with pleasure. Of course, I had to recreate the recipe. My version is considerably less fatty, prepared with only a sparing amount of clarified butter.

2 teaspoons Clarified Butter (page 346) or ghee
20 whole button mushrooms, cleaned and trimmed
3 tablespoons fresh parsley, chopped
sea salt and freshly ground black pepper, to taste

Heat a nonstick skillet over medium heat. Add Clarified Butter. Place mushrooms in the skillet, caps facing upward. For optimal even cooking, wet an *otoshibuta and place it on top of mushrooms. Cook until mushrooms soften all the way through. Remove otoshibuta. Sprinkle mushrooms with chopped parsley. Season with salt and pepper.

[serves 4]

*Note: If you do not have an otoshibuta, you can weight the mushrooms with a lid that fits inside your skillet.

Nutrition Per Serving: Calories 105, Total Fat 3g, Saturated Fat 2g, Cholesterol 6mg, Sodium 16mg, Potassium 1311mg, Total Carbohydrate 18g, Dietary Fiber 5g, Protein 7g, Calcium 22mg, Iron 42mg, Zinc 3mg, Vitamin C 18mg, Vitamin A 231 IU, Vitamin B6 .3mg, Thiamin B1 .4mg, Riboflavin B2 1.6mg, Folacin 78mcg, Niacin 14mg

Laurie's Tomato Sauté

The Diet Doctor's Wife: When I was a child and my parents would go out of town, I would stay with Auntie Helen and Uncle Stan. It was always great fun as Auntie Helen treated me like her little friend. We laughed, talked and even sang together. And mealtime was very special, as Auntie Helen is a marvelous cook. One dish that has stayed with me is her sautéed tomatoes, a favorite of her brother Laurie, as the story goes. Auntie Helen would serve her sautéed tomatoes with eggs; I serve mine with scrambled tofu.

2 teaspoons extra virgin olive oil or Clarified Butter (page 346)
4 large tomatoes, peeled, seeded and chopped
1/4 cup fresh parsley, chopped
sea salt and freshly ground black pepper, to taste

Heat oil in a skillet. Add tomatoes and half the parsley. Sauté 4-5 minutes. Season to taste. Sprinkle with remaining chopped parsley.

[serves 4]

Nutrition Per Serving: Calories 47, Total Fat 3g, Saturated Fat trace, Cholesterol 0mg, Sodium 13mg, Potassium 294mg, Total Carbohydrate 6g, Dietary Fiber 1g, Protein 1g, Calcium 11mg, Iron 1mg, Vitamin C 28mg, Vitamin A 961 IU, Vitamin B6 .1mg, Thiamin B1 .1mg, Riboflavin B2 .1mg, Folacin 24mcg, Niacin 1mg

Cauliflower Mochi Gratin

2 tablespoons tahini
1 1/2 tablespoons ume vinegar
2 teaspoons low sodium tamari
2 tablespoons water
1 1/2 ounces mochi, grated
1 head cauliflower

Preheat oven to 350 F.

To make the sauce, combine the first 5 ingredients and set aside.

Blanch whole cauliflower in salted boiling water for 5 minutes. Drain. Place cauliflower in a baking dish. Cover with the sauce. Bake for 25 minutes, covered with foil. Remove foil and bake for another 20 minutes.

[serves 6]

Nutrition Per Serving: Calories 54, Total Fat 3g, Saturated Fat trace, Cholesterol 0mg, Sodium 340mg, Potassium 75mg, Total Carbohydrate 6g, Dietary Fiber 1g, Protein 2g, Calcium 25mg, Iron 1mg, Vitamin C 8mg, Vitamin A 7 IU, Thiamin B1 .1mg, Folacin 15mcg

Greek Baked Vegetables

The Diet Doctor's Wife: I'm crazy about Greek Baked Vegetables. To me, it's the ultimate comfort food. I shared my feelings with my friend and colleague, Sue Vlangos, who passed on her tried and true recipe. Knowing that I am sensitive to high fat foods, she assured me that I could reduce the amount of olive oil considerably and still get a great result. She was right.

1 pound green beans, trimmed
1 pound potatoes, cut in chunks
1 pound zucchini, cut in chunks
1 pound tomatoes, peeled, seeded and chopped
1 large onion, cut in chunks
3 cloves garlic, halved
1/4 cup fresh parsley, chopped
sea salt and freshly ground black pepper, to taste
1 sprig fresh dill
1 sprig fresh oregano
2 tablespoons extra virgin olive oil
1 1/2 cups water

Preheat oven to 375 F.

Place vegetables in a Dutch oven. Sprinkle with salt, pepper and parsley. Add dill, oregano, extra virgin olive oil and water. Cover and bake for 1 1/2 hours.

[serves 6]

Nutrition Per Serving: Calories 156, Total Fat 5g, Saturated Fat 1g, Cholesterol 0mg, Sodium 20mg, Potassium 942mg, Total Carbohydrate 26g, Dietary Fiber 6g, Protein 5g, Calcium 58mg, Iron 2mg, Zinc 1mg, Vitamin C 52mg, Vitamin A 1369 IU, Vitamin B6 .4mg, Thiamin B1 .2mg, Riboflavin B2 .1mg, Folacin 70mcg, Niacin 2mg

Simmered Potatoes and Olives

The Diet Doctor's Wife: I don't make potatoes very often, but when those delicious fingerlings are in season, I just can't resist. This dish is just as good prepared with Jerusalem artichokes.

2 teaspoons extra virgin olive oil
2 cloves garlic, chopped
1 pound potatoes, cut in large cubes or 1 pound Jerusalem artichokes, peeled and cut in large cubes
1/3 cup black olives, pitted if desired
1/4 cup fresh parsley, chopped
1/2 cup white wine
1/2 cup water
chopped fresh parsley, for garnish

Combine all ingredients in a heavy sauté pan. Cover and simmer on low heat about 40 minutes, until potatoes are tender. Add water throughout cooking if the pan gets too dry. Garnish with chopped parsley.

[serves 4]

Nutrition Per Serving: Calories 146, Total Fat 4g, Saturated Fat trace, Cholesterol 0mg, Sodium 109mg, Potassium 668mg, Total Carbohydrate 22g, Dietary Fiber 2g, Protein 3g,

Calcium 28mg, Iron 2mg, Zinc 1mg, Vitamin C 28mg, Vitamin A 240 IU, Vitamin B6 .3mg, Thiamin B1 .1mg, Folacin 20mcg, Niacin 2mg

Mashed Jerusalem Artichokes and Greens

2 teaspoons extra virgin olive oil
2 cloves garlic, minced
1 pound Jerusalem artichokes, peeled and cut in large chunks
1/2 cup Basic Vegetable Stock (page 94) or water
8 ounces Swiss chard leaves (stems removed), chopped
juice of 1/2 lemon
sea salt and freshly ground black pepper, to taste

Heat oil in a sauté pan on medium low. Add garlic and sauté 2-3 minutes. Add artichokes and sauté 1-2 minutes. Add stock and bring to a boil. Reduce heat and simmer on low for 1/2 hour until artichokes are tender. Mash artichokes to a coarse puree. Add greens and simmer another 10 minutes. Add more water or stock, if necessary. Add lemon juice and continue simmering 1-2 minutes. Season to taste.

[serves 4]

Nutrition Per Serving: Calories 121, Total Fat 2g, Saturated Fat trace, Cholesterol 0mg, Sodium 107mg, Potassium 815mg, Total Carbohydrate 23g, Dietary Fiber 3g, Protein 3g, Calcium 49mg, Iron 5mg, Vitamin C 26mg, Vitamin A 1896 IU, Vitamin B6 .2mg, Thiamin B1 .2mg, Riboflavin B2 .1mg, Folacin 24mcg, Niacin 2mg

Jerusalem Artichoke Chips

The Diet Doctor's Wife: The first year I grew Jerusalem artichokes, I was surprised and frankly overwhelmed by the bounty of my harvest. I grew enough chokes to stock a grocery store for an entire week. No kidding. I gave chokes as gifts to whomever would accept them. I canned and pickled them and basically tried to get away with serving them at every meal. As you can imagine, I spent a great deal of time thinking about creative ways to turn a choke. This recipe is one example.

1 pound Jerusalem artichokes
2 cloves garlic, finely minced
2 tablespoons extra virgin olive oil
juice of 1/2 lemon
sea salt and freshly ground black pepper, to taste

Preheat oven to 325 F.

Peel Jerusalem artichokes. Using a mandoline, cut in 1/16-inch slices. Place artichoke slices in a bowl with garlic, 1 tablespoon extra virgin olive oil and lemon juice. Toss to combine. Allow mixture to sit for 15-30 minutes.

Brush the surface of 2 baking sheets with the remaining extra virgin olive oil. Place baking sheets in the oven for 10 minutes.

Place artichoke slices on the hot baking sheets, making sure that the slices do not overlap. Sprinkle slices with salt and pepper.

Bake for 8-10 minutes. Rotate the pans and bake for another 8-10 minutes. Turn each chip over and then bake for another 5 minutes until golden brown. Watch carefully, so that the chips do not burn. Allow to cool on paper towels.

Repeat with the remaining artichoke slices.

Jerusalem Artichoke Chips can be served hot or cold.

[serves 6]

Nutrition Per Serving: Calories 100, Total Fat 5g, Saturated Fat 1g, Cholesterol 0mg, Sodium 3mg, Potassium 336mg, Total Carbohydrate 14g, Dietary Fiber 1g, Protein 2g, Calcium 14mg, Iron 3mg, Vitamin C 6mg, Vitamin A 17 IU, Vitamin B6 .1mg, Thiamin B1 .2mg, Folacin 11mcg, Niacin 1mg

Sea Vegetables

SEA VEGETABLES

We try to include sea vegetables in our daily diet as they contain a lot of essential nutrients and help to tone down our cravings for sweets. Sea vegetables can be eaten on their own or added to soups, stews or grain dishes. Dried sea vegetables are readily available in any Asian market or health food store. Prepared sea vegetable salads can be found in Japanese and gourmet fish markets. The sea vegetables used in this cookbook are agar agar, arame, hijiki, kombu, nori and wakame.

Agar agar

Agar agar is a gelling agent extracted from red sea algae. It is used to make puddings, aspics and jelly molds. It contains no calories and is a good source of calcium, iron and dietary fiber. Agar agar comes in four forms: flakes, powder, strips and bars. We recommend flakes as they are good quality, readily available and easy to use. Four tablespoons of agar agar flakes will set approximately 3 cups of liquid. Just add the flakes to simmering liquid and stir continuously until they are completely dissolved.

Arame

Arame is a mild tasting sea vegetable that comes in thin strips. It is lovely in salads, soups, grain dishes and stir-fries.

Hijiki

Hijiki is a strong tasting sea vegetable that comes in irregular strips. It is high in calcium and iron. Hijiki goes well with sweet vegetables like carrots or sweet potatoes.

Kombu

Kombu or kelp is a flat, wide, dark green sea vegetable. It is used in stocks, soups and pickles. Kombu tenderizes high protein foods like beans, making them easier to digest. Just add a 4-inch strip of kombu to bean cooking water and cook as directed. You will not have to add salt.

Nori

Nori, also known as sea laver, is pressed into thin sheets. The sheets are generally toasted and used to make sushi or condiments. Sushi nori is nori that has already been toasted.

Wakame

Wakame is a mild-flavored, leafy sea vegetable with a high calcium content. It is used in soups, salads and pickles.

NUTRITIONAL CONTENT

We recommend that you have at least one serving of sea vegetables every day. Sea vegetables are a rich source of calcium, iron, Vitamin A, Vitamin C, niacin and iodine. On a dairy-free mostly vegetarian diet, like the one presented in this book, it is especially important that you eat foods with a high calcium and iron content.

If you have a thyroid problem, please consult your physician before eating sea vegetables that are high in iodine such as arame and kombu.

Nutritional Content of Sea Vegetables Per 100 Grams*

	Calcium	Iron
Agar Agar	540mg	2mg
Arame	1160mg	12mg
Hijiki	1400mg	29mg
Kombu	800mg	43mg
Nori	260mg	21mg
Wakame	1300mg	13mg

*Information sources: U.S. Department of Agriculture and food suppliers and manufacturers.

WASHING SEA VEGETABLES

Most sea vegetables need to be washed before use. Arame and wakame can be quickly rinsed under cold water. Hijiki needs to be washed more carefully as it can be gritty. Just pick through hijiki for tiny shells or clumps of dirt, and immerse in a bowl of clean water. Drain and repeat this washing process until the water runs clear. Kombu just needs to be wiped with a damp cloth or paper towel. Nori and agar agar require no washing at all.

SOAKING SEA VEGETABLES

Some sea vegetables need to be soaked after they are washed. Wakame requires 5-10 minutes of soaking. After wakame is soaked, the coarse stems can be easily cut away and discarded. Instant wakame flakes contain no coarse stems and need less than one minute of soaking. Arame and kombu require no soaking, if they are to be cooked. Otherwise, they need to be soaked for about 10 minutes. Hijiki must be soaked for at least 10 minutes before it is cooked. Nori and agar agar require no soaking (or washing) at all. Refer to recipes or the instructions on the package for more details.

Do not discard the soaking water. Use it to water plants instead. They will surely benefit from the nutritional boost provided by the infusion of vitamins and minerals.

STORAGE

Sea vegetables usually come dried and should be stored in airtight containers in a dark, cool place. Prepared sea vegetable salads should be refrigerated.

Arame Salad

The Diet Doctor: This dish is jammed packed with nutrition. Arame salad is a high source of Calcium, Vitamin A, Zinc and Dietary Fiber. For those of you watching your sodium intake, this salad is still a healthy choice. Just make sure to choose less sodium rich dishes for the rest of the day and remember to drink your water.

1/2 cup dried arame
1 carrot, julienned
1 cup red cabbage, shredded
3 tablespoons scallions, minced
1 tablespoon low sodium tamari
2 tablespoons brown rice vinegar
2 teaspoons Sesame Salt (page 327)

Wash arame and soak in water for about 10 minutes. Drain. Combine arame, carrots, cabbage and scallions.

Stir together tamari and vinegar. Add Sesame Salt and mix to incorporate. Pour dressing on arame mixture and toss to combine.

[serves 4]

Nutrition Per Serving: Calories 107, Total Fat trace, Saturated Fat trace, Cholesterol 0mg, *Sodium 524mg, Potassium 655mg, Total Carbohydrate 24g, Dietary Fiber 22g, Protein 4g, Calcium 315mg, Iron 2mg, Zinc 3mg, Vitamin C 8mg, Vitamin A 6582 IU, Riboflavin B2 .2mg, Folacin 14mcg

*Note: The sodium content of this dish is a bit high. Watch sodium intake for the rest of the day and remember to drink plenty of water.

Braised Arame

1/2 cup dried arame, loosely packed
1 carrot, julienned
1 cup onion, sliced in half-moons

2 teaspoons low sodium tamari
1/4 teaspoon fresh ginger root, grated
*2 tablespoons toasted sesame seeds

Soak arame in water to cover for 10 minutes. Drain.

Place arame, carrots, onions and 1 cup of water in a saucepan, and bring to a boil. Lower heat, cover and simmer for 45 minutes. Add more water throughout cooking, if necessary

When arame is cooked, add tamari and squeeze juice from the grated ginger into the pot. Simmer a few minutes longer and cook off excess liquid. Toss with sesame seeds.

[serves 4]

Nutrition Per Serving: Calories 132, Total Fat 2g, Saturated Fat trace, Cholesterol 0mg, Sodium 464mg, Potassium 658mg, Total Carbohydrate 26g, Dietary Fiber 22g, Protein 4g, Calcium 312mg, Iron 3mg, Zinc 3mg, Vitamin C 4mg, Vitamin A 6545 IU, Vitamin B6 .1mg, Thiamin B1 .1mg, Riboflavin B2 .2mg, Folacin 12mcg, Niacin 1mg

*Note: Refer to the recipe for Sesame Salt on page 327 for instructions on how to toast sesame seeds.

Braised Hijiki with Carrots and Shitake Mushrooms

1/2 cup dried hijiki
8 dried shitake mushrooms, soaked in warm water for 30 minutes
2 teaspoons toasted sesame oil
1 carrot, julienned
1 tablespoon low sodium tamari

Submerge hijiki in several changes of cold water to remove sand, dirt and tiny seashells. Discard washing water and then soak hijiki in 2 cups of fresh cold water for 10 minutes.

Bring hijiki and soaking water to a boil and cook for 5 minutes. Add 1/2 cup water, cover and simmer for 20 minutes. Drain.

Drain mushrooms, reserving soaking liquid. Strain soaking liquid through a cheesecloth-lined, wire-mesh strainer to remove grit. Remove and discard mushroom stems. Slice caps into 1/8-inch strips.

Heat oil in a skillet on medium low. Add hijiki, carrots and mushrooms. Sauté for 1 minute. Add 1/4 cup of mushroom soaking liquid and tamari. Cover and gently simmer for 10 minutes. Remove cover and boil off remaining liquid. Season to taste.

[serves 4]

Nutrition Per Serving: Calories 140, Total Fat 2g, Saturated Fat trace, Cholesterol 0mg, *Sodium 571mg, Potassium 1478mg, Total Carbohydrate 25g, Dietary Fiber 1g, Protein 4g, Calcium 450mg, Iron 16mg, Zinc 1mg, Vitamin C 2mg, Vitamin A 5063 IU, Vitamin B6 .1mg, Riboflavin B2 .1mg, Folacin 15mcg, Niacin 1mg

*Note: The sodium content in this dish is relatively high. Watch sodium intake for the rest of the day and make sure to drink a lot of water. To lower sodium content, use less tamari.

Hijiki Salad

1/2 cup dried hijiki
2 tablespoons mirin
1/2 teaspoon toasted sesame oil
1 tablespoon low sodium tamari or low sodium soy sauce
2 teaspoons Sesame Salt (page 327)

Submerge hijiki in several changes of cold water to remove sand, dirt and tiny seashells. Discard washing water and then soak hijiki in enough fresh cold water to cover for 15 minutes.

Put hijiki and soaking liquid in a pot. Add water to cover. Bring to a boil. Cover and simmer gently for 30 minutes, adding water throughout cooking, if necessary. Drain. Place hijiki in a serving bowl.

In a small bowl, whisk together mirin, sesame oil and tamari, and add to the hijiki. Toss to combine. Sprinkle with Sesame Salt.

[serves 4]

Nutrition Per Serving: Calories 107, Total Fat 1g, Saturated Fat trace, Cholesterol 9mg, *Sodium 573mg, Potassium 1312mg, Total Carbohydrate 18g, Protein 3g, Calcium 447mg, Iron 16mg, Folacin 1mcg

*Note: The sodium content in this dish is relatively high. Watch sodium intake for the rest of the day and make sure to drink a lot of water. To lower sodium content, use less tamari or Sesame Salt.

Hijiki Sweet Potato Stir-Fry

1/2 cup dried hijiki
1 medium sweet potato or 2 medium carrots
2 teaspoons grapeseed oil
1 cup Basic Vegetable Stock (page 94), Japanese Stock (page 95) or water
2 teaspoons maple syrup
1 tablespoon mirin
1 tablespoon low sodium tamari
1 1/2 teaspoons Sesame Salt (page 327)

Submerge hijiki in several changes of cold water to remove sand, dirt and tiny seashells. Discard washing water and then soak hijiki in enough fresh cold water to cover for 15 minutes. Drain.

Peel sweet potato and cut into 1/4-inch thick julienne strips. (If using carrots, peel and cut into 1/4-inch diagonal slices.) Heat oil in a nonstick wok or pan on medium low. Stir-fry sweet potato strips 3 minutes until lightly browned. Add hijiki. Stir-fry for another minute. Add stock, maple syrup, mirin and tamari. Bring to a boil and cover. Reduce heat to low and simmer gently for 20-30 minutes. Uncover and boil away liquid. Sprinkle with Sesame Salt.

[serves 6]

Nutrition Per Serving: Calories 107, Total Fat 2g, Saturated Fat trace, Cholesterol 0mg, Sodium 385mg, Potassium 923mg, Total Carbohydrate 19g, Dietary Fiber 1g, Protein 2g, Calcium 305mg, Iron 11mg, Vitamin C 5mg, Vitamin A 4347 IU, Vitamin B6 .1mg, Folacin 4mcg

Wakame and Glass Noodles

*1 cucumber, sliced in 1/4–inch rounds
sea salt
8 ounces glass noodles
1 ounce dried wakame
1 carrot, cut in julienne strips
1 cup red cabbage, thinly shredded
2 tablespoons scallion, minced
1 teaspoon toasted sesame oil
1 tablespoon tamari
1 tablespoon brown rice vinegar
1 teaspoon Sesame Salt (page 327)

Place cucumber slices in a colander and sprinkle lightly with salt. Allow to drain over a bowl for 30 minutes.

Place glass noodles in a separate bowl. Pour boiling water over the noodles. Allow to sit for 20 minutes. Drain and set aside.

Soak wakame in water for 5 minutes. Drain. Cut out the coarse veins and discard. Chop wakame leaves in 1-inch squares and set aside.

Mix together noodles, cucumber slices, wakame, carrot strips and cabbage.

To make the dressing, whisk together scallion, oil, tamari and vinegar. Toss noodle mixture with dressing.

[serves 4]

Nutrition Per Serving: Calories 237, Total Fat 2g, Saturated Fat trace, Cholesterol 0mg, Sodium 231mg, Potassium 224mg, Total Carbohydrate 58g, Dietary Fiber 3g, Protein 1g, Calcium 81mg, Iron 1mg, Vitamin C 16mg, Vitamin A 5269 IU, Vitamin B6 .1mg, Riboflavin B2 .1mg, Folacin 33mcg, Niacin 1mg

*Note: I prefer to use thin-skinned cucumbers with small seeds.

Wakame Salad

1 ounce dried wakame or dried instant wakame flakes
1 teaspoon toasted sesame oil
1 tablespoon low sodium tamari
1 tablespoon brown rice vinegar

Soak wakame in water for 5 minutes. Drain. Cut out the coarse veins and discard. Chop wakame leaves into 1-inch squares. If using instant wakame flakes, simply soak for one or two minutes and drain.

Whisk together the rest of the ingredients and toss with the wakame.

[serves 4]

Nutrition Per Serving: Calories 16, Total Fat 1g, Saturated Fat trace, Cholesterol 0mg, Sodium 212mg, Potassium 12mg, Total Carbohydrate 1g, Calcium 11mg, Vitamin A 26 IU, Folacin 15mcg

Korean Sea Laver Chips

The Diet Doctor's Wife: I was introduced to this treat by a Korean woman whose son I used to tutor in English. After every lesson, she would insist on feeding me to express her gratitude for the boy's progress. I happily obliged and particularly enjoyed her sea laver chips, which she served with ginseng tea.

6 nori sheets
1 tablespoon toasted sesame oil
sea salt, to taste

Brush one side of each nori sheet with toasted sesame oil and then sprinkle lightly with salt. Heat a gas or electric burner on medium. With a pair of tongs, hold a nori sheet 1-2 inches over the burner. Toast one side for a few seconds. Turn to the other side and toast a few more seconds. Repeat the same procedure with the other nori sheets. Allow to cool and cut each sheet into bite-size squares.

[serves 12]

Nutrition Per Serving: Calories 12, Total Fat 1g, Saturated Fat trace, Cholesterol 0mg, Sodium 2mg, Potassium 18mg, Calcium 4mg, Vitamin C 2mg, Vitamin A 260 IU, Folacin 7mcg

Intense Kombu Condiment

The Diet Doctor's Wife: A small amount of this kombu condiment is terrific with plain brown rice. Believe it or not, the 1/2 teaspoon serving size is quite generous. As the name suggests, the flavor is very intense.

6-inch piece dried kombu, soaked in cold water until softened
3 tablespoons brown rice vinegar
5 tablespoons low sodium tamari
1 tablespoon mirin
2 teaspoons Sesame Salt (page 327)

Cut kombu into 1/2-inch squares. Put kombu squares, 4 cups of water and 1 tablespoon of vinegar in a saucepan. Bring to a boil. Cover saucepan and reduce heat to low. Simmer 2 hours.

Add tamari, mirin and the 2 remaining tablespoons of vinegar. Boil, uncovered, until liquid reduces to 2 tablespoons. Turn off heat. Add Sesame Salt. Put mixture in a small container and allow to cool. Kombu Condiment can be refrigerated for up to 1 month.

[makes 1/4 cup, 24 servings]

Nutrition Per 1/2 Teaspoon Serving: Calories 3, Total Fat trace, Saturated Fat trace, Cholesterol 0mg, Sodium 127mg, Potassium 9mg, Calcium 2mg, Folacin 1mcg

Other recipes with sea vegetables: Basic Vegetable Stock (page 94), Japanese Stock (page 95), Bonito Dashi (page 96), Cool Weather Miso Soup (page 118), Warm Weather Miso Soup (page 119), Bonito Miso (page 120), Inside-Out Sushi (page 134), California Sushi Bowl (page 135), Thin Cucumber Rolls (page 136), Mah Zeh Rice (page 139), Japanese Simmered Tofu (page 213)

Pickles

Lebanese Turnip Pickles

The Diet Doctor's Wife: These pickles are addictive. If you find them too salty, just rinse them with water or use less salt in the pickling preparation.

1 pound small white turnips
1 raw beet, peeled and sliced
2 cups water
1 1/2 tablespoons sea salt
2 tablespoons white wine vinegar or brown rice vinegar

Peel turnips and cut in 1/2-inch thick slices. Place slices in a 2-quart jar. Intersperse with beet slices.

Boil water with salt and vinegar. When cooled, pour liquid over turnips. Cover and store at room temperature for 6 days. Then store in the refrigerator for up to 6 weeks.

[serves 16]

Nutrition Per Serving: Calories 9, Total Fat trace, Saturated Fat trace, Cholesterol 0mg, Sodium 548mg, Potassium 62mg, Total Carbohydrate 2g, Dietary Fiber 1g, Calcium 8mg, Vitamin C 5mg, Vitamin A 2 IU, Folacin 9mcg

Rich Onion Pickles

1 cup onions, sliced in half-moons
2 tablespoons low sodium tamari or low sodium soy sauce
1 tablespoon brown rice vinegar
1 tablespoon water

Combine ingredients and refrigerate for at least 2 hours. Eat within 3 days.

[serves 8]

Nutrition Per Serving: Calories 10, Total Fat trace, Saturated Fat trace, Cholesterol 0mg, Sodium 151mg, Potassium 41mg, Total Carbohydrate 2g, Protein 1g, Calcium 5mg, Vitamin C 1mg, Folacin 5mcg

Note: If you find these pickles too salty, use less soy sauce or rinse the pickles with water before eating.

Quick Cucumber and Onion Pickles

1 cup cucumber, seeded and sliced
1 small onion, cut in half-moons
1/2 teaspoon sea salt

Sprinkle vegetables with salt. Put in a *pickle press and allow to rest at room temperature for 1/2 hour. Drain and serve. If pickles are too salty, rinse gently with water and drain before serving.

[serves 4]

Nutrition Per Serving: Calories 18, Total Fat trace, Saturated Fat trace, Cholesterol 0mg, Sodium 237mg, Potassium 128mg, Total Carbohydrate 4g, Dietary Fiber 1g, Protein 1g, Calcium 14mg, Vitamin C 5mg, Vitamin A 127 IU, Folacin 13mcg

*Note: If you do not have a pickle press, place ingredients in a bowl. Cover ingredients with a plate that fits inside the bowl. Weight the plate down with a couple of 28-ounce cans or with a mason jar filled with water.

Variation: For a less salty pickle, substitute 1 tablespoon ume vinegar for the sea salt. Allow pickle to sit for 1-2 days before serving.

Spicy Korean Cucumber Pickles

1 1/2 pounds Japanese or pickling cucumbers
2 teaspoons sea salt
1 teaspoon red pepper flakes
1 tablespoon brown rice vinegar
1 teaspoon Sesame Salt (page 327)
1 teaspoon garlic, finely minced
1 teaspoon toasted sesame oil
1 tablespoon maple syrup

Slice cucumbers in thin rounds and place them in a colander. Sprinkle rounds with salt and cover with a couple of handfuls of ice cubes. Allow to sit for 20 minutes. Squeeze cucumber rounds to release excess water or pat gently with a paper towel. After the excess water has been removed, place cucumber rounds in a mixing bowl.

In a separate bowl, whisk together the remaining ingredients. Add to the cucumber rounds and toss with your hands until the dressing is well incorporated. Chill for at least 1/2 hour.

[serves 6]

Nutrition Per Serving: Calories 31, Total Fat 1g, Saturated Fat trace, Cholesterol 0mg, *Sodium 635mg, Potassium 169 mg, Total Carbohydrate 5g, Dietary Fiber 1g, Protein 1g, Calcium 21mg, Vitamin C 6mg, Vitamin A 254 IU, Folacin 14mcg

*Note: The sodium content in this dish looks deceptively high. Although 2 teaspoons of sea salt are used in this preparation, much of the salt is washed away by the melting ice cubes. If you still find the pickle too salty, rinse it with cold water and drain.

Meyer Lemon Pickles

The Diet Doctor's Wife: Try these pickles with Moroccan Root Vegetable Tagine (page 169) or Grilled Halibut Steak with Chermoula (page 240). Just use a very little bit, no more than a 1/2 teaspoon of pickle per serving. If you are watching your salt intake, rinse the pickle with water first. Note that you can use regular lemons if Meyer lemons are not available. I chose Meyer lemons for this recipe because they have a sweet, tangerine-like quality, which adds a little something special.

4 organic Meyer lemons, washed and dried
1/4 cup coarse sea salt
1/2 cup freshly squeezed Meyer lemon juice
1/4 cup extra virgin olive oil

Cut each lemon lengthwise into 8 wedges. Toss lemon wedges with salt and juice. Transfer to a glass-top canning jar, pressing down so that the lemon wedges are squashed together. Seal jar and allow lemons to sit at room temperature for 1 week. Shake jar once daily. Top lemons with olive oil and refrigerate. This pickle will keep up to 6 months.

[serves 60]

Nutrition Per 1/2 Teaspoon Serving: Calories 9, Total Fat 1g, Saturated Fat trace, Cholesterol 0mg, Sodium 376mg, Potassium 8mg, Calcium 4mg, Vitamin C 3mg, Vitamin A 2 IU, Folacin 1mcg

Pressed Salad

1 cup red or green cabbage, shredded
1 carrot, cut in thin matchsticks
2 scallions, cut in thin diagonal slices
1 tablespoon ume vinegar
1 tablespoon brown rice vinegar
1 tablespoon mirin

Put ingredients in a *pickle press. Leave to rest at room temperature 1-24 hours. Refrigerate until ready to serve. Pressed Salad will keep in the refrigerator for up to 3 days.

To serve, remove the pickled vegetables with a slotted spoon. If a less salty taste is preferred, rinse the pickled vegetables gently with water and drain.

[serves 4]

Nutrition Per Serving: Calories 22, Total Fat trace, Saturated Fat trace, Cholesterol 0mg, Sodium 274mg, Potassium 134mg, Total Carbohydrate 4g, Dietary Fiber 1g, Protein 1g, Calcium 21mg, Vitamin C 10mg, Vitamin A 5122 IU, Folacin 17mcg

*Note: If you do not have a pickle press, place ingredients in a bowl. Cover ingredients with a plate that fits inside the bowl. Weight the plate down with a couple of 28-ounce cans or with a mason jar filled with water.

Mixed Japanese Pickles

*1 cup cucumber, cut in 1/4-inch slices
1 cup daikon, cut in 1/4-inch slices

1 carrot, cut in 1/4-inch slices
1 teaspoon sea salt

Place a handful of vegetables in a **pickle press. Sprinkle with sea salt. Continue layering and salting. Close the press and apply maximum pressure. Let stand overnight. To reduce salt content, rinse with water before eating.

[serves 6]

Nutrition Per Serving: Calories 22, Total Fat trace, Saturated Fat trace, Cholesterol 0mg, Sodium 331mg, Potassium 214mg, Total Carbohydrate 4g, Dietary Fiber 1g, Calcium 19mg, Vitamin C 13mg, Vitamin A 5807 IU, Folacin 19mcg

*Note 1: I prefer to use thin-skinned cucumbers with small seeds.

**Note 2: If you do not have a pickle press, place ingredients in a bowl. Cover ingredients with a plate that fits inside the bowl. Weight the plate down with a couple of 28-ounce cans or with a mason jar filled with water.

Speedy Sauerkraut

The Diet Doctor's Wife: This moderately fermented sauerkraut is so easy to prepare with a pickle press. And the flavor is terrific. All you need is a couple of tablespoons to jazz up plain ol' brown rice.

1 cabbage, finely shredded
1 tablespoon sea salt
1 tablespoon caraway seeds

Put a handful of cabbage in a *pickle press and sprinkle with some sea salt and caraway seeds. Continue layering. Close the press and apply maximum pressure. Let stand at room temperature for 2-4 days until bubbles form. After the first day, you may have to adjust the pressure to make sure that the cabbage is submerged in the brine that develops in the pickling process.

Remove cabbage from the press and put in an airtight container. Refrigerate.

[serves 16]

Nutrition Per Serving: Calories 16, Total Fat trace, Saturated Fat trace, Cholesterol 0mg, Sodium 363mg, Potassium 145mg, Total Carbohydrate 3g, Dietary Fiber 1g, Protein 1g, Calcium 30mg, Vitamin C 18mg, Vitamin A 77 IU, Vitamin B6 .1mg, Folacin 24mcg

*Note: If you do not have a pickle press, put ingredients in a bowl and place a weighted plate on top. You may have to add more weight over time to apply maximum pressure and to make sure that the cabbage is submerged in the brine that develops during the pickling process.

Desserts

The desserts in this section are made with very little saturated fat, practically no refined sugar and absolutely no dairy or eggs. Organic and natural ingredients are used whenever possible to create delicious and nutritious treats that can be enjoyed guilt-free.

WHOLE GRAIN FLOUR

I use organic, whole grain flour whenever possible. Whole grain flour is much less processed and contains more nutrients and flavor than refined white flour. I prefer to bake with whole wheat pastry flour as it is a bit lighter than regular whole wheat flour. To create an even lighter texture, I often combine whole wheat flour with unbleached, non-chemically processed white flour. For added interest, I experiment with flours made from whole grains other than whole wheat such as spelt (a relative of whole wheat), corn, barley, oats, brown rice, buckwheat and rye.

Whole grain flours and unbleached, non-chemically processed white flour are readily available in health food markets, gourmet shops, and some grocery stores as well as through mail order baker's catalogues.

SWEETENERS

Americans are huge consumers of sugar. We eat a lot of cookies, cakes, candy, muffins, pies and ice cream. We put sugar in our coffee, sprinkle it on top of our grapefruit and add it to our cereal. Sugar is a hidden ingredient in many of our packaged crackers, breads, salad dressings and even seasonings. It's no wonder that the average American consumes between 120 and 143 pounds of sugar each year.

The sugar that we most commonly use is refined from sugar cane or beets. This refined sugar is quickly absorbed by the bloodstream, which results in a quick burst of energy. The energy high is soon followed by an energy low, which creates a craving for more sugar. Once this craving is satisfied, the cycle repeats itself. Over the long haul, over-consumption of refined sugar affects the body chemistry to such a degree that there is increased risk of mood disorders, diabetes, fungal conditions, digestive problems, tooth decay, eczema and acne.

Artificial sweeteners are not the answer to this problem. In spite of being practically calorie-free, artificial sweeteners give many people headaches and digestive problems.

But, do not despair. There are many natural sweeteners that can be used as healthy alternatives to refined sugar. Natural sweeteners are usually made from organically grown food sources that are produced through chemical-free processing techniques. Natural sweeteners contain complex carbohydrates, which break down slowly into simple sugars. As a result, you don't get the quick highs and lows that you do with refined sugar.

The natural sweeteners that I use in this cookbook are brown rice syrup, barley malt, maple syrup, unsulphured blackstrap molasses and fruit (fresh, juiced, dried and pureed). Honey is a natural sweetener that I rarely use as it is 70 percent sweeter than refined sugar. All of the mentioned natural sweeteners can be purchased in any health food market.

Most of the desserts in this chapter are made with natural sweeteners. The only exceptions are the sorbet recipes, which are made with sugar syrup. To date, I have not been able to create the desired effect without using refined sugar.

BAKING WITHOUT BUTTER

The recipes in this section are made without any butter or margarine. The consumption of butter, a saturated fat, is linked with high cholesterol and heart disease. Margarine, a manufactured saturated fat, is associated with the same health risks. There may be evidence to suggest that margarine is even more harmful due to the extensive processing techniques required for its production.

The type of fat I prefer to use for baking is nut oil, usually walnut or almond. I also use light vegetable oil. My preference is grapeseed oil as it does not impart a particular flavor. If you are worried about nut allergies, just substitute grapeseed oil or any other light vegetable oil for the nut oils called for in a given recipe.

BAKING WITHOUT MILK

Baking without milk is very simple. In many cases, the addition of milk is really just to add liquid volume more than flavor. I find that if I add water, fruit juice, soy milk, rice milk or amasake, the recipes come out beautifully.

THICKENING AGENTS

To create puddings, gels or pie fillings, most cooks rely on thickening agents such as eggs, gelatin or cornstarch. That is not the case in this cookbook. There is no need to add the saturated fat from eggs or the cocktail of chemicals used to manufacture gelatin and refined cornstarch. There are healthier alternatives. Natural thickening agents, such as agar agar, arrowroot and kuzu, are fat-free and processed without chemicals. Agar agar and kuzu even have medicinal properties.

Agar Agar

Agar agar is a sea vegetable that is used as a gelling agent. It has a subtle taste that Bill and I don't particularly like.

However, I find that when I combine agar agar with highly flavored ingredients, the unpleasant taste seems to disappear.

Agar agar is rich in iodine, calcium, iron, phosphorus and vitamins A, B complex, C, D and K. It also has mild laxative properties. Agar agar can be purchased in the macrobiotic section of any health food market.

Arrowroot

Arrowroot powder is derived from a rhizome. It works beautifully for thickening pie filling.

Kuzu

Kuzu is derived from the root of a vine that grows in Japan and the Southern U.S. It comes in white chalky chunks that need to be dissolved in water.

Kuzu is used to thicken sauces, puddings and pie fillings. It also has medicinal value, aiding in digestion and inhibiting cravings for alcohol. Kuzu can be purchased in the macrobiotic section of any health food market.

LEAVENING AGENTS

Most bakers use eggs, yeast, baking powder and baking soda to leaven batters and doughs. As discussed in the section What We Eat, I try to omit eggs whenever possible because of fat content, food sensitivities and other health risks. I rarely bake with yeast, which triggers allergic reactions in many of the members of my family.

I do use aluminum-free baking powder (which is available in most grocery stores and health food markets) and baking soda.

Almond Pastry Cream

2 cups soy milk or rice milk
6 tablespoons maple syrup
1 vanilla bean pod, halved, seeds scraped out and set aside, or
1 teaspoon vanilla extract
pinch of sea salt
3 tablespoons kuzu, dissolved in 1/4 cup water
1/4 teaspoon almond extract

Put soy milk, maple syrup, vanilla bean pod halves and seeds, and salt in a pot. Bring to a slow boil. Remove vanilla bean pod halves. Lower heat to simmer. Add kuzu mixture and stir to combine. Simmer, stirring continuously, until thickened, about 3 minutes. Remove from heat and add almond extract (and vanilla extract, if not using vanilla bean). Stir to combine. Allow to cool, then cover with plastic wrap, and refrigerate for at least 1 hour.

[2 cups, 6 servings]

Nutrition Per Serving: Calories 103, Total Fat 2g, Saturated Fat trace, Cholesterol 0mg, Sodium 31mg, Potassium 155mg, Total Carbohydrate 21g, Dietary Fiber 1g, Protein 2g, Calcium 24mg, Iron 1mg, Vitamin A 26 IU, Thiamin B1 .2mg, Riboflavin B2 .1mg, Folacin 1mcg

Tofu Cream

12-ounce package silken tofu
1 tablespoon almond butter or sesame seed paste
4 tablespoons brown rice syrup or barley malt
grated zest of 1 lemon or 1/2 orange
1 teaspoon vanilla extract

Combine tofu, almond butter, rice syrup, zest and vanilla in a food processor. Puree. Chill until ready to serve.

[4 servings]

Nutrition Per Serving: Calories 135, Total Fat 6g, Saturated Fat 1g, Cholesterol 0mg, Sodium 8mg, Potassium 133mg, Total Carbohydrate 13g, Dietary Fiber 1g, Protein 7g, Calcium 101mg, Iron 5mg, Zinc 1mg, Vitamin C 1mg, Vitamin A 73 IU, Thiamin B1 .1mg, Riboflavin B2 .1mg, Folacin 15mcg

Walnut Crisp Topping

1/2 cup whole wheat flour
1 cup rolled oats
1/4 teaspoon cinnamon
1/4 teaspoon sea salt
*2 tablespoons crushed walnuts
*2 tablespoons walnut oil
2 tablespoons maple syrup
1/2 teaspoon vanilla extract

To make topping, lightly roast flour and oats in a dry skillet over medium heat just until heated through. Continually stir with a wooden spoon to avoid burning. Do not allow to brown. Transfer to a medium bowl. Add cinnamon, salt and nuts. Stir to combine. In a separate bowl, whisk oil, maple syrup and vanilla. Add wet ingredients to the dry mixture. Mix together until consistency is sticky. Bake according to recipe instructions (see page 302).

[serves 6]

Nutrition Per Serving: Calories 120, Total Fat 5g, Saturated Fat 1g, Cholesterol 0mg, Sodium 60mg, Potassium 86mg, Total Carbohydrate 16g, Dietary Fiber 2g, Protein 3g, Calcium 15mg, Iron 1mg, Zinc 1mg, Vitamin A 16 IU, Thiamin B1 .1mg, Folacin 6mcg, Niacin 1mg

*Note: For nut allergies, eliminate the nuts and substitute light vegetable oil for the nut oil.

Almond Crisp Topping

1/2 cup whole wheat flour
1 cup rolled oats
1/4 cup cornmeal
1/4 teaspoon cinnamon
1/4 teaspoon sea salt
*2 tablespoons crushed almonds

*2 tablespoons almond oil
2 tablespoons maple syrup

In a dry skillet, roast flour, oats and cornmeal over medium heat for 3 minutes until a nutty aroma is released. Continually stir with a wooden spoon to avoid burning. Transfer to a medium bowl. Add remaining dry ingredients and stir to combine. In a smaller bowl, whisk together wet ingredients. Add to the dry mixture and stir to combine. Bake according to recipe instructions (see pages 304 and 305).

[serves 8]

Nutrition Per Serving: Calories 136, Total Fat 5g, Saturated Fat 1g, Cholesterol 0mg, Sodium 60mg, Potassium 99mg, Total Carbohydrate 19g, Dietary Fiber 3g, Protein 3g, Calcium 20mg, Iron 1mg, Zinc 1mg, Vitamin A 28 IU, Thiamin B1 .1mg, Riboflavin B2 .1mg, Folacin 9mcg, Niacin 1mg

*Note: For nut allergies, eliminate the nuts and substitute light vegetable oil for the nut oil.

Single Crust Almond Pastry

3/4 cup whole wheat pastry flour
3/4 cup unbleached white flour
*1/4 cup ground almonds
1/8 teaspoon fine sea salt
*1/4 cup almond oil
4 tablespoons brown rice syrup

Place dry ingredients in a food processor. Pulse for a few seconds. Add oil and pulse a few more seconds. Add rice syrup. Pulse again until dough begins to form, adding a tablespoon or two of water if necessary. Do not over-mix. Remove dough and place on a lightly floured surface and form into a smooth flattened disk.

Place dough between two sheets of plastic wrap. Roll out dough between the plastic wrap and form into a circle to fit a 9-inch pie plate or tart pan.

Peel off top layer of wrap. Flip pastry onto greased pie plate or tart pan. Bake according to recipe instructions or cover with plastic wrap and refrigerate until ready to use. Dough can be frozen as well.

[serves 10]

Nutrition Per Serving: Calories 149, Total Fat 7g, Saturated Fat 1g, Cholesterol 0mg, Sodium 25mg, Potassium 74mg, Total Carbohydrate 19g, Dietary Fiber 2g, Protein 3g, Calcium 13mg, Iron 1mg, Thiamin B1 .1mg, Riboflavin B2 .1mg, Folacin 6mcg, Niacin 1mg

*Note: For nut allergies, eliminate the nuts and substitute light vegetable oil for the nut oil.

Single Crust Walnut Pastry

3/4 cup whole wheat pastry flour
3/4 cup unbleached white flour
*1/4 cup ground toasted walnuts
1/8 teaspoon sea salt
*1/4 cup walnut oil
2 tablespoons brown rice syrup, maple syrup or barley malt
1/4 cup water

Place dry ingredients in a food processor. Pulse for a few seconds. Add oil and pulse for a few more seconds. Add rice syrup. Pulse again. Then gradually add water, pulsing, until dough begins to form. Do not over-mix. Remove from processor and place dough on a lightly floured surface and form into a smooth flattened disk.

Place dough between two sheets of plastic wrap. Roll out dough between the plastic wrap and form into a circle to fit a 9-inch pie plate or tart pan.

Peel off top layer of wrap. Flip pastry onto a greased pie plate or tart pan. Bake according to recipe instructions or cover in plastic wrap and refrigerate until ready to use. Dough can be frozen as well.

[serves 10]

Nutrition Per Serving: Calories 133, Total Fat 7g, Saturated Fat 1g, Cholesterol 0mg, Sodium 25mg, Potassium 57mg, Total Carbohydrate 16g, Dietary Fiber 2g, Protein 3g, Calcium 6mg, Iron 1mg, Vitamin A 6 IU, Thiamin B1 .1mg, Riboflavin B2 .1mg, Folacin 6mcg, Niacin 1mg

*Note: For nut allergies, eliminate the nuts and substitute light vegetable oil for the nut oil.

Single Crust Pecan Pastry

3/4 cup whole wheat pastry flour
3/4 cup unbleached white flour
*1/4 cup ground pecans
1/8 teaspoon sea salt
*1/4 cup walnut oil
2 tablespoons maple syrup
1/4 cup water

Place dry ingredients in a food processor. Pulse for a few seconds. Add oil and pulse a few more seconds. Add syrup. Pulse again. Then gradually add water, pulsing, until dough begins to form. Do not over-mix. Remove from processor and place dough on a lightly floured surface and form into a smooth flattened disk.

Place dough between two sheets of plastic wrap. Roll out dough between the plastic wrap and form into a circle to fit a 9-inch pie plate or tart pan.

Peel off top layer of wrap. Flip pastry onto a greased pie plate or tart pan. Bake according to recipe instructions or cover in plastic wrap and refrigerate until ready to use. Dough can be frozen as well.

[serves 10]

Nutrition Per Serving: Calories 136, Total Fat 7g, Saturated Fat 1g, Cholesterol 0mg, Sodium 25mg, Potassium 62mg, Total Carbohydrate 17g, Dietary Fiber 2g, Protein 2g, Calcium 9mg, Iron 1mg, Vitamin A 3 IU, Thiamin B1 .1mg, Riboflavin B2 .1mg, Folacin 6mcg, Niacin 1mg

*Note: For nut allergies, eliminate the nuts and substitute light vegetable oil for the nut oil.

Dried Fruit Puree

1 cup prunes, pitted
1/2 cup prune juice or water
1 teaspoon vanilla extract
pinch of sea salt

Put fruit in a saucepan with enough juice to barely cover. Bring to a boil and then lower heat to simmer, uncovered, until no liquid remains. Puree.

[3/4 cup]

Nutrition Per Tablespoon: Calories 42, Total Fat trace, Saturated Fat trace, Cholesterol 0mg, Sodium 11mg, Potassium 134mg, Total Carbohydrate 11g, Dietary Fiber 1g, Calcium 8mg, Vitamin C 1mg, Vitamin A 278 IU, Vitamin B6 .1mg, Folacin 1mcg

Note: You can substitute dried apricots or dried pears for the prunes. If making such substitutions, omit the prune juice. Use apricot nectar, pear juice or water instead.

Sugar Syrup

*The Diet Doctor's Wife: I hardly ever use sugar, unless absolutely necessary. And sugar (in the form of sugar syrup) is absolutely necessary in a fresh fruit sorbet. I have tried to use other sweeteners and have been gravely disappointed. Fresh fruit sorbets are included in this cookbook because they contain no dairy products or *fat, and they satisfy ice cream cravings. So as long as you don't eat sorbet everyday, the little bit of sugar won't hurt you.*

3 cups sugar
3 cups water

In a medium saucepan, heat sugar and water on medium until sugar has completely dissolved. Bring to a boil and cook for 2 minutes. Remove from the heat and allow to cool. Store in the refrigerator in an airtight container for up to 1 week.

[yields approximately 4 1/2 cups]

Nutrition Per Tablespoon: Calories 32, Total Fat 0g, Saturated Fat 0g, Cholesterol 0mg, Total Carbohydrate 8g

*Note: The coconut sorbets are made with reduced fat coconut milk, which still contains fat.

Earl Grey Tea Infused Citrus Terrine

The Diet Doctor's Wife: When in Paris a few years ago, Bill and I had dinner at the famous Guy Savoy. The meal was wonderful from start to finish. We particularly enjoyed the light grapefruit terrine, which we had for dessert. My rendition is quite a bit less complicated and prepared without gelatin. I use the vegetarian gelling agent, agar agar, instead.

2 oranges
1/2 grapefruit
1/2 cup brewed Earl Grey tea
1/2 cup white dessert wine
1/2 cup freshly squeezed grapefruit juice
1/2 cup freshly squeezed orange juice
pinch of sea salt
*1/4 cup agar agar flakes

Peel the oranges and grapefruit, and separate in sections. Remove the pits, pith and thin membrane protecting the individual sections. Slice fruit sections thinly and set aside.

In a saucepan, heat tea, wine, juices and salt. Bring to a boil. Reduce heat to simmer and add agar agar flakes, whisking constantly until the flakes are completely dissolved. This will take about 5 minutes.

Place fruit in a terrine or mold. Pour hot liquid on top. Allow to cool. Refrigerate to set, at least 1 hour.

[serves 8]

Nutrition Per Serving: Calories 62, Total Fat trace, Saturated Fat trace, Cholesterol 0mg, Sodium 19mg, Potassium 286mg, Total Carbohydrate 11g, Dietary Fiber 1g, Protein 1g, Calcium 20mg, Vitamin C 36mg, Vitamin A 184 IU, Thiamin B1 .1mg, Folacin 24mcg

*Note: This dessert contains agar agar, which is a mild laxative.

Panna Cotta with Strawberry Coulis

1 cup reduced fat coconut milk
3/4 cup soy milk, rice milk or water
1/4 cup maple syrup
pinch of sea salt
*2 tablespoons agar agar
1 1/2 teaspoons vanilla extract

In a saucepan, combine first 5 ingredients. Bring to a boil, stirring continuously. Reduce heat to simmer. Continuing to stir, simmer until agar agar flakes are completely dissolved. This will take 5-15 minutes. Remove from the heat and stir in vanilla. Pour hot liquid in 4 ramekins. Cool to room temperature. Refrigerate to set, about 1 hour.

Strawberry Coulis

1 1/2 cups strawberries, hulled
2-3 tablespoons brown rice syrup or maple syrup
pinch of sea salt or splash of freshly squeezed lemon juice

Puree ingredients. Pass through a strainer. Refrigerate.

To serve, unmold each panna cotta on individual serving plates. Drizzle 2 tablespoons of coulis around each panna cotta.

[serves 4]

Nutrition Per Serving: Calories 148, Total Fat 4g, Saturated Fat trace, Cholesterol 0mg, Sodium 69mg, Potassium 218mg, Total Carbohydrate 26g, Dietary Fiber 2g, Protein 3g, Calcium 31mg, Iron 1mg, Vitamin C 31mg, Vitamin A 35 IU, Thiamin B1 .1mg, Riboflavin B2 .1mg, Folacin 11mcg

*Note: This dessert contains agar agar, which is a mild laxative.

Apple Sauce I

The Diet Doctor's Wife: Apple sauce is a light, low-calorie dessert or snack. It can also be used in baking to sweeten muffins, cakes and cookies.

The Diet Doctor: Cooked fruit is not only tasty but also far gentler on the digestive system than it's fresh counterpart. The reason is that some of the sugars are broken down in the cooking process, giving you sweetness without an intense sugar jolt. If you are prone to arthritis, as I am, switching to cooked fruit can alleviate inflammation in the joints. Believe it or not, the sugar in fresh fruit can aggravate your symptoms.

*6 apples, peeled, cored and sliced
1/4-1/2 cup water
pinch of sea salt
1 tablespoon brown rice syrup (optional)

Combine ingredients in a saucepan. Simmer over moderate heat for 10 minutes. Puree.

[serves 8]

Nutrition Per Serving: Calories 61, Total Fat trace, Saturated Fat trace, Cholesterol 0mg, Sodium 15mg, Potassium 119mg, Total Carbohydrate 16g, Dietary Fiber 3g, Calcium 7mg, Vitamin C 6mg, Vitamin A 55 IU, Folacin 3mcg

*Note: The sweetness of the apple sauce will depend on the type of apples you choose.

Apple Sauce II

*6 apples, cored and cut in chunks
1/2 cup apple juice
1/2 teaspoon cinnamon
pinch of sea salt

Place apples in a medium saucepan. Add juice and bring to a boil. Lower heat, cover and simmer for 5 minutes, until apples are soft but not mushy. Add cinnamon. Stir gently. Allow to cool.

[serves 8]

Nutrition Per Serving: Calories 69, Total Fat trace, Saturated Fat trace, Cholesterol 0mg, Sodium 15mg, Potassium 138mg, Total Carbohydrate 18g, Dietary Fiber 3g, Calcium 10mg, Vitamin C 6mg, Vitamin A 55 IU, Folacin 3mcg

*Note: The sweetness of the apple sauce will depend on the type of apples you choose.

Apple Pudding with Tofu Cream

*6 apples, peeled, cored and chopped in chunks
6 tablespoons brown rice syrup
pinch of sea salt
1/2 cup apple juice
1/2 teaspoon cinnamon
1 1/2 teaspoons kuzu, dissolved in 2 tablespoons of water
1 recipe Tofu Cream (page 293)

Combine the first 5 ingredients in a saucepan. Bring to a boil. Reduce heat to simmer and cook until apples soften but still retain their shape. Add dissolved kuzu to the apple mixture. Stir in gently. Lower heat and cook a couple of minutes longer until mixture thickens. Remove from the heat and allow to cool. Refrigerate until ready to use.

Place apple pudding in serving bowls. Top with tofu cream.

[serves 8]

Nutrition Per Serving: Calories 171, Total Fat 4g, Saturated Fat trace, Cholesterol 0mg, Sodium 20mg, Potassium 205mg, Total Carbohydrate 33g, Dietary Fiber 3g, Protein 4g, Calcium 60mg, Iron 3mg, Vitamin C 6mg, Vitamin A 92 IU, Vitamin B6 .1mg, Thiamin B1 .1mg, Folacin 11mcg

*Note: The sweetness of the apple pudding will depend on the type of apples you choose. Adjust the amount of brown rice syrup accordingly.

Apple Crisp

1/2 cup apple juice
*6 apples, peeled, cored and chopped in chunks
6 tablespoons brown rice syrup
pinch of sea salt
1/2 teaspoon cinnamon
1 1/2 teaspoons kuzu, dissolved in 2 tablespoons of water
1 recipe Walnut Crisp Topping (page 294)

Preheat oven to 350 F.

To make filling, bring apple juice to a boil. Add apples, syrup, sea salt and cinnamon. Lower heat to simmer and cook until apples soften but still retain their shape. Add dissolved kuzu to the apple mixture, stirring gently and continuously. Lower heat and cook a couple of minutes longer until mixture thickens. Pour into a square 8" x 8" baking pan. Distribute Walnut Crisp Topping over the top of the apple mixture. Bake 30-40 minutes.

[serves 8]

Nutrition Per Serving: Calories 217, Total Fat 6g, Saturated Fat 1g, Cholesterol 0mg, Sodium 76mg, Potassium 214mg, Total Carbohydrate 41g, Dietary Fiber 4g, Protein 3g, Calcium 22mg, Iron 1mg, Zinc 1mg, Vitamin C 4mg, Vitamin A 59 IU, Vitamin B6 .1mg, Thiamin B1 .1mg, Folacin 7mcg, Niacin 1mg

*Note: The sweetness of the apple crisp will depend on the type of apples you choose. Adjust the amount of brown rice syrup accordingly.

Super Easy Apple Crisp

The Diet Doctor: I am totally addicted to Super Easy Apple Crisp, especially during the fall when apples are at their best. And I suffer no guilt, as this fruit crisp is very low in fat and packed with essential nutrients. Better yet, it's "super easy" to make, even for me. And I'll let you in on a little secret; I don't follow the directions exactly as written. My version is "super super easy." Before going to bed, I just preheat the oven to 400 F, pop the crisp in and immediately turn off the heat. When I get up the next morning, the crisp is done.

*4 apples, cored and thinly sliced
1/2 cup raisins
cinnamon
1 cup apple cider or apple juice
2/3 cup rolled oats
1/3 cup whole wheat flour
1/4 teaspoon cinnamon
pinch of sea salt

Preheat oven to 350 degrees F.

Cover the bottom of an 8-inch soufflé dish with a single layer of apple slices. Add a sprinkle of cinnamon and a couple of tablespoons of raisins. Continue layering. Pour 1/3 cup of apple cider over the apples and raisins.

In a separate bowl, mix together oats, flour, 1/4 teaspoon cinnamon and a pinch of sea salt. Add 1/3 cup of apple cider. Mix until topping binds together.

Sprinkle topping over the apple and raisin mixture. Pour the remaining apple cider over the crisp.

Bake for 40 minutes. Allow to cool before serving.

[6 servings]

Nutrition Per Serving: Calories 168, Total Fat 1g, Saturated Fat trace, Cholesterol 0mg, Sodium 23mg, Potassium 305mg, Total Carbohydrate 39g, Dietary Fiber 5g, Protein 3g, Calcium 25mg, Iron 1mg, Zinc 1mg, Vitamin C 6mg, Vitamin A 60 IU, Vitamin B6 .1mg, Thiamin B .1mg, Folacin 8 mcg, Niacin 1mg

*Note: The sweetness of the crisp will depend on the type of apples you choose.

Pear and Ginger Crisp

6 pears, peeled, cored and chopped in chunks
6 tablespoons brown rice syrup
pinch of sea salt
1/2 teaspoon cinnamon
1 1/2 teaspoons kuzu, dissolved in 2 tablespoons of water
1 tablespoon fresh ginger root, grated
1 teaspoon vanilla extract
1 recipe Almond Crisp Topping (page 294)

Preheat oven to 350 degrees F.

Bring 1/2 cup water to a boil. Add pears, rice syrup, sea salt and cinnamon. Reduce heat to a simmer and cook until pears are tender, still retaining their shape. Add dissolved kuzu to pear mixture, stirring gently and continuously. Roll grated ginger into a ball and squeeze juice into pear mixture. Discard ginger pulp. Cook 1-2 minutes until pear mixture thickens. Remove from heat. Add vanilla and stir to incorporate. Pour mixture into a square 8" x 8" baking pan. Crumble Almond Crisp Topping on top of fruit. Bake 30-40 minutes.

[serves 8]

Nutrition Per Serving: Calories 247, Total Fat 6g, Saturated Fat 1g, Cholesterol 0mg, Sodium 76mg, Potassium 260mg, Total Carbohydrate 47g, Dietary Fiber 6g, Protein 4g, Calcium 35mg, Iron 1mg, Zinc 1mg, Vitamin C 5mg, Vitamin A 53 IU, Thiamin B1 .2mg, Riboflavin B2 .1mg, Folacin 17mcg, Niacin 1mg

Summer Peach and Berry Crisp

4 cups peaches, peeled and sliced
2 cups blueberries
juice of 1/2 lemon
5 tablespoons brown rice syrup
pinch of sea salt
1 1/2 teaspoons kuzu, dissolved in 2 tablespoons of water
1 teaspoon vanilla extract
1 recipe Almond Crisp Topping (page 294)

Preheat oven to 350 F.

Bring 1/2 cup of water to a boil. Add peaches, berries, lemon juice, rice syrup and sea salt. Reduce heat and simmer for 3 minutes. Add dissolved kuzu, stirring gently and continuously until fruit mixture thickens, about 2 minutes. Remove from heat. Add vanilla and stir to incorporate. Pour mixture into a square 8" x 8" baking pan. Crumble Almond Crisp Topping on top of fruit. Bake 30-40 minutes.

[serves 8]

Nutrition Per Serving: Calories 225, Total Fat 6g, Saturated Fat 1g, Cholesterol 0mg, Sodium 78mg, Potassium 304mg, Total Carbohydrate 42g, Dietary Fiber 5g, Protein 4g, Calcium 27mg, Iron 1mg, Zinc 1mg, Vitamin C 12mg, Vitamin A 518 IU, Vitamin B6 .1mg, Thiamin B1 .2mg, Riboflavin B2 .1mg, Folacin 14mcg, Niacin 2mg

Apple Tea Cake

The Diet Doctor's Wife: This recipe is a healthful adaptation of a delicious tea cake that I used to make before Bill and I shifted our way of eating. This version is far less fatty than the original, but still tastes great. The big chunks of apple are delightful.

3/4 cup whole wheat pastry flour
3/4 cup unbleached white flour
1 teaspoon cinnamon
1/4 teaspoon sea salt
2 1/2 teaspoons aluminum-free baking powder
2 large cooking apples, peeled, cored and cut in large chunks
1/2 cup barley malt syrup
1/4 cup walnut oil or grapeseed oil
3/4 cup apple juice

Preheat oven to 350 F. Grease a 7-inch spring-form pan. Line the bottom with parchment paper. Lightly grease the parchment paper.

In a medium bowl, combine dry ingredients. Add apple chunks and toss until coated and evenly distributed throughout the dry mixture.

In a separate bowl, whisk together wet ingredients.

Add wet ingredients to the dry mixture. Mix together until well incorporated. The batter should be sticky. Add a little water, if needed.

Pour batter into prepared spring-form pan and smooth out.

Bake 45-60 minutes until tester comes out clean.

[serves 8]

Nutrition Per Serving: Calories 174, Total Fat 7g, Saturated Fat 1g, Cholesterol 0mg, Sodium 213mg, Potassium 128mg, Total Carbohydrate 26g, Dietary Fiber 3g, Protein 3g, Calcium 98mg, Iron 1mg, Vitamin C 2mg, Vitamin A 19 IU, Thiamin B1 .2mg, Riboflavin B2 .1mg, Folacin 7mcg, Niacin 1mg

Banana Bread with Coconut Streusel

The Diet Doctor's Wife: This tea bread is based on a treasured recipe by David Wood, a former caterer, cookbook writer and gourmet shop owner of 1980s Toronto. I hear that he has since moved to British Columbia to pursue cheese making.

1 1/2 cups whole wheat pastry flour
1 1/2 teaspoons aluminum-free baking powder
1/4 teaspoon sea salt
*1/2 cup walnut meats, coarsely chopped
1 cup mashed ripe bananas
*1/4 cup almond oil or walnut oil
1/4 cup maple syrup
1 1/2 teaspoons vanilla extract
2 tablespoons water

Preheat oven to 350 degrees F. Grease a 9" x 5" x 3" loaf pan and place parchment paper on the bottom of the pan.

In a medium bowl, combine dry ingredients. Stir in nuts.

In a small bowl, whisk together wet ingredients.

Add wet ingredients to dry ingredients and stir until you get a thick batter. Add water if needed.

Pour batter into prepared loaf pan and smooth out.

Streusel

1 tablespoon whole wheat pastry flour
1 cup unsweetened shredded coconut
1/4 cup maple syrup
1/2 teaspoon nutmeg
*2 tablespoons almond oil or walnut oil

Combine streusel ingredients in a small bowl. Mix until well incorporated. Sprinkle streusel on top of cake batter.

Bake for 1 hour, until tester comes out clean.

[serves 10]

Nutrition Per Serving: Calories 267, Total Fat 15g, Saturated Fat 3g, Cholesterol 0mg, Sodium 124mg, Potassium 259mg, Total Carbohydrate 32g, Dietary Fiber 4g, Protein 5g, Calcium 70mg, Iron 1mg, Zinc 1mg, Vitamin C 3mg, Vitamin A 37 IU, Vitamin B6 .2mg, Thiamin B1 .1mg, Riboflavin B2 .1mg, Folacin 15mcg, Niacin 1mg

*Note: For nut allergies, eliminate the nuts and substitute light vegetable oil for the nut oil.

Gingerbread

1 cup whole wheat pastry flour
1 cup unbleached white flour
1 tablespoon aluminum-free baking powder
1 tablespoon ground ginger
1 teaspoon ground cinnamon
1 teaspoon ground cloves
1/4 teaspoon sea salt
1/2 cup maple syrup
1/2 cup unsulphured blackstrap molasses
1/2 cup grapeseed oil
1/2 cup apple juice

Preheat oven to 350 degrees F. Grease an 8-inch square baking pan.

In a large bowl, mix together dry ingredients.

In a separate bowl, whisk together wet ingredients. Add wet ingredients to dry ingredients and fold together until well incorporated.

Pour batter into the greased baking pan. Bake 35-40 minutes until tester comes out clean.

[serves 12]

Nutrition Per Serving: Calories 227, Total Fat 9g, Saturated Fat 1g, Cholesterol 0mg, Sodium 171mg, Potassium 441mg, Total Carbohydrate 34g, Dietary Fiber 2g, Protein 3g, Calcium 208mg, Iron 4mg, Zinc 1mg, Vitamin A 2 IU, Vitamin B6 .1mg, Thiamin B1 .1mg, Riboflavin B2 .1mg, Folacin 6mcg, Niacin 1mg

Spiced Pumpkin Pie

1 recipe Single Crust Pecan Pastry (page 297)
3 tablespoons kuzu
1 cup amasake
1 teaspoon ground cinnamon
1/2-3/4 teaspoon ground ginger
1/2 teaspoon sea salt
1/2 cup maple syrup
*1 3/4 cups pureed pumpkin
1 tablespoon brown rice syrup mixed with 1 teaspoon water

Preheat oven to 350 degrees F.

Roll out pastry in a circle large enough to line an 8 or 9-inch pie plate. Make sure the pastry meets the edge of the plate. Roll out the remaining pastry, and use a cookie cutter to make autumn leaf shapes. Using a little water, attach pastry leaves to the edge of the pie crust, so that they rest on the lip of the pie plate. Pierce the pastry on the bottom of the pie plate with a fork several times. Bake for 10 minutes.

To make the filling, first dissolve the kuzu in 1/3 cup amasake and whisk to remove lumps. Place dissolved kuzu, remaining amasake, cinnamon, ginger, salt and maple syrup in a saucepan. Bring to a boil, stirring continuously. Reduce heat and simmer for 3 minutes until liquid thickens.

Whisk together hot kuzu-mixture and pumpkin puree. Pour pumpkin filling into the pie shell. Brush leaves with the rice syrup and water mixture. Bake pie for an additional 8-10 minutes.

[serves 10]

Nutrition Per Serving: Calories 236, Total Fat 7g, Saturated Fat 1g, Cholesterol 0mg, Sodium 125mg, Potassium 186mg, Total Carbohydrate 42g, Dietary Fiber 3g, Protein 3g, Calcium 41mg, Iron 2mg, Zinc 1mg, Vitamin C 2mg, Vitamin A 9460 IU, Thiamin B1 .2mg, Riboflavin B2 .1mg, Folacin 11mcg, Niacin 1mg

*Note: You can buy pureed pumpkin or make it yourself. To make pureed pumpkin, cut pumpkin in half and remove seeds. Cut pumpkin halves into large chunks. Steam chunks over boiling water for 30 minutes until tender. Remove skin and puree pumpkin flesh.

Winter Fruit Compote

3 cups water
1/3 cup Earl Grey or Lap Sang Souchong tea leaves
1/2 cup white dessert wine
1/4 cup brown rice syrup
pinch of sea salt
4 pears, peeled, cored and halved
1/3 cup dried unsulphured sultanas
1/3 cup dried unsulphured currants
3 ounces dried unsulphured apricots
3 ounces dried unsulphured prunes

In a large saucepan, bring water to a boil. Remove from the heat. Add tea leaves and allow to steep for 3 minutes. Strain tea and pour liquid back into the saucepan. Add the wine, rice syrup and sea salt. Bring to a simmer.

Poach the pears in the simmering liquid for 15-20 minutes until they are tender yet still retaining their shape. Remove pears from the poaching liquid with a slotted spoon. Cut pear halves in half lengthwise.

Poach the sultanas for 4 minutes and remove with a slotted spoon. Then poach the currants for 4 minutes and remove with a slotted spoon. Poach the apricots for 4 minutes and remove with a slotted spoon. Poach the prunes for 10 minutes and remove with a slotted spoon.

Continue cooking the syrup until reduced to 1 1/2 cups.

Pour syrup over the fruit and chill.

To serve, arrange each serving dish with an assortment of each type of fruit. Add a few spoonfuls of the syrup.

[serves 8]

Nutrition Per Serving: Calories 214, Total Fat trace, Saturated Fat trace, Cholesterol 0mg, Sodium 36mg, Potassium 1279mg, Total Carbohydrate 50g, Dietary Fiber 5g, Protein 3g, Calcium 36mg, Iron 2mg, Zinc 1mg, Vitamin C 4mg, Vitamin A 1005 IU, Vitamin B6 .1mg, Riboflavin B2 .1mg, Folacin 21mcg, Niacin 2mg

Not So Sweet Oatmeal Raisin Cookies

1 cup whole wheat flour
2 cups rolled oats
1/2 cup cornmeal
1/2 teaspoon ground cinnamon
1/2 teaspoon sea salt
*1/2 cup almonds or walnuts, chopped
1/2 cup raisins
*1/3 cup almond oil or walnut oil
1/4 cup maple syrup or brown rice syrup

1 tablespoon vanilla extract
1/2 cup water

Preheat oven to 350 degrees F. Grease 2 baking sheets or line 2 dry baking sheets with parchment paper.

Dry-roast whole wheat flour, oats and cornmeal in a skillet over medium heat just until warmed through. Continually stir with a wooden spoon to avoid burning. Do not allow to brown. Pour dry-roasted ingredients into a bowl. Add cinnamon, salt, nuts and raisins. Mix to incorporate.

In a separate bowl, whisk together oil, maple syrup, vanilla and water. Add wet ingredients to dry mixture. Mix together until incorporated. Add water if necessary. Shape into cookies and place on baking sheet. Bake for 20-25 minutes until golden brown around the edges.

[30 cookies]

Nutrition Per Cookie: Calories 94, Total Fat 4g, Saturated Fat trace, Cholesterol 0mg, Sodium 33mg, Potassium 81mg, Total Carbohydrate 13g, Dietary Fiber 2g, Protein 2g, Calcium 15mg, Iron 1mg, Vitamin A 15 IU, Thiamin B1 .1mg, Folacin 5mcg, Niacin 1mg

*Note: For nut allergies, eliminate the nuts and substitute light vegetable oil for the nut oil.

Oatmeal Raisin Cookies

2 cups whole wheat pastry flour
1 cup rolled oats
1 cup quick cooking oats
*1/2 cup chopped nuts
1/2 cup raisins
1/4 teaspoon sea salt
1/2 teaspoon ground cinnamon
*1/4 cup almond oil
1 cup brown rice syrup
1 tablespoon vanilla extract
1 cup water

Preheat oven to 350 degrees F. Grease 2 baking sheets or line 2 dry baking sheets with parchment paper.

Mix together dry ingredients. In a separate bowl, whisk together wet ingredients and then add to the dry mixture. Mix together until batter is formed. Add water if necessary. Shape into cookies and place on baking sheet. Bake for 20-25 minutes until edges are golden brown.

[30 cookies]

Nutrition Per Serving: Calories 108, Total Fat 3g, Saturated Fat trace, Cholesterol 0mg, Sodium 20mg, Potassium 81mg, Total Carbohydrate 17g, Dietary Fiber 2g, Protein 3g, Calcium 9mg, Iron 1mg, Vitamin A 12 IU, Thiamin B1 .1mg, Folacin 5mcg, Niacin 1mg

*Note: For nut allergies, eliminate the nuts and substitute light vegetable oil for the nut oil.

Mandelbroit with Walnuts

The Diet Doctor's Wife: This is a vegan adaptation of my Grandma Libby's mandelbroit recipe.

1 1/2 cups whole wheat pastry flour
1 1/2 cups unbleached white flour
1 tablespoon aluminum-free baking powder
1/2 teaspoon sea salt
1 cup walnut meats, coarsely chopped
1/2 cup walnut oil or grapeseed oil
2/3 cup maple syrup
1/3 cup water
1 teaspoon vanilla extract

Preheat oven to 350 degrees F. Line a dry baking sheet with parchment paper.

Combine dry ingredients in a large bowl. In a smaller bowl, whisk together wet ingredients and add to the dry mixture. Stir until a batter is formed. Divide batter in half and shape each half into a log (about 15 inches long and 2-3 inches wide). Place logs on the baking sheet.

Bake 25-30 minutes until golden around the edges. Allow to cool. Then cut loaves into 1-inch thick diagonal slices. Transfer slices to baking sheet. Bake 10 minutes per side.

[36 biscotti]

Nutrition Per Biscotti: Calories 100, Total Fat 5g, Saturated Fat trace, Cholesterol 0mg, Sodium 68mg, Potassium 56mg, Total Carbohydrate 12g, Dietary Fiber 1g, Protein 2g, Calcium 33mg, Iron 1mg, Vitamin A 10 IU, Thiamin B1 .1mg, Folacin 5mcg, Niacin 1mg

Orange Biscotti

The Diet Doctor's Wife: This recipe is based on the yummy orange-flavored cookies sold at Zingerman's Delicatessen in Ann Arbor, Michigan.

1 1/2 cups whole wheat pastry flour
1 1/2 cups white unbleached flour
1 tablespoon aluminum-free baking powder
1/2 teaspoon sea salt
*1 cup blanched almonds
1/2 cup sultanas
*1/2 cup almond oil or grapeseed oil
1/3 cup maple syrup
1/3 cup brown rice syrup
1/3 cup freshly squeezed orange juice
1 tablespoon orange zest, grated
1 teaspoon vanilla extract
1 teaspoon almond extract

Preheat oven to 350 degrees F. Line a dry baking sheet with parchment paper.

Combine dry ingredients in a large bowl. In a smaller bowl, whisk together wet ingredients and add to the dry mixture. Stir until a batter is formed. Divide batter in half and shape each half into a log (about 15 inches long and 2-3 inches wide). Place logs on the baking sheet.

Bake 25-30 minutes until golden around the edges. Allow to cool, about 10 minutes. Then cut loaves into 3/4-inch thick diagonal slices. Transfer slices to baking sheet. Bake 10 minutes per side.

[36 biscotti]

Nutrition Per Biscotti: Calories 109, Total Fat 5g, Saturated Fat trace, Cholesterol 0mg, Sodium 68mg, Potassium 84mg, Total Carbohydrate 14g, Dietary Fiber 1g, Protein 2g, Calcium 40mg, Iron 1mg, Vitamin C 1mg, Vitamin A 6 IU, Thiamin B1 .1mg, Riboflavin B2 .1mg, Folacin 6mcg, Niacin 1mg

*Note: For nut allergies, eliminate the nuts and use grapeseed oil instead of almond oil.

Chocolate Chip Cookies

The Diet Doctor's Wife: This is an awesome treat for the lactose intolerant. If you want to be holy, use malt-sweetened chocolate chips.

1 cup whole wheat pastry flour
1 cup spelt flour
1 3/4 cups semi-sweet chocolate chips or malt-sweetened chocolate chips
*1/2 cup walnuts, chopped
1 teaspoon aluminum-free baking powder
1/2 teaspoon baking soda
1/4 teaspoon sea salt
*1/2 cup walnut oil or grapeseed oil
3/4 cup maple syrup
1/4 cup water
1 tablespoon vanilla extract

Preheat oven to 350 degrees F. Line two dry baking sheets with parchment paper.

In a large bowl, combine dry ingredients. In a smaller bowl, whisk together wet ingredients. Pour wet ingredients into the dry mixture. Stir to incorporate. Using a tablespoon, spoon batter onto baking sheet.

Bake 15-20 minutes, until edges are lightly browned.

[36 cookies]

Nutrition Per Cookie: Calories 117, Total Fat 7g, Saturated Fat 2g, Cholesterol 0mg, Sodium 46mg, Potassium 79mg, Total Carbohydrate 15g, Dietary Fiber 1g, Protein 2g, Calcium 20mg, Iron 1mg, Vitamin A 22 IU, Folacin 3mcg

*Note: For nut allergies, eliminate the nuts and use grapeseed oil instead of walnut oil.

Bran Muffins

1 cup bran
2 1/2 cups whole wheat pastry flour
1 1/2 cups whole wheat, barley, rye or buckwheat flour
1 tablespoon flax seeds
1 1/2 teaspoons aluminum-free baking powder
1/2 teaspoon sea salt
1/4 cup grapeseed oil
1 1/2 cups apple juice or water
*1/2 cup barley malt
2 bananas, mashed or 2 apples, cut in chunks
1/2-1 cup dried currants

Preheat oven to 350 F. Grease a muffin tin.

Mix together dry ingredients. In a separate bowl, whisk together wet ingredients, and then add to dry ingredients. Add fruit and mix. Spoon batter into muffin tin. Bake 50-60 minutes.

[12 muffins]

Nutrition Per Muffin: Calories 240, Total Fat 6g, Saturated Fat 1g, Cholesterol 0mg, Sodium 143mg, Potassium 393mg, Total Carbohydrate 45g, Dietary Fiber 8g, Protein 7g, Calcium 61mg, Iron 3mg, Zinc 2mg, Vitamin C 2mg, Vitamin A 21 IU, Vitamin B6 .2mg, Thiamin B1 .2mg, Riboflavin B2 .1mg, Folacin 21mcg, Niacin 3mg

*Note: If you like a sweeter muffin, you can substitute maple syrup for the barley malt.

Mincemeat Tartlets

The Diet Doctor's Wife: Miso gives vegetarian mincemeat a traditional meaty flavor. Mulled cider and cognac add special touches as well.

1/2 cup raisins
1/2 cup dried currants
mulled apple cider, apple cider or apple juice
1 recipe Dried Fruit Puree (page 298)
4 cups apple, peeled and cut into 1/2-inch cubes
zest and juice of 1/2 lemon
zest and juice of 1/2 orange
1 teaspoon cinnamon
1/4 teaspoon ground cloves
1/4 teaspoon ground ginger
1 tablespoon barley miso
3 tablespoons cognac
double recipe Single Crust Walnut Pastry (page 296)

Preheat oven to 350 degrees F. You will need 1-5 nonstick mini muffin tins.

Soak raisins and currants in mulled apple cider to cover until softened. Drain raisins and currants, reserving liquid.

In a saucepan, combine raisins, currants, dried fruit puree, apple pieces, lemon zest and juice, orange zest and juice, cinnamon, cloves and ginger. Add 1/4 cup reserved mulled apple cider. Bring mixture to a boil. Reduce heat and simmer for 10 minutes. Dilute miso in a few tablespoons of cider or cooking liquid. Add diluted miso to the fruit mixture. Remove from the heat and stir in cognac.

Roll out pastry and cut out 3-inch circles. Line mini muffin tins with the circles. Spoon 1 tablespoon of mincemeat filling into each pastry shell. Bake for 15-20 minutes.

[serves 60]

Nutrition Per Serving: Calories 66, Total Fat 2g, Saturated Fat trace, Cholesterol 0mg, Sodium 21mg, Potassium 84mg, Total Carbohydrate 10g, Dietary Fiber 1g, Protein 1g, Calcium 6mg, Vitamin C 2mg, Vitamin A 167 IU, Folacin 3mcg

Variation: Roll out any left over dough and use the small end of a melon-baller to make 3/4-inch circles. Place circles on top of the filled tartlets. Bake for 15 minutes. Glaze the mini circles with a mixture of 1/2 brown rice syrup and 1/2 water. Bake 5 minutes more.

Blueberry Tart

1 Single Crust Almond Pastry (page 295)
1 cup Almond Pastry Cream (page 293)
2 cups fresh blueberries
1/4 cup apricot jam

Preheat oven to 350 degrees F.

Flip pastry onto greased 9-inch tart pan. Pierce the pastry shell with a fork several times. Bake for 20 minutes. Allow pastry shell to cool. Spread pastry cream on bottom of pastry shell. Top with berries. Heat jam until it starts to boil. Strain. Brush strained jam on top of berries.

[serves 10]

Nutrition Per Serving: Calories 211, Total Fat 8g, Saturated Fat 1g, Cholesterol 0mg, Sodium 45mg, Potassium 154mg, Total Carbohydrate 34g, Dietary Fiber 3g, Protein 4g, Calcium 22mg, Iron 1mg, Vitamin C 4mg, Vitamin A 53 IU, Thiamin B1 .1mg, Riboflavin B2 .1mg, Folacin 9mcg, Niacin 1mg

Strawberry Tart

1 Single Crust Almond Pastry (page 295)
1 cup Almond Pastry Cream (page 293)
2-3 cups fresh strawberries, hulled
1/4 cup apricot jam

Preheat oven to 350 degrees F.

Flip pastry onto greased 9-inch tart pan. Pierce the pastry shell with a fork several times. Bake for 20 minutes. Allow pastry shell to cool. Spread pastry cream on bottom of pastry shell. Top with berries. Heat jam until it starts to boil. Strain. Brush strained jam on top of berries.

[serves 10]

Nutrition Per Serving: Calories 204, Total Fat 8g, Saturated Fat 1g, Cholesterol 0mg, Sodium 44mg, Potassium 177mg, Total Carbohydrate 32g, Dietary Fiber 2g, Protein 4g, Calcium 25mg, Iron 1mg, Vitamin C 17mg, Vitamin A 32 IU, Thiamin B1 .1mg, Riboflavin B2 .1mg, Folacin 12mcg, Niacin 1mg

Rhubarb and Strawberry Cobbler

2 cups rhubarb, cut in 1/2-inch slices
2 cups strawberries, halved
1 tablespoon freshly squeezed lemon juice
3/4 cup maple syrup
3/4 cup plus 1 tablespoon unbleached white flour
3/4 cup whole wheat flour or oat flour
2 1/4 teaspoons aluminum-free baking powder
1/2 teaspoon ground cinnamon
1 teaspoon lemon or orange zest, grated
1/4 teaspoon sea salt
1/4 cup grapeseed oil
3 tablespoons water or rice milk

Preheat oven to 375 degrees F.

In a medium-size bowl, combine rhubarb, strawberries, lemon juice, 1/2 cup of maple syrup and 1 tablespoon of white unbleached flour. Mix through until well combined and set aside.

In another medium-size bowl, combine the remaining white flour, whole wheat flour, baking powder, cinnamon, zest and sea salt. In a separate bowl, whisk together the rest of the maple syrup, oil and water. Add to dry ingredients and stir to combine until a dough is formed. Roll out the dough into an 8-inch square.

Place the rhubarb mixture in an 8-inch square baking pan. Top with the dough. Using a fork, pierce the dough every few inches.

Cover the dish with aluminum foil and bake for 1/2 hour. Uncover and continue baking for 10-15 minutes until the cobbler is lightly browned and the juices bubble up around the edges.

[serves 9]

Nutrition Per Serving: Calories 215, Total Fat 7g, Saturated Fat 1g, Cholesterol 0mg, Sodium 179mg, Potassium 243mg, Total Carbohydrate 38g, Dietary Fiber 3g, Protein 3g, Calcium 130mg, Iron 2mg, Vitamin C 22mg, Vitamin A 37 IU, Vitamin B1 .2mg, Riboflavin B2 .1mg, Folacin 14mcg, Niacin 1mg

Strawberry Parfait

2 pints strawberries
3 cups apple cider or apple juice
*1/4 cup agar agar flakes
1 tablespoon kuzu or arrowroot, dissolved in 2 tablespoons apple cider or apple juice
1 recipe Tofu Cream (page 293)

Blend half the strawberries with 1 cup of apple cider. Add more cider to create a volume of 4 cups. Bring cider-strawberry mixture and agar agar to a boil, stirring continuously. Reduce heat and simmer, continuing to stir until agar agar flakes are completely dissolved. This will take about 5 minutes. Add the dissolved kuzu. Stir to combine and simmer for 1 more minute.

Cut the rest of the strawberries in half and place in a shallow pan. Pour the hot liquid over the fruit. Allow to cool.

Refrigerate for at least 1/2 hour. Break up strawberry gel with a potato masher.

To serve, take out 6 clear wine glasses. Add 2 tablespoons of strawberry gel to each wine glass. Add 1 tablespoon of Tofu Cream. Top with 1-2 tablespoons of strawberry gel and another 1-2 tablespoons of Tofu Cream.

[serves 6]

Nutrition Per Serving: Calories 190, Total Fat 5g, Saturated Fat 1g, Cholesterol 0mg, Sodium 10mg, Potassium 414mg, Total Carbohydrate 33g, Dietary Fiber 3g, Protein 6g, Calcium 92mg, Iron 4mg, Zinc 1mg, Vitamin C 57mg, Vitamin A 76 IU, Vitamin B6 .1mg, Thiamin B1 .1mg, Riboflavin B2 .1mg, Folacin 31mcg

*Note: This dessert contains agar agar, which is a mild laxative.

Rice Pudding

The Diet Doctor's Wife: This is a completely dairy-free variation of a favorite old standard.

1 cup sweet brown rice
6 cups water
1 vanilla bean
1/4 teaspoon sea salt
1 tablespoon orange zest, grated
1/4 cup brown rice syrup
1/4 cup maple syrup
Tofu Cream (page 293) (optional)
ground cinnamon or nutmeg (optional)

Put rice and water in a pressure cooker and let stand for 5 hours.

Take a sharp knife and cut vanilla bean in half lengthwise. Scrape out seeds. Add seeds and pod to the rice. Add salt, orange zest, rice syrup and maple syrup. Secure lid. Allow rice mixture to come up to pressure over high heat. Reduce heat to low and cook for 45 minutes. Turn off heat and let pressure cooker sit with the lid on for 20 minutes. Remove vanilla bean. Allow to cool to room temperature and then chill in the refrigerator until ready to serve. Add tofu cream and a sprinkle of cinnamon or nutmeg, if desired.

[serves 6]

Nutrition Per Serving: Calories 178, Total Fat 1g, Saturated Fat trace, Cholesterol 0mg, Sodium 82mg, Potassium 114mg, Total Carbohydrate 40g, Dietary Fiber 1g, Protein 2g, Calcium 26mg, Iron 1mg, Zinc 1mg, Vitamin C 1mg, Vitamin A 4 IU, Vitamin B6 .2mg, Thiamin B1 .1mg, Folacin 7mcg, Niacin 1mg

Coconut Sorbet

The Diet Doctor's Wife: This is a serious treat. The reduced fat coconut milk creates the creaminess of ice cream without the use of dairy. Note that I have chosen to use sugar syrup in this recipe since I couldn't get a good result with a natural sweetener.

14 ounces reduced fat coconut milk
1/2 cup Sugar Syrup (page 298)
pinch of sea salt
1/4 teaspoon vanilla extract

Combine ingredients in a bowl and mix together. Chill in the refrigerator. Process in an ice cream maker as per manufacturer's instructions.

[serves 4]

Nutrition Per Serving: Calories 130, Total Fat 5g, Saturated Fat 0g, Cholesterol 0mg, Sodium 30mg, Total Carbohydrate 23g, Protein 1g

Decadent Coconut Sorbet

The Diet Doctor: The "decadent" shredded coconut in this sorbet creates interesting texture and explosive flavor.

14 ounces reduced fat coconut milk

1/2 cup Sugar Syrup (page 298)
pinch of sea salt
1 cup unsweetened shredded coconut
1/4 teaspoon vanilla extract

Place all ingredients except for the vanilla in a saucepan. Heat on low until coconut flakes are soft, about 30 minutes. Remove from the heat and stir in the vanilla. Place pan in an ice bath and allow to cool to room temperature. Process in an ice cream maker as per manufacturer's instructions.

[serves 6]

Nutrition Per Serving: Calories 134, Total Fat 8g, Saturated Fat 4g, Cholesterol 0mg, Sodium 22mg, Potassium 48mg, Total Carbohydrate 17g, Dietary Fiber 1g, Protein 1g, Calcium 2mg, Folacin 4mcg

Rum and Coconut Sorbet

14 ounces reduced fat coconut milk
1/2 cup Sugar Syrup (page 298)
pinch of sea salt
3 tablespoons rum, chilled in the freezer for at least 1 hour

Whisk the first 3 ingredients together and process in ice cream maker as per manufacturer's instructions. Add rum in the last 5 minutes of processing.

[serves 5]

Nutrition Per Serving: Calories 123, Total Fat 4g, Saturated Fat 0g, Cholesterol 0mg, Sodium 24mg, Total Carbohydrate 18g, Protein 1g

Raspberry Sorbet

1 pound fresh raspberries
1/2 cup Sugar Syrup (page 298)

1 tablespoon freshly squeezed lemon juice
pinch of sea salt

Combine ingredients and puree. Strain to remove seeds. Process in an ice cream maker as per manufacturer's instructions.

[serves 8]

Nutrition Per Serving: Calories 63, Total Fat trace, Saturated Fat 0g, Cholesterol 0mg, Sodium 15mg, Potassium 85mg, Total Carbohydrate 16g, Dietary Fiber 4g, Calcium 12mg, Vitamin C 14mg, Vitamin A 71 IU, Folacin 14mcg

Grapefruit Sorbet

2 1/2 cups freshly squeezed grapefruit juice
1/4 cup Sugar Syrup (page 298)
1/4 cup dry white wine, chilled

Combine ingredients and process in an ice cream maker as per manufacturer's instructions.

[serves 6]

Nutrition Per Serving: Calories 78, Total Fat trace, Saturated Fat trace, Cholesterol 0mg, Sodium 4mg, Potassium 161mg, Total Carbohydrate 16g, Protein 1g, Calcium 8mg, Vitamin C 30mg, Vitamin A 7 IU, Folacin 11mcg

Meyer Lemon Sorbet

The Diet Doctor's Wife: Meyer lemons taste like an exquisite hybrid of tangerine and lemon. They are available in specialty food markets November through March.

1/2 cup freshly squeezed Meyer lemon juice
2/3 cup water
1/2-2/3 cup Sugar Syrup (page 298)
pinch of sea salt

Combine ingredients. Taste for sweetness and make any adjustments, if necessary. Process in an ice cream maker as per manufacturer's instructions.

[serves 4]

Nutrition Per Serving: Calories 83, Total Fat trace, Saturated Fat trace, Cholesterol 0mg, Sodium 30mg, Potassium 47mg, Total Carbohydrate 22g, Calcium 4mg, Vitamin C 12mg, Vitamin A 68 IU, Folacin 3mcg

Mango Sorbet

2 ripe mangoes
6 tablespoons Sugar Syrup (page 298)
3 tablespoons freshly squeezed lemon juice
pinch of sea salt

Peel mangoes and cut into chunks. Puree mango pieces together with the rest of the ingredients. Process in an ice cream maker as per manufacturer's instructions.

[serves 5]

Nutrition Per Serving: Calories 104, Total Fat trace, Saturated Fat trace, Cholesterol 0mg, Sodium 25mg, Potassium 141mg, Total Carbohydrate 27g, Dietary Fiber 2g, Calcium 9mg, Vitamin C 27mg, Vitamin A 3226 IU, Vitamin B6 .1mg, Thiamin B1 .1mg, Folacin 13mcg

Basics

Sesame Salt (Gomasio)

The Diet Doctor's Wife: A wonderful condiment to go with brown rice.

16 tablespoons black or tan sesame seeds
1 tablespoon sea salt

Wash seeds in a fine mesh strainer. Drain and allow to dry.

Put sea salt in a stainless steel skillet over medium heat. Roast until the color turns grayish and a chlorine smell is released, about 3 minutes. Turn off heat and pour salt into a suribachi or mortar.

In a circular motion use the surikogi or pestle to grind the salt to a fine powder.

Dry-roast seeds over medium low heat. Stir continuously with a wooden spoon so that the seeds don't burn. The seeds are done when they begin to pop or release a nutty aroma, about 5 minutes. Immediately remove from the heat.

Add seeds to the ground salt in the suribachi. In a circular motion, use the surikogi to grind the seeds until each seed is half-crushed and coated with salt. Do not over-grind. Pour mixture into an airtight container.

[96 servings]

Nutrition Per Serving: Calories 9, Total Fat 1g, Saturated Fat trace, Cholesterol 0mg, Sodium 59mg, Potassium 7mg, Calcium 15mg, Zinc trace, Folacin 1mcg

Toasted Almonds

Preheat oven to 350 F. Place 1 cup of raw whole almonds on a baking sheet and bake for 10 minutes. Allow to cool.

[16 servings]

Nutrition Per Serving: Calories 51, Total Fat 4g, Saturated Fat trace, Cholesterol 0mg, Sodium 1mg, Potassium 66mg, Total Carbohydrate 2g, Dietary Fiber 1g, Protein 1g, Calcium 24mg, Riboflavin B2 .1mg, Folacin 6mcg

Tamari Toasted Almonds

Preheat oven to 350 F. Place 1 cup of raw whole almonds on a baking sheet and bake for 8-10 minutes. Put almonds in a bowl and sprinkle with 1/2 teaspoon of tamari. Stir to coat. Allow to cool.

[16 servings]

Nutrition Per Serving: Calories 51, Total Fat 4g, Saturated Fat trace, Cholesterol 0mg, Sodium 11mg, Potassium 67mg, Total Carbohydrate 2g, Dietary Fiber 1g, Protein 1g, Calcium 24 mg, Riboflavin B2 .1mg, Folacin 6 mcg

Tamari Toasted Pumpkin Seeds

Heat a dry medium-size skillet on medium low. Place 1 cup of raw shelled pumpkin seeds in the skillet. Dry-roast the seeds, stirring continuously with a wooden spoon so that the seeds don't burn. When the seeds begin to pop or a nutty fragrance is released, remove from the heat. This should take 3-5 minutes.

Pour seeds into a bowl. Add 1/2 teaspoon of tamari. Stir to coat. Allow to cool.

[16 servings]

Nutrition Per Serving: Calories 18, Total Fat 1g, Saturated Fat trace, Cholesterol 0mg, Sodium 11mg, Potassium 37mg, Total Carbohydrate 2g, Dietary Fiber 1g, Protein 1g, Calcium 2mg, Vitamin A 2 IU

Tamari Toasted Sunflower Seeds

Heat a dry medium-size skillet on medium low. Place 1 cup of raw shelled sunflower seeds in the skillet. Dry-roast the seeds, stirring continuously with a wooden spoon so that the seeds do not burn. When a nutty fragrance is released or when the seeds begin to pop, remove from the heat. This should take 3-5 minutes.

Pour the seeds into a bowl. Add 1/2 teaspoon of tamari. Stir to coat. Allow to cool.

[16 servings]

Nutrition Per Serving: Calories 52, Total Fat 5g, Saturated Fat 1g, Cholesterol 0mg, Sodium 11mg, Potassium 41mg, Total Carbohydrate 1g, Dietary Fiber 1g, Protein 2g, Calcium 5mg, Iron 1mg, Vitamin A 4 IU, Vitamin B6 .1mg, Folacin 20 mcg

Zen Salsa

The Diet Doctor's Wife: This is more delicate than the average salsa, but still very flavorful.

1/4 cup tomato, peeled, seeded and chopped
*2 tablespoons Japanese cucumber, seeded and chopped
1 tablespoon onion, finely chopped
splash of freshly squeezed lemon juice
pinch of sea salt
1/2 teaspoon fresh coriander leaves, chopped

Gently combine ingredients. Let sit for 10 minutes before serving.

[serves 2]

Nutrition Per Serving: Calories 8, Total Fat trace, Saturated Fat trace, Cholesterol 0mg, Sodium 61mg, Potassium 72mg, Total Carbohydrate 2g, Calcium 3mg, Vitamin C 5mg, Vitamin A 153 IU, Folacin 6mcg

*Note: If using a regular thick-skinned cucumber, peel and seed before chopping.

Variation: Use fresh dill instead of coriander and add 1 teaspoon of extra virgin olive oil.

Mexican Salsa

The Diet Doctor's Wife: Homemade salsa is well worth the effort. Use it to jazz up Mexican beans and guacamole, or serve it as a dip with tortilla chips.

2 medium tomatoes, peeled, seeded and chopped
1/4 cup onion, minced
1/4 teaspoon fresh chili pepper, chopped
pinch of sea salt
splash of freshly squeezed lime juice
1 tablespoon coriander leaves, chopped

Combine ingredients.

[serves 2]

Nutrition Per Serving: Calories 37, Total Fat trace, Saturated Fat trace, Cholesterol 0mg, Sodium 72mg, Potassium 349mg, Total Carbohydrate 8g, Dietary Fiber 2g, Protein 1g, Calcium 22mg, Iron 1mg, Vitamin C 31mg, Vitamin A 822 IU, Vitamin B6 .1mg, Thiamin B1 .1mg, Riboflavin B2 .1mg, Folacin 25 mcg, Niacin 1mg

Basic Tomato Sauce

2 teaspoons extra virgin olive oil
1/2 cup onion, finely chopped
28-ounce can Italian plum tomatoes, drained
sea salt and freshly ground black pepper, to taste

In a heavy saucepan, heat oil on medium. Add onions and sauté until soft and translucent. Add drained tomatoes, breaking them up with the back of a wooden spoon. Bring to a boil. Reduce heat and gently simmer for 30 minutes.

Pass sauce through a food mill. Season to taste with salt and pepper.

[serves 4]

Nutrition Per Serving: Calories 65, Total Fat 3g, Saturated Fat trace, Cholesterol 0mg, Sodium 294mg, Potassium 470mg, Total Carbohydrate 10g, Dietary Fiber 2g, Protein 2g, Calcium 64mg, Iron 1mg, Vitamin C 29mg, Vitamin A 1181 IU, Vitamin B6 .2mg, Thiamin B1 .1mg, Riboflavin .1mg, Folacin 19mcg, Niacin 1mg

Tomato Confit

The Diet Doctor's Wife: Tomato confit is wonderfully rich. It adds marvelous flavor to soups, sauces and sandwiches.

2 pounds Italian tomatoes, peeled, seeded and quartered
1 tablespoon extra virgin olive oil
sea salt and freshly ground white pepper, to taste
1/2 teaspoon maple syrup
4 cloves garlic, finely sliced
2 tablespoons fresh thyme leaves

Preheat oven to 200 degrees F. Lightly grease a non-metal baking dish.

Place tomatoes in a bowl. In a separate bowl, whisk together oil, sea salt, white pepper and maple syrup. Add mixture to the tomatoes and toss together until all tomato pieces are coated.

Arrange tomato pieces on the baking dish without any overlap.

Place a garlic slice and a sprinkle of thyme leaves on top of each piece of tomato.

Bake tomatoes for 2 hours, turning them every 1/2 hour. Allow to cool to room temperature and store in a jar with cooking juices. Tomato Confit will keep in the refrigerator for 5 days.

[16 servings or 2 cups]

Nutrition Per Serving: Calories 20, Total Fat 1g, Saturated Fat trace, Cholesterol 0mg, Sodium 5mg, Potassium 118mg, Total Carbohydrate 3g, Dietary Fiber 1g, Calcium 4mg, Vitamin C 10mg, Vitamin A 322 IU, Folacin 8mcg

Onion Confit

The Diet Doctor's Wife: The lovely caramelized richness of Onion Confit enhances soups, stews and sauces. Onion Confit also makes a nice sandwich spread.

4 pounds onions, cut in 1/4-inch slices
2 bay leaves
2 tablespoons fresh thyme leaves
1 teaspoon freshly ground black pepper
3 tablespoons extra virgin olive oil

Preheat oven to 300 degrees F. Lightly grease a large, shallow baking dish with a drizzle of oil. Combine ingredients directly in the baking dish. Toss to coat. Spread out onions evenly. Bake for 1 to 1 1/2 hours, turning onions every 15 minutes. Onions should reduce by half and turn a light golden brown. Allow to cool. Store in the refrigerator for up to 1 week.

[4 cups, 32 servings]

Nutrition Per Serving: Calories 31, Total Fat 1g, Saturated Fat trace, Cholesterol 0mg, Sodium 2mg, Potassium 82mg, Total Carbohydrate 4g, Dietary Fiber 1g, Protein 1g, Calcium 11mg, Vitamin C 4mg, Vitamin A 8 IU, Vitamin B6 .1mg, Folacin 10mcg

Cranberry Sauce

The Diet Doctor's Wife: This is a simple, no-nonsense cranberry sauce. It is not too sweet and not too tart.

4 cups fresh cranberries
1/3-1/2 cup maple syrup

1/4 cup water
juice of 1 orange
zest of 1 orange
pinch of sea salt

Rinse cranberries, discarding any bruised or soft fruit.

In a medium saucepan, combine ingredients. Bring to a boil over medium heat. Immediately reduce heat to a gentle simmer. Stir often to prevent berries from sticking to the pan. Cook berries until they begin to pop, approximately 7-10 minutes. Remove from heat. Allow to cool. Refrigerate to chill.

[serves 8]

Nutrition Per Serving: Calories 66, Total Fat trace, Saturated Fat trace, Cholesterol 0mg, Sodium 16mg, Potassium 91mg, Total Carbohydrate 17g, Dietary Fiber 2g, Calcium 24mg, Iron trace, Vitamin C 15mg, Vitamin A 56 IU, Folacin 6mcg

Guacamole

1 avocado, peeled, pitted and mashed
1 tablespoon onion, minced
1 teaspoon freshly squeezed lemon juice
1/8 teaspoon sea salt
1-3 drops Tabasco® sauce

Mix all ingredients together until smoothly blended. Check for seasoning.

[serves 4]

Nutrition Per Serving: Calories 82, Total Fat 8g, Saturated Fat 1g, Cholesterol 0mg, Sodium 65mg, Potassium 307mg, Total Carbohydrate 4g, Dietary Fiber 1g, Protein 1g, Calcium 6mg, Iron 1mg, Vitamin C 5mg, Vitamin A 308 IU, Vitamin B6.1mg, Thiamin B1 .1mg, Riboflavin B2 .1mg, Folacin 32mcg, Niacin 1mg

Avocado Pate

1 avocado, peeled, pitted and mashed
1 tablespoon onion, minced
1/8 teaspoon sea salt
2 teaspoons freshly squeezed lemon juice

Combine ingredients and mash with a fork to create a smooth puree.

[serves 4]

Nutrition Per Serving: Calories 82, Total Fat 8g, Saturated Fat 1g, Cholesterol 0mg, Sodium 64mg, Potassium 308mg, Total Carbohydrate 4g, Dietary Fiber 1g, Protein 1g, Calcium 6mg, Iron 1mg, Vitamin C 5mg, Vitamin A 308 IU, Vitamin B6 .1mg, Thiamin B1 .1mg, Riboflavin B2 .1mg, Folacin 32mcg, Niacin 1mg

Couscous Seasoning

1/2 teaspoon whole cloves
1/2 cinnamon stick
1 teaspoon coriander seeds
1 teaspoon allspice berries
1 teaspoon cumin seeds
1 teaspoon caraway seeds
1 teaspoon fennel seeds
1 teaspoon black peppercorns
1 teaspoon white peppercorns
1 dime-size piece dried ginger or 1/4 teaspoon ground ginger
1/2 teaspoon ground turmeric

Combine cloves and cinnamon stick in an electric spice or coffee grinder and grind for a few seconds. Add the rest of the ingredients and grind to a fine powder. Store spice mixture in an airtight spice jar. Couscous Seasoning keeps up to 6 months.

[3 tablespoons, approximately 36 servings]

Nutrition Per Serving: Calories 3, Total Fat trace, Saturated Fat trace, Cholesterol 0mg, Potassium 8mg, Total Carbohydrate 1mg, Calcium 6mg, Vitamin A 2 IU

Harissa

2 tablespoons cumin seeds
1/2 tablespoon caraway seeds
1/2 tablespoon coriander seeds
2 tablespoons ground cayenne pepper
sea salt, to taste
2 cloves garlic
2 tablespoons extra virgin olive oil

In a heavy mortar and pestle, grind seeds to a fine powder. Add cayenne pepper, sea salt and garlic. Pound to a paste. Slowly add olive oil and blend. (If you do not have a mortar and pestle, you can use a food processor.) Refrigerate for up to 3 months.

[6 tablespoons, serves 18]

Nutrition Per Serving: Calories 15, Total Fat 2g, Saturated Fat trace, Cholesterol 0mg, Potassium 7mg, Calcium 3mg, Vitamin C 1mg, Vitamin A 35 IU

My Zatar

The Diet Doctor's Wife: Zatar is a Middle Eastern condiment. Sprinkle it over rice or use it as a topping for bread. Bill loves to dip bread in a dish of fruity olive oil and then again in a dish of zatar.

2 tablespoons Sesame Salt (page 327)
2 tablespoons dried thyme
1/2 teaspoon ground sumac

Put Sesame Salt and thyme in an electric spice or coffee grinder. Grind to a powder. Add sumac. Stir to combine. Store in an airtight container. Keeps up to 6 months.

[serves 24 or more]

Nutrition Per Serving: Calories 1, Total Fat trace, Saturated Fat trace, Cholesterol 0mg, Sodium 2mg, Potassium 3mg, Calcium 7mg, Vitamin A 14 IU, Folacin 1mcg

Sesame Dipping Sauce

The Diet Doctor's Wife: Use this dipping sauce to perk up steamed vegetables, particularly greens.

1 tablespoon tahini
1 tablespoon low sodium tamari
1 tablespoon brown rice vinegar
1/4 teaspoon ginger juice (squeezed from grated fresh ginger)

Whisk ingredients together.

[serves 2]

Nutrition Per Serving: Calories 50, Total Fat 4g, Saturated Fat 1g, Cholesterol 0mg, Sodium 309mg, Potassium 51mg, Total Carbohydrate 3g, Dietary Fiber 1g, Protein 2g, Calcium 34mg, Iron 1mg, Vitamin A 5 IU, Thiamin B1 .1mg, Folacin 9mcg, Niacin 1mg

Ginger Soy Dipping Sauce

1 tablespoon ginger juice (squeezed from grated fresh ginger)
4 tablespoons low sodium tamari or low sodium soy sauce
2-4 tablespoons hot water or Japanese Stock (page 95)

Warm ingredients in a small saucepan over medium low heat.

[serves 4]

Nutrition Per Serving: Calories 12, Total Fat trace, Saturated Fat trace, Cholesterol 0g, *Sodium 600mg, Potassium 45mg, Total Carbohydrate 2g, Protein 1g, Calcium 4mg, Folacin 3mcg, Niacin 1mg

*Note: This dipping sauce is relatively high in sodium. Watch sodium intake for the rest of the day and remember to drink a lot of water.

Soy Garlic Dipping Sauce

4 tablespoons low sodium soy sauce
3 tablespoons brown rice vinegar
1/2 teaspoon toasted sesame oil
5 1/2 teaspoons grapeseed oil or other light vegetable oil
1 teaspoon garlic, minced
1 teaspoon scallion, minced
1 teaspoon maple syrup

Warm ingredients in a small saucepan over medium low heat.

[serves 6]

Nutrition Per Serving: Calories 50, Total Fat 5g, Saturated Fat trace, Cholesterol 0mg, Sodium 400mg, Potassium 27mg, Total Carbohydrate 2g, Protein 1g, Calcium 4mg, Vitamin A 1 IU, Folacin 2mcg

Soy Garlic Sherry Dipping Sauce

1 tablespoon grapeseed oil
1 scallion, finely minced
1 clove garlic, smashed with the side of a knife
3 tablespoons low sodium soy sauce
1 tablespoon maple syrup
2 tablespoons sherry

Combine ingredients. Allow to sit for 1 hour. Remove garlic clove.

[serves 4]

Nutrition Per Serving: Calories 61, Total Fat 3g, Saturated Fat trace, Cholesterol 0mg, Sodium 452mg, Potassium 52mg, Total Carbohydrate 5g, Protein 1g, Calcium 12mg, Vitamin C 1mg, Vitamin A 14 IU, Folacin 5mcg

Basic Japanese Dipping Sauce

3 tablespoons low sodium soy sauce
2 tablespoons mirin
1 teaspoon toasted sesame oil
2 tablespoons Japanese Stock (page 95)

Combine ingredients. Heat on medium low and simmer gently until warmed through.

[serves 4]

Nutrition Per Serving: Calories 27, Total Fat 1g, Saturated Fat trace, Cholesterol 0mg, Sodium 451mg, Potassium 28mg, Total Carbohydrate 2g, Protein 1g, Calcium 3mg, Folacin 2mcg

Variation: Add a few slivers of garlic and/or a few drops of ginger juice.

Korean Dipping Sauce

The Diet Doctor's Wife: This sauce really jazzes up brown rice and steamed vegetables. It is very intense so a little goes a long way.

2 tablespoons low sodium soy sauce
1 teaspoon garlic, crushed
1 teaspoon red pepper flakes
1 teaspoon Sesame Salt (page 327)
1 teaspoon maple syrup
1 teaspoon toasted sesame oil

Whisk together ingredients. Let sit for at least 1/2 hour.

[serves 4]

Nutrition Per Serving: Calories 22, Total Fat 1g, Saturated Fat trace, Cholesterol 0mg, Sodium 309mg, Potassium 24mg, Total Carbohydrate 2g, Protein 1g, Calcium 7mg, Vitamin C 1mg, Vitamin A 26 IU, Folacin 2mcg

Eggless Rouille

1 red bell pepper
1/2 cup soft whole wheat breadcrumbs
1/3-1/2 cup Basic Vegetable Stock (page 94)
1 fresh hot chili pepper, stem and seeds removed, sliced
3 cloves garlic
pinch of saffron
1/4 teaspoon sea salt
freshly ground black pepper, to taste
1/2 teaspoon red wine vinegar
1-2 tablespoons extra virgin olive oil

Grill whole pepper over an open flame until flesh is completely blistered on all sides. Place grilled pepper in a sealed plastic bag and let sit for 1/2 hour. This allows the flesh to soften thoroughly. Remove pepper from the bag and peel off skin. It should come off easily. Scrape out seeds. Place flesh and any cooking juices in a small bowl and set aside.

Put breadcrumbs in a separate bowl. Add stock and any juices from the grilled pepper. Stir to combine. Set aside.

Place chili pepper, garlic and saffron in a mortar and grind to a paste. Add grilled pepper and blend evenly. Add breadcrumb mixture and continue to blend until you get a grainy paste. Add sea salt, black pepper, vinegar and extra virgin olive oil. Stir to combine.

[serves 8]

Nutrition Per Serving: Calories 50, Total Fat 2g, Saturated Fat trace, Cholesterol 0mg, Sodium 124mg, Potassium 77mg, Total Carbohydrate 7g, Dietary Fiber 1g, Protein 1g, Calcium 12mg, Iron 1mg, Vitamin C 42mg, Vitamin A 891 IU, Vitamin B6 .1mg, Folacin 10mcg, Niacin 1mg

Tahini Sauce

1/4 cup tahini
1/4 cup water
1 clove garlic, minced
1 1/2 teaspoons cider vinegar

Whisk together tahini, water, garlic and vinegar.

[serves 4]

Nutrition Per Serving: Calories 91, Total Fat 8g, Saturated Fat 1g, Cholesterol 0mg, Sodium 17mg, Potassium 67mg, Total Carbohydrate 4g, Dietary Fiber 1g, Protein 3g, Calcium 65mg, Iron 1mg, Zinc 1mg, Vitamin A 10 IU, Thiamin B1 .2mg, Riboflavin B2 .1mg, Folacin 15mcg, Niacin 1mg

Dijon Vinaigrette

3/4 cup extra virgin olive oil
1 tablespoon Dijon mustard
1/4 cup red wine vinegar
sea salt and freshly ground black pepper, to taste

Whisk together oil and mustard until slightly thickened. Add vinegar and whisk until well incorporated. Season to taste.

[16 tablespoons]

Nutrition Per Tablespoon: Calories 91, Total Fat 10g, Saturated Fat 1g, Cholesterol 0mg, Sodium 12mg, Potassium 5mg, Calcium 1mg

Balsamic Vinaigrette

3 tablespoons extra virgin olive oil
1/2 teaspoon Dijon mustard

1 tablespoon balsamic vinegar
sea salt and freshly ground black pepper, to taste

Whisk together oil and mustard until slightly thickened. Add vinegar and whisk until well incorporated. Season to taste.

[4 tablespoons]

Nutrition Per Tablespoon: Calories 91, Total Fat 10g, Saturated Fat 1g, Cholesterol 0mg, Sodium 8mg, Potassium 5mg, Calcium 1mg

Lemon Vinaigrette

3/4 cup extra virgin olive oil
3 tablespoons fresh parsley leaves, chopped
1/4 cup freshly squeezed lemon juice
sea salt and freshly ground black pepper, to taste

Whisk together oil, parsley and lemon juice. Season to taste.

[16 tablespoons]

Nutrition Per Tablespoons: Calories 91, Total Fat 10g, Saturated Fat 1g, Cholesterol 0mg, Potassium 9mg, Calcium 1mg, Vitamin C 3mg, Vitamin A 37 IU, Folacin 2mcg

Maple Walnut Vinaigrette

1/4 cup walnut oil
1 teaspoon Dijon mustard
3 tablespoons maple syrup
1/4 teaspoon sea salt
1 tablespoon fresh tarragon leaves, finely chopped
1/4 cup sherry vinegar

Whisk together first 5 ingredients until slightly thickened. Add vinegar and whisk until well incorporated. Taste for seasoning.

[12 tablespoons]

Nutrition Per Tablespoon: Calories 55, Total Fat 5g, Saturated Fat trace, Cholesterol 0mg, Sodium 50mg, Potassium 28mg, Total Carbohydrate 4g, Calcium 11mg, Vitamin A 17 IU, Folacin 1mcg

Garlic and Chive Vinaigrette

1/3 cup extra virgin olive oil
1 clove garlic, peeled and smashed with the side of a knife
2 tablespoons freshly squeezed lemon juice
1 tablespoon fresh chives, finely chopped
sea salt and freshly ground black pepper, to taste

Place garlic clove in the olive oil and let sit at room temperature for 1/2 hour. Whisk in lemon juice and chives. Season to taste. Remove garlic clove.

[8 tablespoons]

Nutrition Per Tablespoon: Calories 81, Total Fat 9g, Saturated Fat 1g, Cholesterol 0mg, Potassium 7mg, Calcium 1mg, Vitamin C 2mg, Vitamin A 17 IU, Folacin 1mcg

Basic Vinaigrette

3/4 cup extra virgin olive oil
1/4 cup red wine vinegar or balsamic vinegar
sea salt and freshly ground black pepper, to taste

Place oil in a small bowl. Add vinegar and whisk together until fully incorporated. Season to taste.

[16 tablespoons]

Nutrition Per Tablespoon: Calories 90, Total Fat 10g, Saturated Fat 1g, Cholesterol 0mg, Potassium 4mg

Mustard Oil

The Diet Doctor's Wife: This oil has an intense, rich flavor that almost seems non-vegetarian. When I use it for roasting vegetables, Bill wants to know where I hid the chicken.

1/4 cup mustard seeds
1 cup grapeseed oil
1/4 teaspoon turmeric

Dry-roast mustard seeds in a small pan over medium heat. Stir continuously with a wooden spoon to prevent seeds from burning. When you begin to smell a pleasant, nutty aroma or when the seeds begin to pop (3-5 minutes), remove pan from the heat.

Allow seeds to cool and grind with a mortar and pestle or electric coffee grinder. Place ground seeds in a blender. Blend with the rest of the ingredients. Cover and store in the refrigerator for 24 hours. Pour oil through a fine mesh strainer lined with cheesecloth. The strained oil is now ready to use and can be stored in the refrigerator for up to 2 weeks.

[16 tablespoons]

Nutrition Per Tablespoon: Calories 134, Total Fat 14g, Saturated Fat 1g, Cholesterol 0mg, Potassium 20mg, Total Carbohydrate 1g, Protein 1g, Calcium 15mg, Vitamin A 2 IU, Folacin 2mcg

Gingery Vinaigrette

3 tablespoons ginger juice (squeezed from fresh grated ginger)
1/3 cup freshly squeezed lime juice

2-3 drops Tabasco® sauce
2/3 cup grapeseed oil
1 clove garlic, smashed with the side of a knife
sea salt and freshly ground white pepper, to taste

Whisk together first 4 ingredients. Add garlic. Season to taste and allow to sit for 1/2 hour. Remove garlic.

[18 tablespoons]

Nutrition Per Tablespoon: Calories 74, Total Fat 8g, Saturated Fat 1g, Cholesterol 0mg, Potassium 11mg, Total Carbohydrate 1g, Calcium 1mg, Vitamin C 1mg, Vitamin A 1 IU, Folacin 1mcg

Japanese Vinaigrette

The Diet Doctor's Wife: Bill is always asking me to replicate the salad dressing served in Japanese restaurants. I finally got around to experimenting and came up with the one below.

1 clove garlic, smashed with the side of a knife
1/4 teaspoon Dijon mustard
1/2 cup brown rice vinegar
1/2 teaspoon ginger juice (squeezed from fresh grated ginger)
2 teaspoons tamari
pinch of sea salt
1 teaspoon maple syrup
*1 teaspoon tan sesame seeds, toasted
1/4 cup grapeseed oil
2 tablespoons carrot, finely grated
1 tablespoon onion, finely grated

Combine all ingredients. Allow to sit for at least 30 minutes.

[1 cup, 16 tablespoons]

Nutrition Per Tablespoon: Calories 35, Total Fat 4g, Saturated Fat trace, Cholesterol 0mg, Sodium 51mg, Potassium 16mg, Total Carbohydrate 1g, Calcium 4mg, Vitamin A 283 IU, Folacin 1mcg

*Note: To toast sesame seeds, refer to directions in the recipe for Sesame Salt on page 327.

Sweet Sesame Vinaigrette

2 tablespoons tahini
2 tablespoons grapeseed oil
1 tablespoon sherry vinegar
1 tablespoon maple syrup
sea salt and freshly ground black pepper, to taste

Whisk together ingredients.

[6 tablespoons]

Nutrition Per Tablespoon: Calories 79, Total Fat 7g, Saturated Fat 1g, Cholesterol 0mg, Sodium 6mg, Potassium 30mg, Total Carbohydrate 3g, Protein 1g, Calcium 25mg, Iron 1mg, Vitamin A 3 IU, Thiamin B1 .1mg, Folacin 5mcg

Citrus Vinaigrette

Orange Juice Reduction

3 cups freshly squeezed orange juice

In a nonreactive saucepan, bring orange juice to a boil over medium heat. Continue cooking until juice is reduced to 1/2 cup of syrupy liquid.

3 tablespoons orange juice reduction
3 tablespoons champagne vinegar
3 tablespoons extra virgin olive oil
pinch of sea salt

Whisk ingredients together. Taste for seasoning.

[9 tablespoons]

Nutrition Per Tablespoon: Calories 78, Total Fat 5g, Saturated Fat 1g, Cholesterol 0mg, Sodium 14mg, Potassium 166mg, Total Carbohydrate 9g, Protein 1g, Calcium 9mg, Vitamin C 41mg, Vitamin A 165 IU, Thiamin B1 .1mg, Folacin 45mcg

Ginger-Beet Horseradish

The Diet Doctor's Wife: This condiment goes beautifully with poached, steamed or boiled fish.

1/2 cup fresh horseradish root, peeled and grated
1/2 cup raw beetroot, peeled and grated
1/4 cup brown rice vinegar
1 tablespoon fresh ginger root, peeled and grated

Combine first 3 ingredients. Form grated ginger root into a ball and squeeze the juice into the horseradish mixture. Discard ginger pulp. Stir ginger juice into the mixture until well incorporated.

[1 1/4 cups, serves 10]

Nutrition Per Serving: Calories 10, Total Fat trace, Saturated Fat trace, Cholesterol 0mg, Sodium 19mg, Potassium 72mg, Total Carbohydrate 2g, Calcium 10mg, Vitamin C 3mg, Vitamin A 3 IU, Folacin 8mcg

Clarified Butter (Ghee)

The Diet Doctor's Wife: Clarified butter is much easier to digest than regular butter as the milk solids are removed. Even so, I wouldn't recommend regular use of it. But once in a while, it's a real treat when nothing but butter will do.

1 stick of unsalted butter

In a heavy saucepan, melt butter over low heat. Remove from the heat and let sit 5 minutes to allow the milk solids to sink to the bottom of the saucepan. Skim foam off the surface. Slowly pour the yellow liquid into a container, leaving the milk solids in the saucepan. Alternatively, pour liquid through a fine mesh strainer lined with cheesecloth. Strain 2 or 3 times, if necessary, to make sure that all milk solids are removed. Store in a covered container in the refrigerator. Clarified butter keeps refrigerated for several months.

(Ghee is an Indian version of clarified butter. To make ghee, melt butter over low heat. Allow foam to form on the top surface and the milk solids to sink to the bottom of the saucepan. Continue cooking until the liquid turns clear and golden. Keep an eye on the milk solids. They will brown slightly but do not allow them to burn. Remove from the heat and allow to sit a few minutes. Pour liquid through a fine mesh strainer lined with 3 to 4 layers of cheesecloth. Strain again, if necessary, in order to remove all the foam and milk solids. Store ghee in a covered container. Ghee keeps refrigerated for several months.)

[6 tablespoons, 18 teaspoons]

Nutrition Per Teaspoon: Calories 37, Total Fat 4g, Saturated Fat 3g, Cholesterol 11mg, Vitamin A 160 IU

PART III

Glossary

Adzuki Beans - Small red beans available in Asian or health food stores.

Agar Agar – A gelatin made from sea vegetables, used to make jellies, aspics and molds. Agar agar is a good source of calcium and iron. It also has mild laxative properties. Agar agar is available in most health food stores.

Amasake - A drink made from fermented sweet rice, available in most health food stores.

Arame – A sea vegetable with a mild flavor that comes in fine black strips. Arame is used in soups, salads and pickles, and can be purchased in the macrobiotic section of most health food stores.

Banh Trang - Dried rice flour rounds that are quickly reconstituted and used as the outer wrapping for fresh spring rolls. Banh Trang are available in most Asian markets.

Barley Malt – A natural sweetener made from barley that is used in baking and cooking. Barley malt is available in most health food stores.

Bean Thread Noodles – See Saifun.

Bonito Flakes – Dried, smoked and fermented fish flakes used to make soup stock and to season certain Japanese dishes. Bonito flakes are available in Asian markets and in the macrobiotic section of most health food stores.

Brown Rice Syrup – See Rice Syrup.

Brown Rice Vinegar - Vinegar made from brown rice. It can be purchased in most health food stores.

Burdock - A long, brown root with a sweet, earthy flavor. It is available in Asian and health food markets

Celery Root - A root of a particular variety of celery. It has a delicate flavor that is a cross between celery and parsley.

Chipotle Pepper - A smoked and dried jalapeno pepper.

Couscoussier - A special pot for steaming couscous.

Cremini Mushrooms - Brown-capped mushrooms slightly more flavorful than white button mushrooms.

Curry Leaf - An herb used in Indian cooking. It can be bought fresh or dried at an Indian food market.

Daikon - A long, white radish that may be eaten cooked or raw.

Enoki Mushrooms - Delicate mushrooms with long spaghetti-like stems. They can be purchased in Asian or specialty markets.

Fenugreek – A spice used in Indian cooking. Fenugreek is available in Indian grocery stores.

Flame Deflector – A perforated metal disk that covers a gas burner to lessen the intensity of the heat.

Fu – Dried wheat gluten, available through macrobiotic mail order catalogues.

Garam Masala - An Indian blend of spices, usually including cardamom, cloves and cinnamon. Garam masala can be found in the spice section of most grocery stores.

Ghee or Clarified Butter - Butter with the milk solids removed. Ghee can be purchased at a health food store or Indian grocer, or it can be easily prepared at home.

GimmeLean$_{\text{TM}}$ - A commercial vegetable protein, available in most health food markets and some grocery stores.

Glass Noodles – See Saifun.

Grapeseed Oil - A light oil made from grape seeds.

Ginger Juice - Juice squeezed from fresh grated ginger.

Heat Diffuser – A metal disk that covers a stove burner, used to lessen the intensity of the heat.

Hijiki – A black, stringy, strong tasting sea vegetable, available in the macrobiotic section of most health food stores.

Hoisin Sauce - A sweet, thick, dark, Chinese bean sauce, available in most grocery stores.

Jicama - A Mexican root vegetable, eaten raw or cooked. It is slightly sweet with a texture similar to a very crisp apple.

Kabocha – A winter squash with a dense, dark-orange flesh that is very rich in flavor.

Kaffir Limes and Leaves - Used in Thai cooking. The fruit rind and leaves are extremely aromatic. They are available in Asian and specialty food markets. Kaffir lime trees can be purchased through mail order gardening catalogues.

Kombu or Kelp - A wide, flat, green sea vegetable with a high mineral content. Kombu is used in soups, pickles, bean dishes, and condiments. Kombu can be purchased in the macrobiotic section of most health food stores.

Kuzu - A white starch made from the kuzu root. It is used as a thickening agent and treatment for minor digestive problems. Kuzu can be purchased in the macrobiotic section of most health food stores.

Lavash - A Middle Eastern flat bread, much like a tortilla.

Lemongrass - A tall, stiff grass with a lemon-like flavor that is used in Asian cooking.

Millet - A small round yellow grain, said to have healing properties for the pancreas.

Mirin - A sweet rice wine used in Japanese cooking.

Miso - A fermented bean paste used to flavor soups, stews, grains and sauces. Miso comes in a variety of flavors and strengths. It is available in most health food stores.

Mochi - A rice cake made from pounded, cooked sweet rice. Mochi can be purchased in most health food stores.

Nori or Sea Laver - Marine algae pressed into very thin sheets, sold dried or toasted. Nori is used in sushi or as a condiment. It is available in most grocery stores, Asian markets and health food stores.

Otoshibuta - A wooden drop lid, placed inside a pan to cover simmering food, helping to create even cooking. An otoshibuta can be purchased in Japanese markets and through specialty mail order catalogues.

Pickle Press - A plastic press that is used to make quick pickles and pressed salads. It is available through macrobiotic mail order catalogues.

Red Kuri Squash – A red-fleshed squash with orange skin.

Rice Syrup - A sweet syrup made from brown rice, used to sweeten sauces, vegetable dishes and desserts. It can be purchased in most health food stores.

Rice Vinegar – See Brown Rice Vinegar.

Saifun (Bean Thread or Glass Noodles) - Noodles made from mung bean starch.

Sea Salt – Unrefined salt that is slightly grayish in color, obtained from the evaporation of ocean water. Unrefined sea salt contains no additives. It is available in health food stores and gourmet shops.

Sea Vegetables - Refer to agar agar, arame, hijiki, kombu, nori and wakame.

Seitan - A vegetable protein made from boiled wheat gluten, available in most health food stores.

Somen Noodles – Thin wheat noodles used in Japanese cooking, available in the macrobiotic section of most health food stores.

Soy Sauce or Shoyu - A fermented product made from wheat, soybeans, water and sea salt. Low sodium versions of soy sauce are available.

Spelt – A subspecies of common wheat that many wheat-sensitive people do not react to. Spelt berries and spelt flour are available in most health food stores.

Sumac – A sour spice used in Middle Eastern cooking.

Suribachi - A Japanese mortar with a grooved inner surface. It is used with a surikogi (wooden pestle). A suribachi and surikogi can be purchased in Japanese markets and through macrobiotic mail order catalogues.

Surikogi – A wooden pestle used with a suribachi (Japanese mortar). A surikogi and suribachi can be purchased in Japanese markets and through macrobiotic mail order catalogues.

Sushi Nori – Sea laver that is dried and roasted into a papery texture. Sushi nori is used to make sushi or condiments. Sushi nori can be purchased in Asian markets, most grocery stores as well as in the macrobiotic section of most health food stores.

Tahini – A paste made from hulled sesame seeds. Tahini is used to flavor sauces and desserts. It has a very high calcium content.

Tamari - A wheat-free soy sauce made from soybeans, water and sea salt. Low sodium versions of tamari are available.

Tamarind Paste – A sweet and sour paste made from tamarind seeds, used in Asian and Middle Eastern cuisine.

Taro – A potato-like vegetable with a dark hairy skin, available in Asian markets.

Tat Soi – A Chinese green with small, flat, rounded leaves.

Tempeh – A fermented cake made from soybeans. Tempeh is high in protein and available in health food stores.

Thai Fish Sauce – A thin sauce made from anchovy extract, used in Thai cooking.

Toasted Sesame Oil – An oil made from toasted sesame seeds, available in Asian markets and health food stores.

Tofu - A white cake made from soaked, ground and cooked soybeans. Tofu is high in protein and a good source of calcium. It is available fresh or dried. The fresh form comes in a variety of textures: extra firm, firm, soft and silken.

Tree Ear Fungus – A dried, edible fungus available in Asian markets. Also called cloud ears or wood ears.

Ume Vinegar – A salty vinegar produced in the making of umeboshi plums, available in the macrobiotic section of most health food stores.

Umeboshi – Salty, pickled plums used in Japanese cooking. Umeboshi are available in Asian markets and in the macrobiotic section of most health food stores.

Vegan – A vegetarian who does not eat eggs or dairy products.

Wakame - A thin, leafy sea vegetable used in soups, salads and pickles. Wakame can be purchased in the macrobiotic section of most health food stores.

Wasabi - A Japanese horseradish that is commonly available in the form of a green powder or a ready-made paste. It has a sharp flavor and is used as an accompaniment to fish, especially sushi.

Yucca – A tropical tuber with a sweet, starchy, slightly floral flavor.

Zatar – A Middle Eastern spice blend containing thyme, roasted sesame seeds and sumac.

Shopping Guide

HEALTH FOOD, MACROBIOTIC AND ORGANIC MAIL ORDER

Eden Foods, Inc.
701 Tecumseh Rd.
Clinton MI 49236
1-888-441-3336
www.eden-foods.com

Gold Mine Natural Food Co.
7805 Arjons Drive
San Diego CA 92126
1-800-475-3663
www.goldminenaturalfood.com

Kushi Institute Store
P.O. Box 500
Becket MA 01223
1-800-645-8744
www.macrobiotics.org

SPECIALTY FOOD MAIL ORDER

Oils and vinegars

Dean and Deluca
www.deandeluca.com
1-877-826-9246

Zabar's
2245 Broadway
NY NY 10024
1-800-697-6301
www.zabars.com

Zingerman's
422 Detroit St.
Ann Arbor MI 48108
1-888-636-8162
www.zingermans.com

Grain and nut flours

King Arthur Flour Company
Norwich VT 05055
1-800-827-6836
www.kingarthurflour.com

Dried herbs and spices

Penzeys Spices
19300 West Janacek Court
P.O. Box 924
Brookfield WI 53045
1-800-741-7787
www.penzeys.com

KITCHEN EQUIPMENT

General

Bridge Kitchenware
214 East 52nd Street
New York NY 10022
1-212-688-4220
www.bridgekitchenware.com

Broadway Panhandler
477 Broome Street
New York NY 10013
1-866-COOKWARE
www.broadwaypanhandler.com

Sur La Table
P.O. Box 34707
Seattle WA 98124
1-800-243-0852
www.surlatable.com

Dean and Deluca
1-877-826-9246
www.deananddeluca.com

Williams-Sonoma
1-877-812-6235
www.williams-sonoma.com

Ceramic Knives

CutleryAndMore.com
160 Kelly St.
Elk Grove IL 60007
1-800-650-9866
www.cutleryandmore.com

Professional Cutlery Direct
242 Branford Rd
North Branford CT 06471
1-800-859-6994
www.cutlery.com

Ginger Graters, Pickle Presses, Pressure-Cookers, Suribachi and Surikogi, Sushi Mats

Kushi Institute Store
P.O. Box 500
Becket MA 01223
1-800-645-8744
www.macrobiotics.org

Gold Mine Natural Food Co.
7805 Arjons Drive
San Diego CA 92126
1-800-475-3663
www.goldminenaturalfood.com

ORGANIC SEEDS

Seeds of Change
P.O. Box 15700
Santa Fe NM 87506
1-505-438-6502
www.seedsofchange.com

Menu Ideas

Breakfast

Mochi Waffles (page 159) with Winter Fruit Compote (page 310)

Scrambled Tofu with Spinach (page 214) with Laurie's Tomato Sauté (page 264)

Bill's Oatmeal with Raisins (page 158)

Fish Porridge (page 148)

Pressure Cooked Brown Rice (page 132) with Sesame Salt (page 327), Warm Weather Miso Soup (page 119), Simple Kale (page 251)

Brown Rice Cakes with Tofu Spread (page 211)

Lunch

Beet Salad (page 90), Lentil Salad (page 191), Carrot Salad (page 77), Whole Wheat and Rosemary Beer Bread (page 176), Fresh Fruit

Tofu Frittata (page 214), Pressure Cooked Brown Rice (page 132)

Middle Eastern Lentil Soup (page 97), Middle Eastern Salad (page 83), Tabouleh (page 149), Lebanese Turnip Pickles (page 282), Olives, Whole Wheat Pita

Vegetable Fried Rice (page 143), Hot-and-Sour Soup (page 117), Steamed Greens, Apple Pudding with Tofu Cream (page 302)

Japanese Style Mixed Grains (page 152), Intense Kombu Condiment (279), Cool Weather Miso Soup (page 118), Braised Squash (page 255)

Dinner

Hungarian Cauliflower Soup (page 107), Seitan Paprikash (page 230), Quick Cucumber and Onion Pickles (page 283), Pressure-Cooked Rice (page 132), Steamed Greens

Japanese Fish Nabe (page 122), Hijiki Salad (page 275), Strawberry Parfait (page 320)

Field Greens (page 82), Penne Puttanesca (page 170), Italian Steamed Vegetables (page 259), Orange Biscotti (page 314)

Tofu and Vegetable Cobbler (page 218), Michele's Salad (page 84)

Mexican Beans (page 195), Mexican Rice (page 144), Tamari Toasted Pumpkin Seeds (page 328), Mexican Salsa (page 330), Guacamole (page 333), Mexican Steamed Vegetables (page 260)

High Tea

Inside-Out Sushi (page 134), Baked Millet Samosas (page 155), Rice Cakes with Eggless Salad (page 210) and Black Bean Puree (page 194), Coconut Curry Scones (page 184) and Jam, Blueberry Tart (page 318) or Strawberry Tart (page 318), Tea

Spring Party

Olive Scones (page 183), Snow Peas and Carrots (page 261), Grilled Halibut Steak with Chermoula (page 240), Herbed Basmati Rice (page 145), Rhubarb and Strawberry Cobbler (page 319)

Summer Party

Fresh Spring Rolls (page 165), Gado Gado (page 87), Fresh Fruit Salad, Coconut Sorbet (page 322)

Fall Party

Moroccan Root Vegetable Tagine (page 169), Steamed Couscous the Traditional Way (page 168), Bisteeya (page 222), Steamed Greens, Winter Fruit Compote (page 310)

Winter Party

Seitan Stew (page 227), Cranberry Sauce (page 332), Brown and Wild Rice with Vegetables (page 142), Steamed Greens, Spiced Pumpkin Pie (page 309)

Index

Conversion Tables

This section contains conversion tables for common cooking measurements. Due to practicality, many of the measurements are approximations.

Common Cooking Measurements

1 tbsp = 3 tsp = 15 ml
4 tbsp = 1/4 cup = 2 fl oz = 60 ml
1 cup = 16 tbsp = 8 fl oz = 250 ml
2 cups = 1 pt = 1/2 qt = 16 fl oz = 500 ml
4 cups = 2 pt = 1 qt = 32 fl oz = 1 liter
1 lb = 16 oz = 450 gm

Weights (1 oz = approximately 28.35 gm)

1 oz = 30 gm	5 oz = 140 gm	9 oz = 255 gm	13 oz = 370 gm
2 oz = 60 gm	6 oz = 170 gm	10 oz = 285 gm	14 oz = 400 gm
3 oz = 85 gm	7 oz = 200 gm	11 oz = 310 gm	15 oz = 425 gm
4 oz = 115 gm	8 oz = 225 gm	12 oz = 340 gm	16 oz = 450 gm

Liquid (2 tbsp = 1 fl oz = approximately 29.57 ml)

US	UK	Metric
2 tbsp	1 fl oz	30 ml
1/4 cup	2 fl oz	60 ml
1/3 cup	3 fl oz	80 ml
1/2 cup	4 fl oz	125 ml
2/3 cup	5 fl oz	160 ml
3/4 cup	6 fl oz	180 ml
1 cup	8 fl oz	250 ml

Length (1 in = approximately 2.54 cm)

1 in = 2 ½ cm	5 in = 13 cm	9 in = 23 cm
2 in = 5 cm	6 in = 15 cm	10 in = 25 cm
3 in = 7 ½ cm	7 in = 18 cm	11 in = 28 cm
4 in = 10 cm	8 in = 20 cm	12 in = 30 ½ cm

Oven Temperatures

Degrees Fahrenheit	Degrees Celsius	Gas Mark
250	120	1/2
275	140	1
300	150	2
325	160	3
350	180	4
375	190	5
400	200	6
425	220	7
450	230	8
475	250	9
500	260	10

Other Books, Tapes and CDs from Diet Results

Books

Doctor Nagler's Crash Diet
Doctor Nagler's Super-Saver Injection Program
The Dirty Half Dozen

Cassette Tapes

Hypnosis for Weight Loss
Hypnosis to Stop Smoking
Hypnosis to Stop Drinking
Motivating Implosion 6-Tape Set
Motivating Implosion Single Tape
Positive Implosion for Sweets
Positive Implosion for Starches
Negative Implosion for Sweets
Negative Implosion for Starches
Brainwashing Weight Reduction Seminar

Audio CDs

Hypnosis for Weight Loss
Hypnosis to Stop Smoking
Hypnosis to Stop Drinking
Living Well is the Best Medicine
Brainwashing Weight Reduction Seminar
Brainwashing Graduate Reinforcement

Computer CDs

Hypnosis for Weight Loss
Hypnosis to Stop Smoking
Hypnosis to Stop Drinking

Diet Results
16311 Middlebelt
Livonia MI 48154
800-511-9769 or 734-422-8040
www.dietresults.com

Recommended Reading

I love flipping through cookbooks. Below is a list of some of my favorites:

Brennan, Georgeanne. *The Vegetarian Table: France.* San Francisco: Chronicle Books, 1995.

Ferré, Julia. *Basic Macrobiotic Cooking.* Oroville, CA: George Ohsawa Macrobiotic Foundation, 1987.

Heatter, Maida. *Maida Heatter's Cakes.* New York: Cader Books, 1982.

Jaffrey, Madhur. *Madhur Jaffrey's World-of-the-East Vegetarian Cooking.* New York: Alfred A. Knopf, 1981.

La Place, Viana. *Unplugged Kitchen.* New York: William Morrow and Company, Inc., 1996.

Madison, Deborah. *Vegetarian Cooking for Everyone.* New York: Broadway Books, 1997.

McCarty, Meredith. *Sweet and Natural.* New York: St. Martin's Press, 1999.

Rosengarten, David with Joel Dean and Giorgio DeLuca. *The Dean & DeLuca Cookbook.* New York: Random House, 1996.

Schneider, Sally. *A New Way to Cook.* New York: Artisan, 2001.

Waters, Alice. *Chez Panisse Vegetables.* New York: HarperCollins Publishers Inc., 1996.

Wells, Patricia. *Patricia Wells at Home in Provence.* New York: Scribner, 1996.

Wood, David with Karen Barnaby, Daphna Rabinovitch, Darlene MacDavid, and Krystyna Schmidt. *David Wood Food Book.* Toronto, Canada: Whitecap Books Ltd., 1988.

About the Authors

Gabrielle Nagler, M.A. writes on health and diet. She is a graduate of the University of Toronto and McGill University. In the early nineties, she moved to Singapore where she studied alternative medicine, macrobiotics and shiatsu massage. An avid cook and organic vegetable gardener, she has taught macrobiotic cooking classes in both the United States and Canada. Gabrielle lives with her husband, Bill Nagler, in Ann Arbor, Michigan. She is co-author of *Doctor Nagler's Crash Diet.*

Bill Nagler, M.D. has been practicing weight control medicine for over 20 years. He is a graduate of the University of Michigan, the University of California and a Harvard Fellowship. He is a Diplomate of the American Board of Bariatric (Weight Control) Medicine and a Diplomate of the American Board of Psychiatry and Neurology. Bill Nagler has appeared on Larry King Live, CBS This Morning, Montel Williams, Jenny Jones, Jerry Springer, Phil Donahue, Joan Rivers and Sally Jessy Raphael, and has been featured in USA Today, Cosmopolitan and Self Magazine. He is the author of *Doctor Nagler's Super-Saver Injection Program*, *Doctor Nagler's Crash Diet*, and *The Dirty Half Dozen.*